Integrated Disease Surveillance and Response (IDSR) in Africa

Mogana S. Flomo, Jr.

Published by CEPRES International University, 2024.

INTEGRATED DISEASE SURVEILLANCE AND RESPONSE (IDSR) IN AFRICA

First edition. February 5, 2024.

Copyright © 2024 Mogana S. Flomo, Jr..

ISBN: 979-8224580248

Written by Mogana S. Flomo, Jr..

Table of Contents

Chapter 1. Introduction to communicable diseases, epidemics, and surveillance

1.1 Definition and classification of communicable diseases

1.1.1 Classification of communicable diseases based on types of agents

1.1.2 Classification of Communicable diseases base on severity of illness

1.1.3 The role of epidemiology in understanding disease transmission and control

1.2 Overview of epidemic surveillance and response systems

1.2.1 Surveillance:

1.2.2 Early warning:

1.2.3 Outbreak investigation:

1.2.4 Response:

1.2.5 Evaluation:

1.3 Understanding the epidemiology of common communicable diseases

1.3.1 Tuberculosis (TB):

1.3.2 Malaria:

1.3.3 HIV/AIDS:

1.3.4 Neglected Tropical Diseases (NTDs)

1.4 The role of vectors and hosts in transmission

1.4.1 Vectors:

1.4.2 Hosts:

1.5 Outbreak investigation

1.5.1 Confirm the existence of an outbreak:

1.5.2 Define the case definition:

1.5.3 Documentation

1.5.4 Generate hypotheses:

1.5.5 Implement control measures:

1.5.6 Communicate findings:

1.6 Case study: Malaria in Ghana

1.7 Exercises

Chapter 2. Disease prevention and control

2.1 Prevention strategies for communicable diseases

2.1.1 Vaccination:

2.1.2 Sanitation:

2.1.3 Hygiene measures:

2.1.4 Environmental measures:

2.1.5 Screening and testing:

2.1.6 Isolation and quarantine:

2.2 The use of antibiotics and antivirals in disease control

2.2.1 Antibiotics:

2.2.2 Antivirals:

2.2.3 Overuse and misuse:

2.2.4 Side effects:

2.2.5 Combination therapy:

2.3 The importance of surveillance and early warning systems

2.3.1 Early detection:

2.3.2 Rapid response:

2.3.3 Identification of high-risk populations:

2.3.4 Monitoring of disease trends:

2.3.5 Early warning:

2.3.6 International cooperation:

2.4 Case study: Polio eradication in Nigeria

2.5 Exercises

Chapter 3. Emerging and re-emerging infectious diseases

3.1 Understanding the drivers of emerging infectious diseases

3.1.1 Environmental changes:

3.1.2 Globalization:

3.1.3 Agricultural practices:

3.1.4 Human behavior:

3.1.5 Pathogen evolution:

3.1.6 Health systems and infrastructure:

3.2 The role of climate change and environmental factors

3.2.1 Altering the distribution of disease vectors:

3.2.2 Changing host-pathogen dynamics:

3.2.3 Impacting food and water security:

3.2.4 Displacing populations:

3.2.5 Amplifying extreme weather events:

3.3 The need for preparedness and response plans

3.3.1 Early detection and response:

3.3.2 Coordination and communication:

3.3.3 Resource mobilization:

3.3.4 Capacity building:

3.3.5 Prevention and control:

3.4 Case study: Zika outbreak in Brazil

3.5 Exercises

Chapter 4. Public health surveillance systems

4.1 Overview of surveillance systems in Africa and Europe

4.1.1 Africa:

4.1.2 National Action Plan for Health Security in Liberia:

4.1.3 Europe:

4.2 The role of surveillance in public health decision-making

4.2.1 Detecting outbreaks:

4.2.2 Monitoring disease trends:

4.2.3 Evaluating interventions:

4.2.4 Planning resource allocation:

4.2.5 Informing policy decisions:

4.3 The challenges and opportunities of digital surveillance

4.3.1 Challenges:

4.3.2 Opportunities:

4.4 Case Studies of Surveillance of Communicable diseases in Africa

4.4.1 COVID-19 pandemic in Kenya

4.4.2 COVID-19 Pandemic in South Africa Epidemiology:

4.4.3 COVID-19 Pandemic in Nigeria Epidemiology:

4.4.4 COVID-19 Pandemic in Ethiopia Epidemiology:

4.4.5 COVID-19 Pandemic in Egypt Epidemiology:

4.4.6 COVID-19 Pandemic in Senegal Epidemiology:

4.4.7 COVID-19 Pandemic in Morocco Epidemiology:

4.4.8 Ebola Outbreak in Democratic Republic of the Congo (DRC) Epidemiology:

4.4.9 Malaria Control in Tanzania Epidemiology:

4.4.10 Yellow Fever Outbreak in Nigeria Epidemiology:

4.4.11 Cholera Outbreak in Zambia Epidemiology:

4.4.12 HIV/AIDS Epidemic in South Africa Epidemiology:

4.5 Exercises

Chapter 5. Disease surveillance and response in Europe

5.1 Comparative analysis of disease surveillance systems in Europe

5.1.1 European Centre for Disease Prevention and Control (ECDC):

5.1.2 Health Protection Surveillance Centre (HPSC) in Ireland:

5.1.3 Robert Koch Institute (RKI) in Germany:

5.1.4 National Institute of Public Health and the Environment (RIVM) in the Netherlands:

5.1.5 Comparative analysis:

5.2 The role of the European Centre for Disease Prevention and Control

5.3 Best practices and lessons learned from the response to recent outbreaks

5.3.1 Early detection and rapid response are critical:

5.3.2 Communication and community engagement are essential:

5.3.3 Collaboration and coordination are key:

5.3.4 Preparedness is essential:

5.3.5 Investment in public health infrastructure is crucial:

5.3.6 Health equity and social determinants of health must be addressed:

5.4 Case study: Measles outbreak in Ukraine

5.5 Exercises

Chapter 6. Disease surveillance and response in Africa

6.1 Comparative analysis of disease surveillance systems in Africa

6.2 The role of the Africa Centers for Disease Control and Prevention

6.3 Best practices and lessons learned from the response to recent outbreaks

6.3.1 Early detection and reporting:

6.3.2 Rapid response:

6.3.3 Coordination and collaboration:

6.3.4 Risk communication:

6.3.5 Capacity building:

6.3.6 Sustainable financing:

6.4 Case study: Lassa fever outbreak in Nigeria

6.5 Exercises

Chapter 7. Integrated Disease Surveillance and Response (IDSR)

7.1 Definition of Integrated Disease Surveillance and Response (IDSR)

7.2 Importance of IDSR in Africa

7.2.1 Early detection of disease outbreaks:

7.2.2 Rapid response to outbreaks:

7.2.3 Improved disease surveillance:

7.2.4 Strengthened laboratory services:

7.2.5 Better coordination and collaboration:

7.3 Historical background of IDSR implementation in Africa

7.4 Recap of Definition and classification of communicable diseases

7.4.1 Bacterial infections:

7.4.2 Viral infections:

7.4.3 Fungal infections:

7.4.4 Parasitic infections:

7.4.5 Sexually transmitted infections:

7.4.6 Vector-borne infections:

7.5 The role of epidemiology in understanding disease transmission and control

7.5.1 Identify the agent responsible for the disease:

7.5.2 Determine the mode of transmission:

7.5.3 Identify the populations at risk:

7.5.4 Monitor disease trends:

7.5.5 Evaluate interventions:

7.6 Overview of epidemic surveillance and response systems

7.6.1 Surveillance:

7.6.2 Early warning:

7.6.3 Outbreak investigation:

7.6.4 Response:

7.6.5 Evaluation:

7.7 Case study: Ebola outbreak in Liberia

Exercises

Chapter 8. The IDSR System

8.1 Disease transmission dynamics

8.1.1 Modes of Transmission:

8.1.2 Infectious Period and Incubation Period:

8.1.3 Basic Reproduction Number (R0):

8.1.4 Herd Immunity:

8.1.5 Super-Spreading Events:

8.1.6 Seasonality and Environmental Factors:

8.1.7 Population Factors:

8.2 Transmission patterns in different settings

8.2.1 Person-to-person transmission:

8.2.2 Vector-borne transmission:

8.2.3 Waterborne transmission:

8.2.4 Foodborne transmission:

8.2.5 Airborne transmission:

8.3 The role of social and behavioral factors in transmission

8.3.1 Contact patterns:

8.3.2 Hygiene and sanitation practices:

8.3.3 Health behaviors:

8.3.4 Vaccination:

8.3.5 Knowledge and attitudes:

8.4 Case study: Cholera outbreak in Yemen

8.5 Exercises

Chapter 9. Public health interventions

9.1 Introduction to public health interventions for communicable diseases

9.1.1 Surveillance and early detection:

9.1.2 Containment and control:

9.1.3 Prevention:

9.1.4 Education and communication:

9.1.5 Research:

9.2 Treatment and prevention of common communicable diseases

9.3 The role of mass media and community engagement in promoting public health

9.3.1 Designing mass media programs for prevention and control of communicable diseases

9.4 Case study: HIV/AIDS prevention in South Africa

9.5 Exercises

Chapter 10. Global health security

10.1 Understanding the International Health Regulations

10.1.1 Goals of the IHR

10.1.2 Reporting requirements

10.2 The importance of global cooperation in disease surveillance and response

10.3 Challenges and opportunities in global health security

10.4 Case study: Ebola outbreak in Sierra Leone

10.5 Exercises

Chapter 11. Ethics and governance in disease surveillance and response

11.1 Ethical considerations in disease surveillance and response

11.1.1 Privacy and confidentiality:

11.1.2 Informed consent:

11.1.3 Equity:

11.1.4 Transparency and accountability:

11.1.5 Respect for human rights:

11.1.6 Cultural sensitivity:

11.1.7 Benefit-sharing:

11.1.8 Collaboration and coordination:

11.2 The role of governance and leadership in epidemic control

11.3 Balancing individual rights and public health interests

11.4 Case study: COVID-19 response in Sweden

11.5 Exercises

Chapter 12. The IDSR Framework

12.1 Components of the IDSR framework

12.1.1 Surveillance:

12.1.2 Laboratory services:

12.1.3 Epidemic preparedness and response:

12.1.4 Health information and communication:

12.1.5 Human resource development:

12.1.6 Program management:

12.2 Data collection

12.2.1 Data sources:

12.2.2 Standard case definitions:

12.2.3 Reporting and notification:

12.2.4 Data management:

12.2.5 Data quality assurance:

12.2.6 Data use:

12.3 Reporting and feedback mechanisms

12.3.1 Reporting channels:

12.3.2 Reporting forms:

12.3.3 Data management:

12.3.4 Feedback mechanisms:

12.3.5 Response planning:

12.3.6 Evaluation and monitoring:

12.4 Surveillance system evaluation

12.4.1 Objective setting:

12.4.2 Data sources:

12.4.3 Performance indicators:

12.4.4 Data quality assessment:

12.4.5 Feedback mechanisms:

12.4.6 Stakeholder engagement:

12.4.7 Action planning:

Chapter 13. Disease-specific Surveillance

13.1 Diseases of public health importance in Africa

13.1.1 Malaria:

13.1.2 HIV/AIDS:

13.1.3 Tuberculosis (TB):

13.1.4 Neglected tropical diseases (NTDs):

13.1.5 Cholera:

13.1.6 Measles:

13.1.7 Ebola virus disease (EVD):

13.1.8 Lassa fever:

13.2 Disease-specific surveillance strategies

13.2.1 Malaria surveillance strategies

13.2.2 HIV/AIDS surveillance strategies

13.2.3 Tuberculosis (TB) surveillance strategies

13.2.4 Cholera surveillance strategies

13.2.5 Measles surveillance strategies

13.2.6 Ebola virus disease (EVD) surveillance strategies

13.3 Case studies of successful disease-specific surveillance in Africa

13.3.1 Polio eradication in Nigeria:

13.3.2 Guinea worm eradication in Ghana:

13.3.3 Ebola response in West Africa:

13.4 Exercises

Chapter 14. Response to Disease Outbreaks

14.1 Importance of rapid response to disease outbreaks

14.1.1 Preventing further spread:

14.1.2 Controlling the outbreak:

14.1.3 Saving lives:

14.1.4 Minimizing economic impact:

14.1.5 Building public trust:

14.2 The IDSR response strategy

14.2.1 Early detection:

14.2.2 Rapid response:

14.2.3 Integrated response:

14.2.4 Evidence-based interventions:

14.2.5 Monitoring and evaluation:

14.3 Case studies of effective outbreak response in Africa

14.3.1 Ebola outbreak in Nigeria (2014):

14.3.2 Yellow fever outbreak in Angola (2016):

14.3.3 Lassa fever outbreak in Nigeria (2018):

14.3.4 Ebola outbreak in Liberia (2014-2016):

14.3.5 Measles outbreak in Nigeria (2020):

14.3.6 Meningitis outbreak in Niger (2015):

14.4 Exercises

Chapter 15. The Role of Laboratory Services in IDSR

15.1 The importance of laboratory services in disease surveillance and response

15.1.1 Disease diagnosis:

15.1.2 Disease monitoring:

15.1.3 Disease research:

15.1.4 Public health emergency preparedness:

15.1.5 Quality assurance:

15.2 Laboratory diagnosis in IDSR

15.2.1 Laboratory capacity:

15.2.2 Laboratory network:

15.2.3 Laboratory test menu:

15.2.4 Laboratory data management:

15.3 Case studies of laboratory services supporting IDSR in Africa

15.3.1 Liberia:

15.3.2 Uganda:

15.3.3 Nigeria:

15.4 Exercises

Chapter 16. Capacity Building for IDSR

16.1 Capacity building for IDSR implementation

16.1.1 Training:

16.1.2 Infrastructure development:

16.1.3 Procurement and supply chain management:

16.1.4 Communication and coordination:

16.1.5 Monitoring and evaluation:

16.2 Importance of training and communication in IDSR

16.2.1 Consistent and accurate implementation:

16.2.2 Early detection and response:

16.2.3 Timely reporting:

16.2.4 Coordination:

16.2.5 Sustainability:

16.3 Case studies of successful capacity building for IDSR in Africa including Liberia

16.3.1 Liberia:

16.3.2 Ethiopia:

16.3.3 Ghana:

16.4 Importance of monitoring and evaluating IDSR implementation

16.4.1 Improving system effectiveness:

16.4.2 Measuring progress:

16.4.3 Accountability and transparency:

16.4.4 Identifying best practices:

16.4.5 Resource allocation:

16.5 Evaluation frameworks for IDSR

16.5.1 The World Health Organization's (WHO) Framework for Evaluation of Surveillance Systems:

16.5.2 The Centers for Disease Control and Prevention (CDC) Framework for Program Evaluation:

16.5.3 The Logical Framework Approach:

16.5.4 The Results-Based Monitoring and Evaluation Framework:

16.6 Case studies of successful monitoring and evaluation of IDSR in Africa

16.7 Emerging challenges in IDSR implementation in Africa

16.7.1 Weak health systems:

16.7.2 Disease outbreaks and epidemics:

16.7.3 Inadequate laboratory capacity:

16.7.4 Poor data quality:

16.7.5 Limited community engagement:

16.7.6 Climate change and environmental factors:

16.8 Opportunities for improvement

16.8.1 Strengthening health systems:

16.8.2 Enhancing laboratory capacity:

16.8.3 Increasing community engagement:

16.8.4 Leveraging technology:

16.8.5 Strengthening surveillance and response networks:

16.8.6 Increasing research and innovation:

16.9 Recommendations for the future of IDSR in Africa

16.10 Exercises

16.11 Call to action for continued improvement and implementation of IDSR in Africa.

Appendices

Appendix A: List of diseases of public health importance in Africa:

Appendix B: Sample data collection and reporting forms

Appendix C: List of national and international organizations involved in IDSR implementation in Africa

Appendix D: Training and capacity building resources

Appendix E: List of reference laboratories for disease diagnosis and confirmation

Appendix F: Sample outbreak response plans and guidelines

Appendix G: List of key stakeholders in IDSR implementation in Africa and their roles

Appendix H: Glossary of all key terms and acronyms used in IDSR.

Bibliography

Book description

"*Integrated Disease Surveillance and Response (IDSR) in Africa: A Comprehensive Guide*" is a vital resource that offers a thorough exploration of the integrated approach to disease surveillance and response in the African context. This comprehensive guide delves into various aspects of IDSR implementation, equipping public health professionals, policymakers, and researchers with the knowledge and strategies needed to effectively address communicable diseases and strengthen surveillance systems in Africa.

The book begins by highlighting the importance of IDSR in Africa, emphasizing its role in detecting and responding to communicable diseases that pose significant public health risks. It underscores the need for a robust and integrated surveillance system to monitor the occurrence and distribution of diseases, identify outbreaks, and facilitate timely and effective response efforts.

Drawing on the historical background of IDSR implementation in Africa, the book provides valuable insights into the challenges and lessons learned from past experiences. It explores the evolution of surveillance systems, shedding light on the progress made and the areas that require further improvement. By understanding the historical context, readers gain a deeper appreciation for the development and significance of IDSR in Africa.

The book then delves into the core components of the IDSR framework, outlining the essential elements necessary for its successful implementation. It covers the entire surveillance cycle, from data collection and management to reporting and feedback mechanisms. Readers learn about the different surveillance strategies and techniques employed to collect, analyze, and interpret data, enabling them to make informed decisions and take appropriate actions based on the findings.

A major focus of the book is disease-specific surveillance, addressing communicable diseases that pose significant public health challenges in Africa. It provides an in-depth examination of the epidemiology, transmission, and control strategies for these diseases. Real-world case studies highlight successful disease-specific surveillance initiatives, offering practical examples of how surveillance efforts can be tailored to specific diseases and contexts.

Recognizing the critical role of laboratory services in disease surveillance and response, the book dedicates a chapter to exploring the importance of accurate and timely laboratory diagnosis. It discusses the integration of laboratory testing into surveillance activities, showcases case studies of how laboratory services support IDSR in Africa, and emphasizes the need for strong collaboration between laboratories and surveillance systems.

Capacity building for IDSR implementation is another key theme addressed in the book. It underscores the significance of training and effective communication in strengthening surveillance systems and equipping healthcare workers with the skills and knowledge necessary to carry out surveillance activities. Real-world case studies demonstrate successful capacity building initiatives in Africa, offering practical insights and best practices for enhancing workforce capabilities.

Monitoring and evaluation play a crucial role in ensuring the effectiveness of IDSR implementation. The book highlights the importance of monitoring and evaluating surveillance systems, program performance, and outcomes. It presents evaluation frameworks and methodologies tailored to IDSR, enabling stakeholders to assess progress, identify strengths and weaknesses, and make evidence-based decisions for program improvement.

Looking towards the future, the book addresses emerging challenges in IDSR implementation in Africa and presents opportunities for improvement. It offers recommendations for strengthening the system, fostering collaboration among stakeholders, and adopting innovative approaches to enhance disease surveillance and response. By embracing these recommendations, Africa can proactively address evolving public health threats and ensure the sustainability of IDSR efforts in the long term.

In conclusion, "Integrated Disease Surveillance and Response (IDSR) in Africa: A Comprehensive Guide" provides a wealth of knowledge and practical insights for professionals working in the field of public health in Africa. It covers a wide range of topics, including communicable diseases, surveillance strategies, laboratory services, capacity building, monitoring and evaluation, and future directions for IDSR. By utilizing the information and recommendations in this guide, stakeholders can contribute to strengthening disease surveillance and response efforts, ultimately improving the health outcomes of communities across Africa.

Chapter 1. Introduction to communicable diseases, epidemics, and surveillance

1.1 Definition and classification of communicable diseases

Communicable diseases are illnesses caused by infectious agents such as bacteria, viruses, fungi, and parasites that can be transmitted directly or indirectly from one person to another, from an animal to a person, or from an environmental source to a person.

1.1.1 Classification of communicable diseases based on types of agents

COMMUNICABLE DISEASES can be classified based on the type of agent that causes the disease, the mode of transmission, the severity of illness, and the population affected. Here are some common classifications:

1.1.1.1 Bacterial infections:

BACTERIAL INFECTIONS are a type of infectious disease caused by bacteria. They can manifest in various forms and affect different body systems. Bacterial infections can be transmitted through various means, including contaminated food, water, air, or direct contact with infected individuals or animals. Here, we will expand on some examples of bacterial infections, their modes of transmission, and their impact on human health:

1. ***Tuberculosis (TB):*** Tuberculosis is a bacterial infection caused by the bacterium Mycobacterium tuberculosis. It primarily affects the lungs but can also affect other organs such as the kidneys, bones, and brain. TB is primarily transmitted through the inhalation of airborne droplets containing the bacteria, typically from an infected individual who coughs or sneezes. It is a major global health concern, with millions of new cases and deaths reported annually. Effective diagnosis, treatment, and prevention strategies are crucial in controlling the spread of TB.

2. **Cholera:** Cholera is an acute diarrheal disease caused by the bacterium Vibrio cholerae. It is primarily transmitted through the ingestion of contaminated food or water. Cholera outbreaks often occur in areas with inadequate sanitation and poor access to clean water. The infection can lead to severe dehydration and, if left untreated, can be life-threatening. Prompt administration of oral rehydration therapy and the provision of clean water and sanitation facilities are key interventions for cholera prevention and control.

3. ***Streptococcal infections***: Streptococcal infections are caused by various species of Streptococcus bacteria. They can cause a range of diseases, including strep throat, scarlet fever, and invasive infections such as pneumonia and bloodstream infections. Streptococcal infections are typically transmitted through respiratory droplets from an infected person or through direct contact with infected wounds or skin lesions. Prompt diagnosis and appropriate antibiotic treatment are essential in managing streptococcal infections and preventing complications.

It is important to note that the prevention, diagnosis, and treatment of bacterial infections require a multidimensional approach involving public health interventions, access to healthcare services, proper hygiene practices, and the development of effective antimicrobial strategies. Vaccination, sanitation improvements, infection control measures, and the responsible use of antibiotics are crucial components in the prevention and management of bacterial infections.

1.1.1.2 Viral infections:

VIRAL INFECTIONS ARE a type of infectious disease caused by viruses. Viruses are microscopic pathogens that require host cells to replicate and survive. They can cause a wide range of diseases in humans, ranging from mild respiratory infections to severe and potentially life-threatening illnesses. Here are some examples of viral infections, their modes of transmission, and their impact on human health:

1. **Influenza**: Influenza, commonly known as the flu, is a viral respiratory infection caused by influenza viruses. It is primarily transmitted through respiratory droplets when an infected person coughs, sneezes, or talks. Influenza can cause a wide range of symptoms, including fever, cough, sore throat, body aches, and fatigue. While most people recover without complications, influenza can be severe, especially in young children, older adults, and individuals with underlying health conditions. Annual vaccination is recommended to prevent influenza and reduce its spread.

2. **HIV/AIDS**: Human Immunodeficiency Virus (HIV) is the virus that causes Acquired Immunodeficiency Syndrome (AIDS). HIV is primarily transmitted through

unprotected sexual intercourse, sharing contaminated needles or syringes, and from mother to child during childbirth or breastfeeding. HIV attacks the immune system, gradually weakening it and making individuals more susceptible to opportunistic infections and certain types of cancers. Antiretroviral therapy (ART) is available to manage HIV infection and prevent the progression to AIDS.

3. **Ebola:** Ebola virus disease (EVD) is a severe and often fatal viral infection caused by the Ebola virus. It is transmitted through direct contact with the blood, body fluids, or tissues of infected animals (such as fruit bats, primates) or through direct contact with the blood, body fluids, or contaminated objects of infected humans. Ebola outbreaks have occurred primarily in Central and West African countries. EVD is characterized by fever, severe headache, muscle and joint pain, and can progress to hemorrhagic fever with internal and external bleeding. Strict infection control measures and rapid response are crucial in containing Ebola outbreaks.

4. **COVID-19**: COVID-19 is the infectious disease caused by the novel coronavirus, SARS-CoV-2. It is primarily transmitted through respiratory droplets when an infected person coughs, sneezes, talks, or breathes. COVID-19 has become a global pandemic, resulting in millions of cases and deaths worldwide. Symptoms range from mild respiratory symptoms to severe pneumonia and acute respiratory distress syndrome (ARDS). Non-pharmaceutical interventions such as wearing masks, practicing hand hygiene, maintaining physical distancing, and vaccination have been crucial in preventing the spread of COVID-19.

Effective prevention and control strategies for viral infections include vaccination, public health measures (such as hygiene practices, isolation, and quarantine), antiviral medications (where available), and public awareness campaigns. Ongoing research and surveillance are important for understanding viral infections, developing new treatments, and preventing future outbreaks.

1.1.1.3 Fungal infections:

FUNGAL INFECTIONS, also known as mycoses, are caused by various types of fungi. Fungi are ubiquitous organisms found in the environment, including soil, plants, and even on our skin. While most fungi are harmless, certain species can cause infections in humans. Here are some examples of fungal infections, their modes of transmission, and their impact on human health:

1. ***Ringworm:*** Ringworm, also known as dermatophytosis, is a common fungal infection of the skin, hair, and nails. It is caused by different species of dermatophyte fungi, including Trichophyton, Microsporum, and Epidermophyton. Ringworm is typically transmitted through direct contact with an infected person, animal, or contaminated surfaces such as towels, clothing, or gym equipment. It manifests as circular, itchy, and scaly patches on the skin or scalp. Antifungal medications, both topical and oral, are used to treat ringworm.

2. **Candidiasis**: Candidiasis is an infection caused by the Candida species of fungi, most commonly Candida albicans. Candida is part of the normal flora found in the mouth, intestines, and genital area. However, certain conditions such as weakened immune system, hormonal changes, or antibiotic use can lead to overgrowth and

cause infections. Candidiasis can affect various body parts, including the mouth (oral thrush), genitals (vaginal yeast infection), and skin (cutaneous candidiasis). Antifungal medications are used to treat candidiasis.

3. ***Aspergillosis:*** Aspergillosis is a group of fungal infections caused by Aspergillus species. These fungi are found in the environment, particularly in decaying vegetation and soil. Aspergillosis can affect the respiratory system, causing allergic reactions, fungal balls (aspergillomas) in lung cavities, or invasive lung infections. It primarily affects individuals with weakened immune systems or underlying lung conditions. Treatment may involve antifungal medications and management of underlying health conditions.

Fungal infections can vary in severity, ranging from mild and localized to severe and systemic. Risk factors for fungal infections include weakened immune system, prolonged use of antibiotics, certain medical conditions (e.g., diabetes), and environmental exposures. Prevention measures include practicing good hygiene, avoiding prolonged exposure to damp environments, wearing appropriate footwear in public areas, and maintaining a healthy immune system.

It's important to note that accurate diagnosis of fungal infections often requires laboratory testing, such as microscopic examination of samples or fungal culture. This helps to identify the specific fungal species and guide appropriate treatment.

1.1.1.4 Parasitic infections:

PARASITIC INFECTIONS are caused by various types of parasites and can be transmitted through different routes. These infections occur when parasites, such as protozoa or helminths, enter the body and establish themselves, leading to a range of symptoms and health consequences. Here are some examples of parasitic infections:

1. *Malaria:* Malaria is a life-threatening disease caused by Plasmodium parasites transmitted to humans through the bites of infected female Anopheles mosquitoes. It is prevalent in tropical and subtropical regions. Symptoms include fever, chills, headache, and body aches. If left untreated, malaria can lead to severe complications and death.

2. *Schistosomiasis*: Schistosomiasis, also known as bilharzia, is caused by parasitic worms called schistosomes. People become infected when they come into contact with contaminated freshwater, such as rivers or lakes, that contain the parasite's larvae. The larvae penetrate the skin during water activities. Chronic infection can lead to liver and kidney damage, bladder problems, and other complications.

3. **Lice infestations**: Lice infestations, such as head lice, body lice, and pubic lice, are caused by parasitic insects. These parasites live on the human body and feed on blood. Lice infestations can spread through close personal contact, sharing personal items, or contact with infested clothing or bedding. Symptoms include itching, visible lice or eggs (nits) in the affected areas, and skin irritation.

4. *Toxoplasmosis*: Toxoplasmosis is caused by the parasite Toxoplasma gondii. It can be acquired through the consumption of undercooked or raw meat, contact with contaminated soil, or exposure to infected cat feces. While most people do not experience symptoms, it can be

serious for individuals with weakened immune systems or pregnant women, as it can cause birth defects.

5. ***Intestinal parasites***: Various intestinal parasites, such as roundworms, hookworms, and tapeworms, can cause infections when ingested through contaminated food, water, or soil. These parasites can reside in the intestines, leading to symptoms like abdominal pain, diarrhea, weight loss, and nutritional deficiencies.

It's important to note that prevention, early diagnosis, and appropriate treatment are crucial in managing parasitic infections. Public health measures, such as proper sanitation, clean water supply, and health education, play a significant role in preventing the transmission of parasitic infections.

1.1.1.5 Sexually transmitted infections:

SEXUALLY TRANSMITTED infections (STIs) are infections that are primarily transmitted through sexual contact, including vaginal, anal, or oral sex, as well as through intimate skin-to-skin contact. They are caused by bacteria, viruses, parasites, or fungi and can have significant health consequences if left untreated. Here are some examples of sexually transmitted infections:

1. ***Gonorrhea***: Gonorrhea is caused by the bacterium Neisseria gonorrhoeae. It can be transmitted through unprotected sexual intercourse with an infected person. Symptoms may include genital discharge, pain or burning during urination, and genital itching. If untreated, gonorrhea can lead to serious complications, including pelvic inflammatory disease (PID) in women and epididymitis in men.

2. ***Syphilis:*** Syphilis is caused by the bacterium Treponema pallidum. It can be transmitted through sexual contact with an infected person or from mother to child during pregnancy. Syphilis progresses through stages and can cause a wide range of symptoms, including genital sores (chancres), rashes, fever, fatigue, and neurological problems. If left untreated, syphilis can cause severe health complications, including damage to the heart, brain, and other organs.

3. ***Herpes:*** Herpes infections are caused by the herpes simplex virus (HSV). There are two types: HSV-1, which is primarily associated with oral herpes (cold sores), and HSV-2, which is primarily associated with genital herpes. Both types can be transmitted through sexual contact. Symptoms include painful blisters or sores in the affected areas, along with flu-like symptoms during the initial infection. While there is no cure for herpes, antiviral medications can help manage symptoms and reduce the risk of transmission.

4. **Human papillomavirus (HPV) infection:** HPV is a common viral infection transmitted through sexual contact. It can cause various health problems, including genital warts and certain types of cancers, such as cervical, anal, and oral cancers. Many people with HPV infection do not experience symptoms, and the infection often clears on its own. Vaccines are available to protect against certain high-risk HPV types.

5. **Human immunodeficiency virus (HIV) infection:** HIV is the virus that causes acquired immunodeficiency syndrome (AIDS). It is primarily transmitted through unprotected sexual intercourse with an infected person, sharing contaminated needles, or from mother to child

during childbirth or breastfeeding. HIV weakens the immune system over time, leading to the development of AIDS. Early diagnosis and antiretroviral therapy (ART) can help manage the infection and prevent the progression to AIDS.

Prevention, regular testing, and safe sexual practices, such as condom use and mutual monogamy, are important in reducing the transmission of sexually transmitted infections. Education and awareness campaigns play a significant role in promoting safe sexual behaviors and encouraging early detection and treatment of STIs.

1.1.1.6 Vector-borne infections:

VECTOR-BORNE INFECTIONS are diseases caused by pathogens that are transmitted to humans through the bite of infected vectors, which are typically blood-feeding arthropods such as mosquitoes, ticks, and fleas. These infections are prevalent in many parts of the world and can have significant impacts on public health. Here are some examples of vector-borne infections:

1. *Malaria:* Malaria is a life-threatening disease caused by parasites of the Plasmodium genus. It is transmitted to humans through the bite of infected female Anopheles mosquitoes. Malaria is prevalent in tropical and subtropical regions and can cause symptoms such as high fever, chills, and flu-like illness. If left untreated, it can lead to severe complications and death.

2. *Lyme disease*: Lyme disease is caused by the bacterium Borrelia burgdorferi and is primarily transmitted to humans through the bite of infected black-legged ticks

It is most commonly found in temperate regions. Early symptoms include fever, fatigue, muscle aches, and a characteristic rash called erythema migrans. If left untreated, Lyme disease can affect the joints, heart, and nervous system.

3. ***Dengue fever***: Dengue fever is caused by the dengue virus, which is transmitted to humans by Aedes mosquitoes, primarily the Aedes aegypti species. It is widespread in tropical and subtropical regions. Symptoms may include high fever, severe headache, joint and muscle pain, rash, and in severe cases, it can lead to dengue hemorrhagic fever or dengue shock syndrome, which can be life-threatening.

4. ***Zika virus disease***: Zika virus is primarily transmitted through the bite of infected Aedes mosquitoes, particularly Aedes aegypti. It gained attention during the 2015-2016 outbreak in the Americas. In most cases, Zika virus infection causes mild or no symptoms, but it can cause birth defects if a pregnant woman becomes infected. It has also been associated with Guillain-Barré syndrome in some cases.

5. ***West Nile fever***: West Nile fever is caused by the West Nile virus and is primarily transmitted to humans through the bite of infected mosquitoes, particularly Culex mosquitoes. It is prevalent in many regions of the world, including North America, Europe, and Africa. Most people infected with West Nile virus do not develop any symptoms, but some may experience mild flu-like illness. In rare cases, it can lead to severe neurological complications.

Preventing vector-borne infections involves measures such as vector control (e.g., insecticide-treated bed nets, mosquito control programs), personal protective measures (e.g., wearing long sleeves, using insect repellents), and public health interventions (e.g., surveillance, early detection, and response). Vaccines are available for some vector-borne diseases, such as yellow fever.

1.1.2 Classification of Communicable diseases base on severity of illness

COMMUNICABLE DISEASES can be classified based on the severity of illness they cause. This classification helps in understanding the impact of the disease and implementing appropriate prevention and control measures. Here are two common classifications based on severity of illness and population affected:

1.1.2.1 Mild versus Severe Diseases:

COMMUNICABLE DISEASES can range from mild illnesses that typically resolve on their own to severe diseases that can have significant health consequences. The severity of a disease depends on factors such as the virulence of the infectious agent, the individual's immune response, and the presence of underlying health conditions.

1. *Mild Diseases*: Examples of mild communicable diseases include the common cold, mild forms of influenza, and certain types of rashes. These diseases generally cause mild symptoms, such as cough, runny nose, fever, or skin irritation, and do not typically result in severe complications or long-term health effects.
2. *Severe Diseases*: Severe communicable diseases can cause

significant illness, disability, and even death. Examples include Ebola virus disease, severe acute respiratory syndrome (SARS), and certain strains of avian influenza. These diseases often present with severe symptoms, such as high fever, respiratory distress, organ failure, and require prompt medical intervention.

1.1.2.2 Age-specific or Vulnerable Populations:

COMMUNICABLE DISEASES can also be classified based on the population groups they primarily affect. Some diseases disproportionately affect specific age groups or individuals with weakened immune systems, such as:

1. **Pediatric Diseases**: Certain communicable diseases are more common in children, such as chickenpox, measles, and whooping cough (pertussis). Children are often more susceptible to these diseases due to their developing immune systems and close contact in school or daycare settings.

1. **Elderly Diseases**: Elderly individuals, especially those with underlying health conditions, are more susceptible to severe forms of certain communicable diseases, such as pneumonia and influenza. Age-related declines in immune function and increased vulnerability to complications contribute to the severity of these diseases in older adults.

Understanding the classification of communicable diseases based on severity and population groups helps guide public health efforts, including prevention strategies, targeted vaccination campaigns, and appropriate medical care. It allows healthcare professionals and public health authorities to allocate resources effectively and prioritize interventions based on the specific needs of different populations.

1.1.3 The role of epidemiology in understanding disease transmission and control

EPIDEMIOLOGY PLAYS a critical role in understanding disease transmission and control by providing scientific methods for investigating the patterns, causes, and effects of communicable diseases within populations. Epidemiology helps to:

1.1.3.1 Identify the agent responsible for the disease:

IDENTIFYING THE AGENT responsible for a disease is a crucial step in understanding and controlling the disease. Epidemiologists employ various methods, including laboratory testing and other investigative techniques, to identify the specific agent causing a particular disease. Here's an overview of the process:

1.1.3.1.1 Laboratory Testing:

1. **Microbiological Testing**: Laboratory tests, such as culture, microscopy, and molecular diagnostics, are performed on patient samples (e.g., blood, sputum, swabs) to detect and identify microorganisms. These tests can help determine whether bacteria, viruses, fungi, or parasites are responsible for the disease.
2. **Serological Testing**: Serological tests detect the presence of antibodies produced by the immune system in response to an infection. They can help identify past or current infections and assist in determining the causative agent.

3. **Genetic Sequencing**: Advanced techniques like genetic sequencing can be used to analyze the genetic material of pathogens, such as viruses or bacteria. This helps identify specific strains or subtypes and provides valuable insights into transmission patterns and potential drug resistance.

1.1.3.1.2 Epidemiological Investigation:

1. *Case Investigations*: Epidemiologists conduct detailed investigations of individual cases to gather information about symptoms, exposure history, and potential sources of infection. This helps identify commonalities among cases and provides clues about the causative agent.

2. *Outbreak Investigations*: During outbreaks, epidemiologists investigate patterns of illness, perform contact tracing, and collect environmental samples to identify the source and mode of transmission. These investigations often involve collaboration with laboratory specialists to confirm the presence of the pathogen.

1.1.3.1.3 Collaboration and Surveillance:

1. *Collaboration with Laboratories*: Epidemiologists work closely with laboratory professionals to ensure timely and accurate testing of patient samples. This collaboration facilitates the identification of the disease agent and enables prompt response measures.

2. *Disease Surveillance*: Ongoing surveillance systems monitor the occurrence and spread of diseases. These systems collect data from healthcare facilities, laboratories, and other sources to detect and investigate unusual disease patterns or emerging pathogens.

IDENTIFYING THE AGENT responsible for a disease is
essential for several reasons:

1. ***Developing Effective Control Measures***: Knowledge of
   the specific agent helps in developing targeted control
   strategies, such as vaccines, antimicrobial treatments, or
   vector control measures.
2. ***Understanding Transmission Dynamics***: Identification
   of the agent provides insights into the mode of
   transmission, reservoirs, and potential sources, enabling
   public health authorities to implement appropriate
   preventive measures.
3. ***Monitoring and Surveillance***: Once the agent is
   identified, surveillance systems can be established to
   monitor its prevalence and track any changes, facilitating
   early detection of outbreaks and informing public health
   interventions.

1.1.3.2 Determine the mode of transmission:

DETERMINING THE MODE of transmission is a crucial step
in understanding how a disease spreads from person to person
or from animals to humans. Epidemiologists employ various
methods, including surveillance data analysis and outbreak
investigations, to identify the mode of transmission. Here's an
overview of the process:

1.1.3.2.1 Surveillance Data Analysis:

EPIDEMIOLOGISTS ANALYZE surveillance data collected
from healthcare facilities, laboratories, and other sources to
identify patterns of disease occurrence and transmission. This

includes examining demographic information, geographical distribution, and temporal trends.

By analyzing the data, epidemiologists can identify commonalities among cases, such as shared exposures or demographic characteristics, which provide clues about the mode of transmission.

1.1.3.2.2 Outbreak Investigations:

DURING OUTBREAKS, EPIDEMIOLOGISTS conduct detailed investigations to determine the mode of transmission. This involves interviewing affected individuals to gather information about their activities, locations, and potential exposures.

Epidemiologists perform contact tracing to identify and interview individuals who had close contact with confirmed cases. This helps identify secondary cases and understand the chains of transmission.

Environmental and laboratory investigations are conducted to collect samples and identify potential sources of the pathogen, such as contaminated food, water, or vectors (e.g., mosquitoes, ticks).

1.1.3.2.3 Analyzing Transmission Patterns:

EPIDEMIOLOGISTS ANALYZE the collected data to identify common exposures, locations, or behaviors among cases. They also examine the timing of cases to understand the incubation period and the duration of infectiousness.

By comparing cases and their exposures, epidemiologists can determine whether the disease is transmitted through direct contact, respiratory droplets, contaminated food or water, vectors, or other routes.

Advanced techniques, such as molecular epidemiology and genetic sequencing, can also provide insights into the relatedness of pathogens and their transmission patterns.

1.1.3.2.4 Prevention and Control Strategies:

ONCE THE MODE OF TRANSMISSION is identified, public health authorities can develop targeted strategies to interrupt the transmission chain.

This may include implementing infection prevention and control measures, promoting hygiene practices, implementing vector control strategies, ensuring safe food and water supply, and recommending appropriate vaccination programs.

Understanding the mode of transmission is crucial for several reasons:

1. *Targeted Prevention Measures*: Knowledge of the mode of transmission helps in developing specific prevention strategies to interrupt the transmission chain and reduce the risk of new infections.
2. *Early Detection and Response*: Identifying the mode of transmission allows for early detection of outbreaks and prompt response to control the spread of the disease.
3. *Risk Communication*: Understanding how a disease is transmitted enables public health authorities to communicate accurate information to the public and provide guidance on preventive measures.

1.1.3.3 Identify the populations at risk:

IDENTIFYING THE POPULATIONS at risk is an important aspect of epidemiological analysis. Epidemiologists analyze various data sources to determine which groups of people are more susceptible to a particular communicable disease. Here's an overview of how this is done:

1.1.3.3.1 Demographic Analysis:

EPIDEMIOLOGISTS EXAMINE demographic data to identify population characteristics associated with increased risk. This includes age, sex, occupation, socioeconomic status, and geographic location.

For example, certain age groups, such as infants or the elderly, may be more vulnerable to specific diseases due to differences in immune system development or age-related physiological changes.

Socioeconomic factors, such as poverty or lack of access to healthcare, can also contribute to higher disease risk.

1.1.3.3.2 Surveillance Data Analysis:

EPIDEMIOLOGISTS ANALYZE surveillance data to identify patterns of disease occurrence within different population groups.

They compare disease rates across demographic categories to determine if certain populations have a higher burden of the disease.

This analysis may reveal disparities in disease prevalence and help target interventions towards the affected populations.

1.1.3.3.3 Risk Factor Assessment:

EPIDEMIOLOGISTS STUDY risk factors associated with the disease to identify populations at increased risk.

Risk factors can include behaviors (e.g., smoking, unprotected sex), pre-existing conditions (e.g., diabetes, immunodeficiency), occupational exposure, or environmental factors.

By understanding the risk factors, epidemiologists can identify populations more likely to be exposed to these factors and, consequently, at higher risk of contracting the disease.

1.1.3.3.4 Outbreak Investigations:

DURING OUTBREAK INVESTIGATIONS, epidemiologists identify individuals or groups that have been exposed to the disease and are at risk of infection.

This includes close contacts of confirmed cases, individuals in specific settings (e.g., healthcare facilities, schools, workplaces), or those with shared exposures (e.g., foodborne outbreaks).

By identifying the populations at risk, public health authorities can implement targeted interventions, such as contact tracing, testing, and preventive measures, to control the spread of the disease.

Identifying populations at risk is crucial for several reasons:

1. *Targeted Interventions*: It allows public health authorities to focus preventive measures, such as vaccination campaigns, health education, or screening programs, on the populations most vulnerable to the disease.

2. ***Resource Allocation***: Understanding which populations are at higher risk helps allocate resources, such as healthcare facilities, personnel, and supplies, to areas with the greatest need.

3. ***Health Equity***: Identifying populations at risk contributes to addressing health disparities and promoting equity in access to healthcare and preventive services.

1.1.3.4 Monitor disease trends:

MONITORING DISEASE trends is a fundamental task of epidemiologists to understand the patterns and dynamics of communicable diseases. Here's an overview of how epidemiologists monitor disease trends:

1.1.3.4.1 Surveillance Systems:

1. *Epidemiologists* establish and maintain surveillance systems to collect data on disease incidence, prevalence, and other relevant indicators.

2. These systems can include national or regional databases, laboratory reporting systems, sentinel surveillance sites, or electronic health records.

3. By regularly collecting and analyzing data, epidemiologists can identify trends and changes in disease occurrence.

1.1.3.4.2 Data Analysis and Visualization:

1. Epidemiologists analyze surveillance data using statistical methods to identify patterns, trends, and changes over

time.

2. They use techniques such as time series analysis, data visualization, and statistical modeling to understand disease trends and predict future patterns.
3. Visual representations, such as graphs, charts, and maps, are often used to communicate the trends effectively to public health officials, policymakers, and the general public.

1.1.3.4.3 Outbreak Detection and Response:

1. Epidemiologists actively monitor disease surveillance data for any unusual or unexpected increases in disease cases.
2. They employ statistical algorithms, thresholds, and syndromic surveillance methods to detect outbreaks or clusters of cases.
3. Early detection of outbreaks enables rapid response and implementation of control measures to limit the spread of the disease and minimize its impact.

1.1.3.4.4 Collaboration and Information Sharing:

1. Epidemiologists collaborate with local, national, and international health agencies to share data, information, and best practices.
2. This collaboration allows for the comparison of disease trends across different regions, identification of common risk factors, and the exchange of outbreak response strategies.

1.1.3.4.5 Research and Evaluation:

1. Epidemiologists conduct research studies and evaluations to understand the underlying factors driving disease trends and evaluate the effectiveness of interventions.
2. This research helps identify risk factors, assess the impact of control measures, and inform evidence-based public health policies and strategies.

BY MONITORING DISEASE trends, epidemiologists can:

1. Identify emerging diseases or changes in the epidemiology of existing diseases.
2. Detect outbreaks or clusters of cases early, enabling swift response and control measures.
3. Evaluate the effectiveness of interventions and assess the impact of public health programs.
4. Provide accurate and timely information to guide public health policies and decision-making.

1.1.3.5 Evaluate interventions:

EVALUATING INTERVENTIONS is a crucial step in epidemiology to assess their effectiveness in controlling the spread of communicable diseases. Epidemiologists conduct evaluations to understand the impact of various interventions, such as vaccination programs, quarantine measures, and other control strategies. Here's a breakdown of the process involved in evaluating interventions:

1.1.3.5.1 Study Design:

1. Epidemiologists design studies or evaluations to assess the

effectiveness of interventions.

2. Study designs can include randomized controlled trials (RCTs), quasi-experimental designs, observational studies, or ecological studies, depending on the nature of the intervention and ethical considerations.

3. Control groups are often used to compare the outcomes between those exposed to the intervention and those who are not.

1.1.3.5.2 Data Collection and Analysis:

1. Epidemiologists collect relevant data before and after implementing the intervention.

2. Data can include disease incidence, prevalence, hospitalization rates, mortality rates, and other relevant outcomes.

3. They may use various data sources such as surveillance systems, registries, medical records, or surveys.

4. Statistical analysis techniques, such as hypothesis testing, regression analysis, or mathematical modeling, are employed to evaluate the impact of the intervention.

1.1.3.5.3 Comparisons and Control Groups:

1. Epidemiologists compare the outcomes between the group receiving the intervention (intervention group) and a control group (either non-exposed or receiving an alternative intervention).

2. The comparison helps determine the effectiveness of the intervention in reducing disease transmission or mitigating its impact.

3. Randomization and blinding techniques are often used to

minimize biases and confounding factors.

1.1.3.5.4 Assessment of Outcomes:

1. Epidemiologists assess various outcomes related to disease transmission, severity, morbidity, and mortality to evaluate the impact of the intervention.
2. This can include changes in disease incidence, reduction in transmission rates, decrease in hospitalization or mortality rates, or improvement in overall health outcomes.
3. Multiple outcome measures may be considered to gain a comprehensive understanding of the intervention's effectiveness.

1.1.3.5.5 Cost-effectiveness Analysis:

1. In addition to evaluating the impact on disease transmission, epidemiologists may perform cost-effectiveness analyses to assess the economic efficiency of interventions.
2. This analysis considers the costs associated with implementing the intervention and compares them to the resulting health benefits or reduction in disease burden.
3. Cost-effectiveness analyses help inform policymakers and stakeholders in making decisions about resource allocation and prioritizing interventions.

1.1.3.5.6 Synthesis of Evidence:

1. Epidemiologists contribute to the synthesis of evidence by conducting systematic reviews and meta-analyses.

2. These approaches help combine and analyze data from multiple studies, providing a more robust assessment of intervention effectiveness across different settings and populations.

1.1.3.5.7 Recommendations and Policy Implications:

1. Based on the evaluation findings, epidemiologists make evidence-based recommendations for public health policies, guidelines, and interventions.
2. These recommendations help refine strategies for controlling the spread of communicable diseases and inform decision-making by public health authorities and policymakers.
3. By evaluating interventions, epidemiologists gain insights into the effectiveness of specific measures, contribute to the refinement of control strategies, and inform evidence-based decision-making in public health.

OVERALL, EPIDEMIOLOGY provides critical information to inform public health policy and decision-making, and plays an important role in preventing and controlling communicable diseases.

1.2 Overview of epidemic surveillance and response systems

EPIDEMIC SURVEILLANCE and response systems are designed to detect, track, and respond to outbreaks of communicable diseases. These systems are crucial in preventing and controlling the spread of infectious diseases, particularly in areas where the risk of epidemics is high. Here's an overview of epidemic surveillance and response systems:

1.2.1 Surveillance:

THE FIRST STEP IN AN epidemic surveillance and response system is surveillance. Surveillance involves the systematic collection, analysis, and interpretation of data on the occurrence and distribution of communicable diseases. This information is used to identify outbreaks and to monitor disease trends over time.

1.2.2 Early warning:

EARLY WARNING SYSTEMS are designed to detect outbreaks early, before they become widespread. These systems use a variety of methods, including laboratory testing, clinical surveillance, and disease reporting, to identify potential outbreaks.

1.2.3 Outbreak investigation:

WHEN AN OUTBREAK IS detected, an outbreak investigation is conducted to identify the source of the outbreak, the mode of transmission, and the populations at risk. This information is used to develop targeted interventions to control the outbreak.

1.2.4 Response:

ONCE AN OUTBREAK HAS been identified and investigated, a response is initiated to control the spread of the disease. This may include measures such as quarantine, isolation of infected individuals, contact tracing, and vaccination campaigns.

1.2.5 Evaluation:

AFTER THE OUTBREAK has been controlled, the epidemic surveillance and response system is evaluated to determine its effectiveness in detecting and responding to the outbreak. This information is used to refine the system and to improve future responses to outbreaks.

Epidemic surveillance and response systems can be implemented at various levels, including national, regional, and local levels. These systems require close collaboration between public health officials, healthcare providers, and community members to be effective in preventing and controlling the spread of communicable diseases.

Case study: Ebola outbreak in Liberia

The Ebola outbreak in Liberia, which began in March 2014, was the largest and deadliest outbreak of Ebola virus disease in history. The outbreak resulted in 10,678 confirmed cases and 4,810 deaths in Liberia alone, with a total of 28,646 cases and 11,323 deaths in West Africa.

The outbreak in Liberia was fueled by a number of factors, including limited healthcare infrastructure, cultural practices such as burial practices that involved close contact with the deceased, and a lack of public awareness about the disease. The country had only a few doctors to serve a population of 4.5 million, and there were only a few dozen ambulances available to transport patients.

The initial response to the outbreak was slow, and the Liberian government was criticized for its handling of the crisis. However, the government eventually declared a state of emergency and launched a comprehensive response effort that included measures such as the establishment of Ebola treatment centers and the deployment of healthcare workers to affected areas.

International aid and support also played a key role in the response to the outbreak. The United States and other countries provided financial and logistical support, and healthcare workers from around the world traveled to Liberia to provide assistance.

The response effort was complicated by factors such as mistrust of healthcare workers and resistance to public health messages, as well as the ongoing civil war in the country. However, through a combination of efforts, including improved communication and outreach, the establishment of treatment centers, and the deployment of healthcare workers, the outbreak was eventually brought under control.

The Ebola outbreak in Liberia highlighted the importance of early detection and response in controlling communicable disease outbreaks, as well as the need for strong healthcare infrastructure and public awareness campaigns. The lessons learned from this outbreak have helped to inform the global response to other outbreaks, such as the COVID-19 pandemic.

1.3 Understanding the epidemiology of common communicable diseases

TUBERCULOSIS, MALARIA, and HIV/AIDS are three common communicable diseases that have significant public health impacts worldwide. Here is an overview of the epidemiology of each disease:

1.3.1 Tuberculosis (TB):

TUBERCULOSIS (TB) IS a contagious infectious disease caused by the bacterium Mycobacterium tuberculosis. It primarily affects the lungs but can also affect other parts of the body, such as the kidneys, spine, or brain. TB is transmitted through the air when an infected individual coughs, sneezes, or speaks, releasing respiratory droplets containing the bacteria. When inhaled by others, the bacteria can infect their lungs, leading to TB disease.

The global burden of TB remains a significant public health challenge. In 2019, there were an estimated 10 million new cases of TB worldwide, with approximately 1.4 million deaths attributed to the disease. TB is a leading cause of death from a single infectious agent, surpassing HIV/AIDS. Although TB is a global concern, its impact is particularly pronounced in low- and middle-income countries, where factors such as poverty, overcrowding, malnutrition, and limited access to healthcare contribute to its spread.

Certain regions bear a higher burden of TB than others. Countries in Southeast Asia and sub-Saharan Africa have the highest rates of TB incidence and mortality. Within these regions, socio-economic disparities, weak healthcare systems, and challenges in implementing effective prevention and control measures contribute to the persistence of the disease.

Efforts to combat TB involve a comprehensive approach, including early diagnosis, appropriate treatment, and prevention strategies. Diagnosis typically involves a combination of medical history assessment, physical examination, chest X-rays, and laboratory tests, such as sputum microscopy and molecular tests. Treatment for TB consists of a combination of antibiotics taken over several months to ensure complete eradication of the bacteria. It is essential for patients to adhere to their treatment regimen to prevent the development of drug-resistant strains of TB.

To reduce the burden of TB, several global initiatives and partnerships have been established. The World Health Organization (WHO) leads the global fight against TB through its "End TB Strategy," which aims to reduce TB deaths by 95% and new cases by 90% by 2035. This strategy emphasizes early diagnosis, effective treatment, and the development of new tools, including vaccines and improved diagnostic tests.

Furthermore, TB prevention efforts focus on identifying and treating latent TB infection in individuals who are at high risk of developing active TB disease. Preventive measures include the use of isoniazid preventive therapy (IPT) and the Bacillus Calmette-Guérin (BCG) vaccine, which provides partial protection against severe forms of TB in children.

Figure 1:Top 20 countries in Africa with the highest incidence and death rates of tuberculosis (TB)

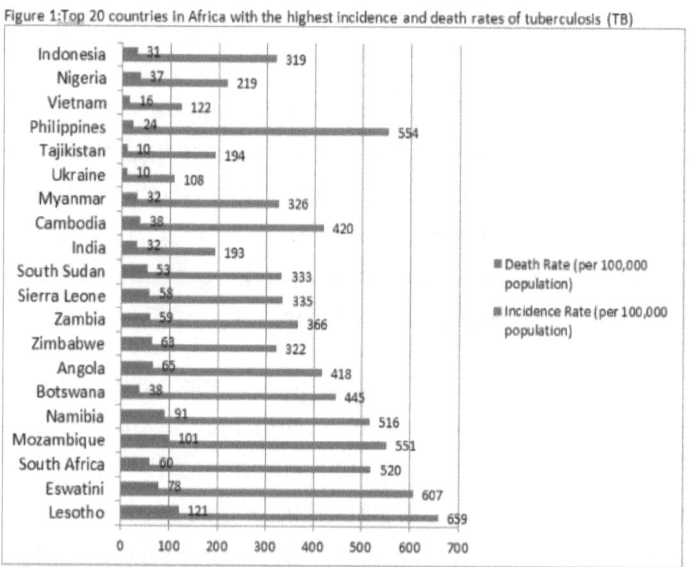

This figure provides a summary of the top 20 countries in Africa with the highest incidence and death rates of tuberculosis (TB).

1.3.2 Malaria:

MALARIA IS A PARASITIC disease that poses a significant global health challenge, particularly in regions with a high prevalence of the disease. It is caused by Plasmodium parasites, with Plasmodium falciparum being the most deadly species responsible for the majority of malaria-related deaths. Other Plasmodium species that can infect humans include Plasmodium vivax, Plasmodium malariae, and Plasmodium ovale.

The transmission of malaria occurs through the bites of infected female Anopheles mosquitoes. When a mosquito carrying the malaria parasite bites a human, the parasites are injected into the bloodstream. Once inside the body, the parasites travel to the liver, where they multiply and mature. They then re-enter the bloodstream and invade red blood cells, leading to the characteristic symptoms of the disease.

The clinical manifestations of malaria can vary depending on the Plasmodium species involved, the individual's immune response, and other factors. The most common symptoms include recurrent episodes of fever, chills, sweats, headache, muscle aches, and fatigue. Malaria can also cause nausea, vomiting, and diarrhea. In severe cases, complications such as organ failure, anemia, cerebral malaria (involving the brain), and death can occur.

According to the World Health Organization (WHO), there were an estimated 229 million cases of malaria worldwide in 2019. Sub-Saharan Africa bears the highest burden of the disease, accounting for approximately 94% of malaria cases and deaths. This region is disproportionately affected due to factors such as a high prevalence of malaria-transmitting mosquitoes, limited access to healthcare services, inadequate infrastructure, and socio-economic challenges.

Certain population groups are particularly vulnerable to malaria. Children under the age of five have reduced immunity to the disease and are at a higher risk of severe illness and death. Malaria during pregnancy also poses significant risks to both the mother and the unborn child, leading to complications such as maternal anemia, low birth weight, and increased infant mortality. Pregnant women are advised to take preventive measures, such as using insecticide-treated bed nets and receiving intermittent preventive treatment.

Preventing and controlling malaria requires a multi-faceted approach. Key strategies include vector control through the distribution and promotion of insecticide-treated bed nets, indoor residual spraying of insecticides, and environmental management to reduce mosquito breeding sites. Prompt diagnosis and effective treatment with appropriate antimalarial drugs are crucial to reduce the severity of illness, prevent complications, and interrupt the transmission cycle.

According to the latest World Malaria Report, published by the World Health Organization (WHO), the global malaria burden remained significant in 2021. The report indicated that there were 247 million cases of malaria in 2021, slightly higher than the 245 million cases reported in 2020. Similarly, the estimated number of malaria deaths in 2021 was 619,000, compared to 625,000 in the previous year.

It is noteworthy that the COVID-19 pandemic had a substantial impact on malaria outcomes during the peak years of 2020 and 2021. The disruptions caused by the pandemic resulted in approximately 13 million additional malaria cases and 63,000 additional malaria deaths.

The WHO African Region continued to bear a disproportionate burden of malaria globally. In 2021, the region accounted for around 95% of all malaria cases and 96% of malaria deaths. Alarmingly, children under the age of 5 accounted for approximately 80% of all malaria-related deaths in the region.

Regarding specific countries, four African nations stood out as major contributors to global malaria mortality. Nigeria had the highest number of malaria deaths worldwide, accounting for 31.3% of the total. The Democratic Republic of the Congo followed, contributing 12.6% of global malaria deaths. The United Republic of Tanzania and Niger accounted for 4.1% and 3.9% of malaria deaths, respectively. Collectively, these four countries were responsible for just over half of all malaria deaths worldwide.

These findings emphasize the persistent burden of malaria in Africa, particularly in the WHO African Region, and the urgent need for intensified efforts to combat this life-threatening disease.

Take a look at the top four countries affected by malaria:

Global efforts to combat malaria have seen significant progress in recent years, with expanded access to interventions and increased funding for prevention and treatment programs. The WHO's Global Malaria Program provides guidance and support to countries in implementing effective control measures, promoting research and innovation, and monitoring the global malaria situation.

Figure 3: estimated death top four countries affected by malaria

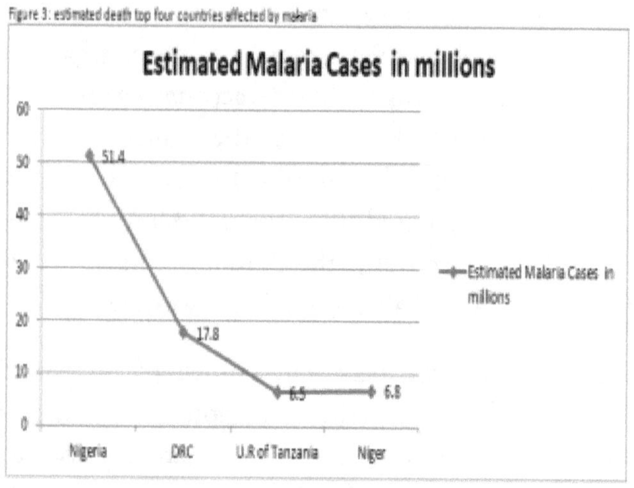

Figure 2: top four countries affected by malaria

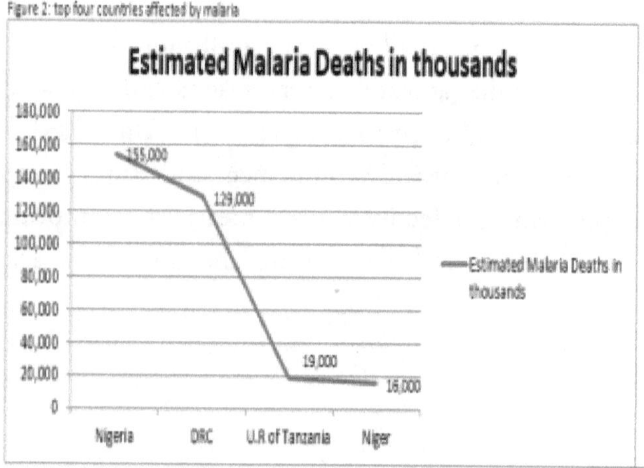

Figure 2 and Figure 3 show the estimate malaria case and deaths in the top four countries mostly affected (Nigeria, Democratic Republic of Congo, United Republic of Tanzania and Niger)

1.3.3 HIV/AIDS:

HIV/AIDS IS A VIRAL disease that attacks the immune system, leaving individuals vulnerable to other infections and illnesses. The disease is primarily spread through unprotected sex, sharing of needles or other drug injection equipment, and mother-to-child transmission during pregnancy, childbirth, or breastfeeding. According to UNAIDS, there were 38 million people living with HIV/AIDS globally in 2019, with an estimated 1.7 million new infections and 690,000 deaths. The disease disproportionately affects vulnerable populations, including men who have sex with men, sex workers, and people who inject drugs.

Understanding the epidemiology of these diseases is critical in developing effective prevention and control strategies. This includes measures such as vaccination campaigns, use of insecticide-treated bed nets to prevent malaria, and early diagnosis and treatment for TB and HIV/AIDS. Public health officials also work to improve surveillance systems to monitor disease trends and detect outbreaks early, and to develop targeted interventions to address the unique challenges posed by each disease.

The burden of HIV/AIDS varies across different countries, with some regions experiencing a higher prevalence and greater impact of the disease. Here are the estimated HIV/AIDS disease burdens for the top 10 countries affected by the epidemic:

South Africa: South Africa has the highest number of people living with HIV/AIDS in the world. It is estimated that around 7.7 million people were living with HIV/AIDS in South Africa in 2020. The country has been severely affected by the epidemic, and efforts are underway to prevent new infections and provide treatment and support to those affected.

Nigeria: Nigeria has the second-highest number of people living with HIV/AIDS globally. It is estimated that around 3.3 million people were living with the disease in Nigeria in 2020. The country faces challenges in terms of prevention, treatment, and stigma associated with HIV/AIDS.

India: India has a significant burden of HIV/AIDS, with an estimated 2.3 million people living with the disease in 2020. The epidemic in India is concentrated in certain states and populations, and efforts are being made to expand prevention and treatment services.

Mozambique: Mozambique has a high prevalence of HIV/AIDS, with an estimated 2.2 million people living with the disease in 2020. The country has made progress in expanding access to antiretroviral therapy (ART) and prevention measures.

Uganda: Uganda has a history of high HIV/AIDS prevalence, but the country has made significant progress in reducing new infections and expanding treatment. It is estimated that around 1.4 million people were living with HIV/AIDS in Uganda in 2020.

Tanzania: Tanzania has a large number of people living with HIV/AIDS, with an estimated 1.4 million in 2020. The country has implemented various prevention and treatment programs to address the epidemic.

Kenya: Kenya has a significant HIV/AIDS burden, with around 1.1 million people living with the disease in 2020. The country has made progress in expanding access to ART and implementing prevention strategies.

Zambia: Zambia has a high prevalence of HIV/AIDS, with an estimated 1.1 million people living with the disease in 2020. The country has implemented various interventions to address the epidemic, including prevention, testing, and treatment programs.

Zimbabwe: Zimbabwe has been severely affected by HIV/AIDS, with an estimated 1.1 million people living with the disease in 2020. The country has made progress in expanding access to treatment and support services.

Ethiopia: Ethiopia has a significant burden of HIV/AIDS, with an estimated 720,000 people living with the disease in 2020. The country has implemented various programs to increase access to prevention, testing, and treatment services.

It's important to note that the numbers provided are estimates and can vary depending on different data sources and methodologies. The burden of HIV/AIDS is dynamic, and efforts are ongoing to track the epidemic and implement effective interventions globally.

Figure 4: Prevalence of HIV/AIDS in the top 20 most affected countries in 2020

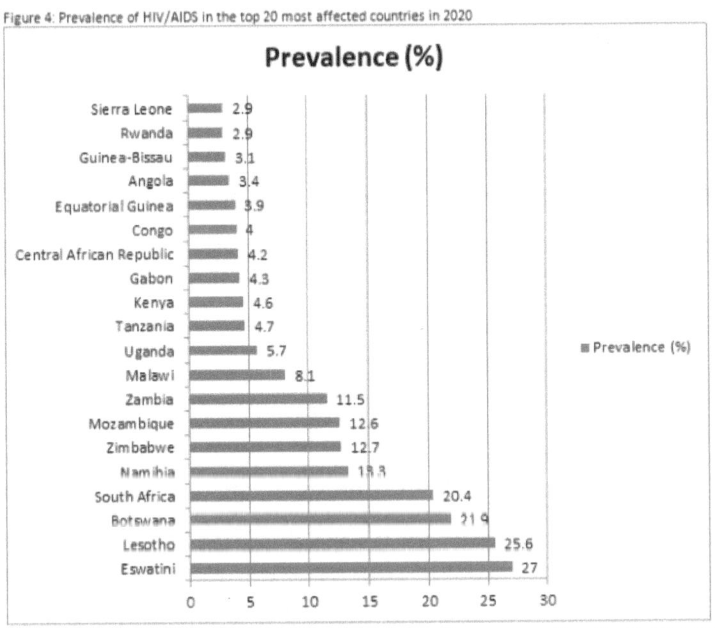

The prevalence rates of HIV/AIDS in the mentioned African countries were sourced from the respective country fact sheets provided by the Joint United Nations Programme on HIV/AIDS (UNAIDS) for the year 2020.

Please note that the prevalence rates represent the estimated percentage of adults (ages 15-49) living with HIV/AIDS in each country. The rates are based on available data and may vary over time as new information becomes available.

1.3.4 Neglected Tropical Diseases (NTDs)

NEGLECTED TROPICAL Diseases (NTDs) encompass a group of diverse communicable diseases that disproportionately afflict impoverished communities residing in tropical and subtropical regions, with Africa bearing a significant burden. These diseases tend to thrive in settings where access to adequate healthcare, clean water, and sanitation facilities is limited, exacerbating the challenges faced by vulnerable populations already grappling with socioeconomic disparities.

Among the prevalent NTDs in Africa, four notable examples are schistosomiasis, lymphatic filariasis, onchocerciasis (commonly known as river blindness), and trachoma. Each of these diseases inflicts substantial morbidity, causing immense suffering and impeding the socioeconomic development of affected communities.

1.3.4.1 Schistosomiasis

SCHISTOSOMIASIS, COMMONLY known as bilharzia, is a neglected tropical disease (NTD) prevalent in many countries in Africa. It is caused by parasitic worms of the genus Schistosoma and is transmitted through contact with freshwater sources contaminated with specific snails that serve as intermediate hosts for the parasite. The burden of schistosomiasis in Africa is significant, with millions of people affected, particularly those living in impoverished communities with limited access to clean water and adequate sanitation facilities.

The disease has a wide-ranging impact on individuals and communities, causing both acute and chronic health problems. When individuals come into contact with contaminated water, the larvae of the Schistosoma parasite can penetrate the skin, leading to an initial acute infection known as swimmer's itch. This acute phase is often asymptomatic or may manifest as a rash, fever, and flu-like symptoms. If left untreated, the infection progresses to the chronic stage, which can have severe consequences.

In the chronic phase of schistosomiasis, the adult worms inhabit the blood vessels surrounding organs such as the intestines, liver, bladder, and genital organs. Prolonged exposure to the parasite can result in significant organ damage and various complications. For example, intestinal schistosomiasis can cause abdominal pain, diarrhea, and blood in the stool, while urogenital schistosomiasis affects the urinary and reproductive systems, leading to conditions such as bladder and kidney damage, urinary tract infections, infertility, and increased susceptibility to HIV/AIDS transmission.

The prevalence of schistosomiasis, or the proportion of individuals infected with the disease, varies across different regions of Africa. It is influenced by factors such as the presence of suitable freshwater habitats for the intermediate snail hosts and human contact with contaminated water sources.

In sub-Saharan Africa, where the majority of schistosomiasis cases occur, the disease is endemic in many countries. The prevalence rates can be high, particularly in areas with limited access to clean water and sanitation facilities. According to the World Health

Organization (WHO), over 90% of the global burden of schistosomiasis is concentrated in Africa.

To provide an overview of the prevalence of schistosomiasis in specific countries, here are some examples:

1. **Nigeria**: In Nigeria, schistosomiasis is highly endemic, with a significant number of individuals affected. A study published in the journal Parasites & Vectors reported a prevalence of 29.3% among school-aged children in selected communities in Nigeria.
2. **Burkina Faso**: In Burkina Faso, schistosomiasis is also endemic. A study conducted in the country found a prevalence of 41.3% among school-aged children.
3. **Tanzania**: Tanzania has a high prevalence of schistosomiasis, particularly in areas near freshwater bodies. A study published in the journal PLOS Neglected Tropical Diseases reported a prevalence of 51.4% among school-aged children in selected districts of Tanzania.

It is important to note that the prevalence of schistosomiasis can vary even within countries, depending on local environmental conditions and population behaviors. Prevalence rates may also differ among different age groups, with higher rates observed among children who have frequent water contact activities.

To combat the prevalence of schistosomiasis, control programs focus on implementing mass drug administration (MDA) campaigns, providing treatment with praziquantel to at-risk populations, particularly school-aged children. Other interventions include health education on the importance of avoiding contact with contaminated water sources and improving water and sanitation infrastructure to minimize transmission.

1.3.4.2 Lymphatic filariasis

LYMPHATIC FILARIASIS, also known as elephantiasis, is a neglected tropical disease caused by thread-like nematode worms of the family Filariidae. The disease is primarily transmitted to humans through the bites of infected mosquitoes, specifically those belonging to the genera Culex, Anopheles, and Aedes. Lymphatic filariasis is endemic in many tropical and subtropical regions, including several countries in Africa.

The disease burden of lymphatic filariasis in Africa is substantial. According to the World Health Organization (WHO), Africa accounts for the highest number of cases globally, with over 30 million people infected. The most affected countries include Nigeria, the Democratic Republic of the Congo, and Ethiopia. These countries bear a significant proportion of the disease burden and are the focus of control and elimination efforts.

Lymphatic filariasis can cause chronic and debilitating symptoms in affected individuals. The parasitic worms infect the lymphatic system, leading to chronic inflammation, lymphedema (swelling), and lymphatic dysfunction. The chronic swelling can affect various body parts, including the limbs, breasts, and genitalia, resulting in significant physical disfigurement and disability. The disease not only causes physical suffering but also has a profound impact on the social, economic, and psychological well-being of individuals and affected communities.

Preventive measures for lymphatic filariasis focus on two main strategies: mass drug administration (MDA) and morbidity management and disability prevention (MMDP). MDA involves the large-scale distribution of antifilarial drugs, such as diethylcarbamazine (DEC) or a combination of DEC with albendazole or ivermectin, to entire at-risk populations. This strategy aims to interrupt transmission by reducing the number of microfilariae (the larvae of the parasites) in the bloodstream of infected individuals.

In terms of disease burden, lymphatic filariasis can have a significant impact on affected communities in Africa. The physical and socioeconomic consequences of the disease can lead to reduced productivity, impaired educational attainment, and increased healthcare costs. Additionally, the stigma associated with the visible disfigurement caused by lymphatic filariasis can further isolate and marginalize affected individuals.

Efforts to combat lymphatic filariasis in Africa and reduce its disease burden have been ongoing. The WHO, in collaboration with national governments and partner organizations, has launched the Global Programme to Eliminate Lymphatic Filariasis (GPELF) with the goal of eliminating the disease as a public health problem. This initiative focuses on scaling up MDA, improving access to healthcare services, and addressing the management of morbidity and disability.

In conclusion, lymphatic filariasis is a debilitating disease prevalent in many African countries. The disease burden is significant, with millions of people affected and experiencing physical and socioeconomic consequences. Control and elimination efforts, including mass drug administration and morbidity management, are crucial in reducing the disease burden and improving the well-being of affected individuals and communities in Africa.

1.3.4.3 Onchocerciasis

ONCHOCERCIASIS, COMMONLY known as river blindness, is a neglected tropical disease caused by the filarial parasite Onchocerca volvulus. It is transmitted to humans through the bites of infected blackflies of the genus Simulium. Onchocerciasis is prevalent in certain regions of Africa, particularly in areas with fast-flowing rivers and close proximity to breeding sites of blackflies.

The disease burden of onchocerciasis in Africa is substantial. According to the World Health Organization (WHO), approximately 99% of the global cases occur in Africa. It is estimated that over 37 million people are infected with the parasite, and around 200 million people are at risk of acquiring the infection. The countries most affected by onchocerciasis in Africa include Nigeria, the Democratic Republic of the Congo, and Sudan.

Onchocerciasis can cause a range of debilitating symptoms and severe manifestations. The most characteristic symptom is intense and persistent itching of the skin, which can be severe and affect the quality of life of affected individuals. Chronic infection with the parasite can lead to the development of nodules under the skin, primarily in the subcutaneous tissues. In addition to skin manifestations, onchocerciasis can also affect the eyes, leading to visual impairment and ultimately blindness in some cases. Eye manifestations include inflammation of the conjunctiva, corneal opacities, and changes in the iris.

Control strategies for onchocerciasis primarily focus on mass drug administration (MDA) of a medication called ivermectin. Ivermectin is an antiparasitic drug that kills the microfilariae (larval forms) of the parasite, thereby reducing the transmission of the disease. MDA involves distributing ivermectin to the at-risk population in endemic areas on an annual or biannual basis. This strategy not only halts the transmission of the disease but also prevents further visual impairment and blindness.

The disease burden of onchocerciasis in Africa extends beyond the physical symptoms experienced by individuals. The disease has a significant impact on affected communities, including reduced productivity and economic development. Visual impairment and blindness can limit educational opportunities, impair social interactions, and lead to increased dependence on others for daily activities. The burden is particularly high in rural areas where access to healthcare and specialized treatment is limited.

Efforts to control and eliminate onchocerciasis in Africa have made significant progress. The African Programme for Onchocerciasis Control (APOC), established by the WHO in 1995, has played a pivotal role in coordinating interventions and distributing ivermectin to endemic communities. The program has achieved remarkable success in reducing the disease burden and preventing blindness in many areas. Additionally, the Expanded Special Project for Elimination of Neglected Tropical Diseases (ESPEN) is working towards the elimination of onchocerciasis as a public health problem.

In conclusion, onchocerciasis, or river blindness, is a parasitic disease prevalent in several African countries. The disease burden is substantial, with millions of people affected and at risk of developing severe skin and eye manifestations. Control strategies involving mass drug administration of ivermectin have been effective in reducing transmission and preventing visual impairment. Continued efforts are necessary to eliminate onchocerciasis as a public health problem in Africa and alleviate its impact on affected individuals and communities.

1.3.4.4 Trachoma

TRACHOMA, AN EYE INFECTION caused by the bacterium Chlamydia trachomatis, spreads through direct and indirect contact with eye and nose discharge from infected individuals. Repeated infections cause scarring of the inner eyelid, turning the eyelashes inward, leading to painful scratching of the cornea and potentially causing irreversible blindness. Trachoma control efforts comprise the SAFE strategy: Surgery to correct eyelid abnormalities, Antibiotics to treat infections, Facial cleanliness, and Environmental improvements to reduce transmission.

To combat the devastating impact of NTDs, various organizations, including the World Health Organization (WHO), local governments, and non-governmental organizations, collaborate to implement integrated control and elimination programs. These initiatives involve not only mass drug administration but also the improvement of sanitation and access to clean water to break the cycle of transmission. Additionally, health education plays a pivotal role in raising awareness about preventive measures, early symptom recognition, and seeking timely medical care.

Addressing Neglected Tropical Diseases in Africa requires sustained commitment, resources, and cooperation from the international community, as these diseases perpetuate cycles of poverty and ill-health. By targeting the root causes and employing a comprehensive approach, it is possible to alleviate the suffering of affected communities and work towards the control and elimination of these debilitating diseases.

Table 1: Prevalence of Neglected Tropical Diseases in Africa

Disease	Description	Prevalence in Africa
Schistosomiasis	Caused by paraitic worms transmitted through contact with contaminated freshwater sources.	Endemic in many African countries. Prevalence rates can be high, particularly in areas with limited access to clean water and sanitation facilities.
Lymphatic	Caused by thread-like nematode worms transmitted through mosquito bites.	Africa accounts for the highest number of cases globally. Most affected countries include Nigeria, the Democratic Republic of the Congo, and Ethiopia.
Filariasis	Results in chronic inflammation, lymphedema (swelling), and lymphatic dysfunction.	Over 30 million people infected in Africa. Significant burden on affected individuals and communities.
Onchocerciasis	Known as river blindness, caused by filarial parasites transmitted through blackfly bites.	Approximately 99% of global cases occur in Africa. Over 37 million people infected. Nigeria, the Democratic Republic of the Congo, and Sudan are most affected.
Trachoma	Eye infection caused by Chlamydia trachomatis, leading to scarring, corneal scratching, and potential blindness.	Prevalent in certain regions of Africa. Control efforts focus on the SAFE strategy: Surgery, Antibiotics, Facial cleanliness, and Environmental improvements.

These neglected tropical diseases disproportionately affect impoverished communities in Africa due to limited access to healthcare, clean water, and sanitation facilities.

1.4 The role of vectors and hosts in transmission

VECTORS AND HOSTS PLAY a critical role in the transmission of many communicable diseases, particularly those caused by viruses, bacteria, and parasites. Here is an overview of the role of vectors and hosts in disease transmission:

1.4.1 Vectors:

VECTORS PLAY A CRUCIAL role in the transmission of various infectious diseases, acting as intermediaries between infected individuals or animals and susceptible hosts. These living organisms, including mosquitoes, ticks, fleas, and flies, serve as vehicles for pathogens, such as bacteria, viruses, and parasites, allowing them to move from one host to another. Understanding the characteristics and behaviors of vectors is essential in developing effective strategies for preventing and controlling vector-borne diseases.

1.4.1.1 Mosquitoes

MOSQUITOES ARE NOTORIOUS vectors for transmitting various diseases, causing significant health burdens worldwide. Malaria, in particular, stands out as a major mosquito-borne disease. It is caused by parasites of the genus Plasmodium and is transmitted when female mosquitoes of the Anopheles genus feed on infected humans and subsequently infect other individuals during subsequent blood meals. Malaria is a global health concern, with Africa shouldering the highest burden of the disease.

According to the World Health Organization (WHO), malaria caused an estimated 229 million cases and 409,000 deaths globally in 2019, with Africa accounting for 94% of malaria cases and deaths. Countries such as Nigeria, the Democratic Republic of the Congo, and Mozambique bear a significant proportion of the malaria burden. These statistics highlight the pervasive impact of mosquitoes and malaria on the African continent.

In addition to malaria, mosquitoes are responsible for transmitting other notable diseases:

1. Dengue fever, caused by the dengue virus, is a mosquito-borne viral infection that affects millions of people annually, primarily in tropical and subtropical regions. Africa is not a primary hotspot for dengue fever, but sporadic cases have been reported in countries such as Cape Verde and Mauritius.
2. The Zika virus, transmitted primarily by the Aedes mosquitoes, gained global attention during the 2015-2016 outbreak in the Americas. While Zika virus transmission is relatively low in Africa, cases have been reported in several countries, including Angola, Guinea-

Bissau, and Cabo Verde. The virus poses a particular risk to pregnant women due to its association with congenital abnormalities, including microcephaly, in newborns.

3. Yellow fever is another mosquito-borne viral disease that is endemic in certain parts of Africa. It is transmitted primarily by the Aedes mosquitoes, particularly Aedes aegypti, which also serves as a vector for dengue and Zika viruses. Yellow fever can cause severe illness, with symptoms ranging from fever and muscle pain to jaundice and organ failure. Vaccination against yellow fever is an important preventive measure, particularly for individuals traveling to or residing in endemic regions.

4. Chikungunya is yet another mosquito-borne viral disease transmitted by Aedes mosquitoes. It causes symptoms such as fever, joint pain, and rash. Although chikungunya has been reported in various African countries, outbreaks have been documented in countries like Kenya, Mauritius, and Comoros.

The impact of mosquito-borne diseases goes beyond health implications. These diseases can have substantial economic consequences, as they contribute to decreased productivity, increased healthcare costs, and strain on healthcare systems. Additionally, outbreaks of mosquito-borne diseases can disrupt tourism and international trade.

Efforts to control mosquito-borne diseases in Africa involve a combination of approaches. These include vector control measures such as insecticide-treated bed nets, indoor residual spraying, and environmental management to reduce mosquito breeding sites. Health education campaigns play a vital role in raising awareness about preventive measures and early recognition of disease symptoms. Vaccination programs, particularly for diseases like yellow fever, are also essential components of control strategies.

1.4.1.2 Ticks

TICKS are another important group of vectors that can transmit various diseases to humans and animals. Lyme disease, caused by the bacterium Borrelia burgdorferi, is one of the most well-known tick-borne illnesses. Ticks become infected with the bacteria by feeding on infected rodents or other small mammals, and then transmit the bacteria to humans during subsequent blood meals. Rocky Mountain spotted fever, caused by the bacterium Rickettsia rickettsii, is another serious tick-borne disease characterized by fever, rash, and potentially life-threatening complications.

1.4.1.3 Fleas

FLEAS, WHILE PRIMARILY known as vectors of diseases among animals, can also pose a risk to human health by transmitting certain pathogens. One of the most significant examples is the bubonic plague, a severe and deadly infectious disease caused by the bacterium Yersinia pestis. Fleas play a crucial role in the transmission of this disease.

The bubonic plague is infamous for its devastating pandemics throughout history, including the Black Death in the 14th century, which caused the deaths of millions of people in Europe. Today, the plague is less common and more localized, with most cases occurring in specific regions such as parts of Africa, Asia, and the Americas.

Fleas become infected with Yersinia pestis when they feed on rodents or other animals that carry the bacteria. Once infected, fleas can transmit the bacteria to humans through their bites. When an infected flea bites a human, the bacteria can enter the bloodstream, leading to the development of the bubonic form of the plague. Symptoms of bubonic plague include painful swollen lymph nodes (buboes), fever, chills, headache, and fatigue.

While the bubonic form is the most well-known, Yersinia pestis can also cause other forms of the plague, such as septicemic and pneumonic plague. Septicemic plague occurs when the bacteria multiply in the bloodstream, leading to sepsis and potential organ failure. Pneumonic plague affects the lungs and is the most severe and contagious form, as it can spread from person to person through respiratory droplets.

Although the bubonic plague remains a serious disease, modern medical advancements have improved its diagnosis and treatment. Antibiotics are effective in treating Yersinia pestis infections, especially when administered early. Prompt identification and reporting of cases, along with effective flea control measures, are crucial for preventing outbreaks and reducing the spread of the disease.

It's important to note that while fleas are primarily associated with the transmission of diseases among animals, such as flea-borne typhus and bartonellosis, their role in transmitting diseases to humans is relatively rare compared to other vectors like mosquitoes and ticks.

1.4.1.4 Flies

FLIES, PARTICULARLY certain species of flies known as tsetse flies, are responsible for transmitting trypanosomes, parasites that cause sleeping sickness in humans and nagana in livestock. Tsetse flies acquire the parasites when they feed on infected humans or animals, and subsequently transmit the parasites to other individuals through their bites.

Controlling vector populations is a vital strategy for preventing the spread of vector-borne diseases. This can be achieved through various approaches, including:

1. ***Insecticide-Treated Bed Nets***: The use of insecticide-treated bed nets provides a physical barrier against mosquitoes, reducing the risk of bites and subsequent transmission of diseases such as malaria. These nets are typically treated with insecticides that repel or kill mosquitoes upon contact.

2. ***Insecticide Spraying***: Indoor residual spraying of insecticides is an effective method to control vector populations. By treating the interior walls of dwellings with insecticides, mosquitoes and other insects that come into contact with the treated surfaces are killed, reducing their numbers and interrupting disease transmission.

3. ***Environmental Management***: Modifying the environment to eliminate or reduce breeding sites for vectors is an important preventive measure. This can involve draining stagnant water, clearing vegetation, and improving sanitation practices to minimize the availability of suitable habitats for mosquitoes, flies, and other vectors.

4. ***Personal Protective Measures***: Individuals can protect themselves from vector bites by wearing appropriate clothing, such as long sleeves and pants, and using insect repellents that contain effective active ingredients. This reduces the risk of direct contact between vectors and potential hosts.

5. ***Vector Control Programs***: Implementing comprehensive vector control programs that integrate multiple strategies, including surveillance, community education, and targeted interventions, is crucial for effective disease prevention and control. These programs aim to identify high-risk areas, monitor vector populations, and implement appropriate measures to reduce vector abundance and disease transmission.

1.4.2 Hosts:

HOSTS ARE THE ORGANISMS that serve as the reservoirs for pathogens, providing a source of infection for vectors and other potential hosts. Hosts can be humans, animals, or both. For example, rodents are the primary hosts for the bacterium that causes plague, while birds serve as the primary hosts for the West Nile virus. In some cases, hosts may be asymptomatic carriers of a pathogen, meaning they do not show any symptoms of disease but can still transmit the pathogen to others. Understanding the ecology of a pathogen and its potential hosts is important in developing effective prevention and control strategies.

Controlling the transmission of communicable diseases often involves targeting both vectors and hosts. This can include measures such as vaccination campaigns, vector control measures such as insecticide spraying and use of bed nets, and public health education campaigns to promote good hygiene and reduce contact between hosts and vectors. By targeting both vectors and hosts, public health officials can work to interrupt the chain of transmission and prevent the spread of disease.

1.5 Outbreak investigation

OUTBREAK INVESTIGATION is a critical component of public health practice, as it allows public health officials to identify and control the spread of communicable diseases. Here is an overview of the steps involved in outbreak investigation:

1.5.1 Confirm the existence of an outbreak:

THE FIRST STEP IN OUTBREAK investigation is crucial for timely recognition and response to a potential public health threat. Confirming the occurrence of an outbreak involves a systematic and thorough analysis of various data sources and reports. Several key activities are undertaken during this phase to establish the presence of an outbreak:

1.5.1.1 Surveillance Data Analysis:

PUBLIC HEALTH AGENCIES routinely collect and analyze surveillance data from various sources, such as hospitals, clinics, laboratories, and disease reporting systems. Epidemiologists examine these data to identify any unusual patterns or increases in the number of cases or deaths compared to the expected baseline. Statistical methods may be applied to determine if the observed numbers are statistically significant.

1.5.1.2 Case and Death Reporting:

HEALTH CARE PROVIDERS and laboratories play a vital role in reporting cases and deaths to public health authorities. During the outbreak investigation, health authorities actively communicate with healthcare facilities and providers to identify any unusual or clustering of cases that may indicate an outbreak.

Public health agencies encourage prompt reporting to ensure timely intervention and control measures.

1.5.1.3 Field Investigations:

FIELD INVESTIGATIONS are often initiated to verify and supplement the information obtained from surveillance data and case reports. This involves on-site visits to affected areas, interviews with affected individuals, and collection of additional data and specimens for laboratory testing. Field investigations aim to gather firsthand information, confirm the presence of the outbreak, and identify potential risk factors or sources of transmission.

1.5.1.4 Outbreak Detection Systems:

SOME REGIONS HAVE ESTABLISHED specific outbreak detection systems, which employ sophisticated algorithms and statistical models to identify unusual patterns in surveillance data automatically. These systems can detect outbreaks earlier than traditional surveillance methods by flagging statistically significant increases in the number of cases or other relevant indicators.

During this initial phase, the focus is on rapidly assessing the situation to determine whether an outbreak is occurring and the potential magnitude of the problem. Once the presence of an outbreak is confirmed, the investigation proceeds to the next phase, which involves a more in-depth examination of the outbreak's characteristics, including its source, mode of transmission, and affected populations.

Confirming an outbreak is crucial as it triggers a coordinated response from public health authorities, healthcare providers, and other relevant stakeholders. It allows for the implementation of targeted interventions, such as case management, infection control measures, contact tracing, and public health education. Timely recognition and confirmation of outbreaks are essential for implementing effective control measures, minimizing the spread of disease, and protecting public health.

1.5.2 Define the case definition:

ONCE AN OUTBREAK HAS been confirmed, the next step in the investigation is to establish a clear case definition. A case definition outlines the criteria used to identify individuals who are considered to be affected by the disease under investigation. This process involves determining both the clinical and laboratory criteria that will be used to classify cases.

1.5.2.1 Clinical Criteria:

THE CLINICAL CRITERIA specify the signs, symptoms, and other clinical features that indicate a probable case of the disease. This includes specific symptoms, such as fever, cough, rash, or gastrointestinal symptoms, that are commonly associated with the disease. The clinical criteria may also consider the duration and severity of symptoms.

1.5.2.2 Laboratory Criteria:

IN SOME CASES, LABORATORY testing is required to confirm the diagnosis or classify cases. The laboratory criteria define the specific laboratory tests or results that are necessary to confirm the presence of the pathogen or its associated markers. This may include tests such as blood cultures, polymerase chain reaction (PCR) assays, serological tests, or other diagnostic methods.

By establishing a clear case definition, public health officials can ensure consistency in identifying and classifying cases, which is essential for accurate surveillance, data collection, and comparison across different settings or time periods.

1.5.3 Documentation

ONCE THE CASE DEFINITION is in place, the next step is to identify and document all cases of the disease in the affected population. This involves conducting thorough case finding activities, which may include:

1.5.3.1 Active Case Finding:

PUBLIC HEALTH OFFICIALS actively search for cases by contacting healthcare providers, hospitals, clinics, and laboratories to identify individuals who meet the case definition. This may involve reviewing medical records, laboratory reports, and other relevant data sources.

1.5.3.2 Passive Case Reporting:

HEALTHCARE PROVIDERS and laboratories are encouraged to report suspected or confirmed cases of the disease to public health authorities promptly. Passive case reporting relies on healthcare professionals recognizing and reporting cases based on their clinical judgment and awareness of the outbreak.

Once cases are identified, a line list is created to systematically track and document the characteristics of each case. The line list includes relevant information such as demographic data (e.g., age, sex, and residence), clinical features, laboratory results, date of onset, and other pertinent details. The line list serves as a valuable tool for analyzing the outbreak data, identifying commonalities or patterns among cases, and informing further investigations.

Establishing a comprehensive line list enables public health officials to monitor the progression of the outbreak, identify risk factors, track the distribution of cases, and evaluate the effectiveness of control measures. It also facilitates data sharing and collaboration among different stakeholders involved in the outbreak response, supporting evidence-based decision-making and timely intervention strategies.

1.5.4 Generate hypotheses:

USING THE LINE LIST and other available data, public health officials utilize the information gathered to generate hypotheses about the possible source and mode of transmission of the disease causing the outbreak. These hypotheses serve as initial theories that guide the subsequent investigations and help in understanding the underlying factors contributing to the outbreak.

1.5.4.1 Source Hypotheses:

PUBLIC HEALTH OFFICIALS propose various potential sources from which the outbreak may have originated. This could include contaminated food or water, specific environmental exposures, animal reservoirs, or human-to-human transmission. The hypotheses are based on patterns observed in the affected individuals, such as common exposures, geographic clustering, or temporal relationships.

1.5.4.2 Transmission Hypotheses:

PUBLIC HEALTH OFFICIALS formulate hypotheses regarding the mode of transmission of the disease. This involves considering the possible routes through which the pathogen could be transmitted from the source to susceptible individuals. Transmission hypotheses may involve direct person-to-person contact, airborne transmission, vector-borne transmission (e.g., through mosquitoes or ticks), or other possible mechanisms based on the characteristics of the disease and available epidemiological evidence.

Once these hypotheses are generated, public health officials proceed to test them through comprehensive epidemiological and laboratory investigations. The aim is to gather additional evidence and data that either support or refute the proposed hypotheses. The investigative process may involve the following steps:

1.5.4.3 Epidemiological Investigations:

EPIDEMIOLOGISTS CONDUCT detailed interviews and questionnaires with affected individuals to gather information about potential exposures, travel history, social interactions, and other relevant factors. Comparisons between affected and non-affected individuals, such as in case-control studies or cohort studies, may be conducted to identify associations between exposures and the disease.

1.5.4.4 Laboratory Investigations:

LABORATORY TESTING plays a crucial role in confirming the diagnosis, identifying the causative agent, and understanding its characteristics. Samples collected from affected individuals, such as blood, respiratory specimens, stool, or environmental samples, are analyzed using various laboratory techniques, including molecular tests, serological assays, culture methods, or other specific diagnostic methods. Laboratory investigations help in confirming the presence of the pathogen, determining its genetic characteristics, and assessing its virulence.

By systematically testing the hypotheses, public health officials can gather solid evidence to support or refine their understanding of the outbreak's source and mode of transmission. This information is critical for implementing appropriate control measures, developing targeted interventions, and preventing further spread of the disease. The investigations also contribute to the overall understanding of the disease and aid in the development of effective prevention and control strategies for similar outbreaks in the future.

1.5.5 Implement control measures:

BASED ON THE RESULTS of the investigations and the confirmed understanding of the source and mode of transmission of the disease, public health officials proceed to implement a range of control measures aimed at preventing further spread of the disease. These measures are essential for containing the outbreak and protecting the health and well-being of the affected population. Some common control measures include:

1.5.5.1 Isolation and Quarantine:

ISOLATION REFERS TO the separation of individuals who have been diagnosed with the disease from healthy individuals to prevent further transmission. Infected individuals are typically isolated in healthcare facilities or designated isolation units, depending on the severity of their condition. Quarantine involves the restriction of movement for individuals who have been exposed to the disease but are not yet showing symptoms. Quarantine helps to monitor and prevent potential transmission during the incubation period.

1.5.5.2 Contact Tracing:

CONTACT TRACING IS a crucial component of outbreak control, particularly for diseases transmitted through person-to-person contact. Public health officials identify and trace individuals who have had close contact with confirmed cases. Contacts are monitored, advised on self-quarantine if necessary, and tested for the disease to identify early cases and interrupt the chain of transmission.

1.5.5.3 Targeted Vaccination Campaigns:

IF AN EFFECTIVE VACCINE is available for the disease, public health officials may initiate targeted vaccination campaigns. This involves vaccinating individuals at high risk of infection or those in close contact with confirmed cases. Vaccination helps to prevent new infections and reduce the overall impact of the outbreak. Vaccine distribution may prioritize vulnerable populations, such as children, the elderly, or individuals with compromised immune systems.

1. *Public Health Education and Awareness*: Public health officials play a crucial role in educating the public about the disease, its transmission, and preventive measures. They provide accurate and up-to-date information

through various communication channels, including public announcements, social media, websites, and community outreach programs. Public education helps to raise awareness, promote preventive behaviors (such as hand hygiene and respiratory etiquette), and reduce anxiety and misconceptions surrounding the disease.

2. ***Environmental and Hygiene Measures***: Public health officials may recommend and implement environmental and hygiene measures to minimize the risk of transmission. This could include disinfection and sanitization of public spaces, water treatment and quality control, proper waste management, and promotion of good hygiene practices in households, schools, and healthcare facilities.

These control measures are implemented in a coordinated manner, involving collaboration between public health agencies, healthcare providers, government authorities, and other stakeholders. Ongoing monitoring and evaluation of the implemented measures are essential to assess their effectiveness and make necessary adjustments as the outbreak evolves.

By implementing these control measures, public health officials aim to limit the spread of the disease, reduce the number of new cases, and ultimately bring the outbreak under control. These measures are crucial in protecting the health and well-being of the population and preventing the outbreak from escalating further.

1.5.6 Communicate findings:

FINALLY, AFTER COMPLETING the outbreak investigation and implementing control measures, public health officials recognize the importance of transparent and effective communication. They understand that clear and timely communication is crucial for ensuring that the affected population, healthcare providers, and other stakeholders are well-informed about the disease, the ongoing investigation, and the measures being taken to control the outbreak. Effective communication fosters trust, promotes cooperation, and enables the adoption of preventive behaviors, ultimately contributing to the success of outbreak control efforts.

Public health officials engage in various communication strategies to disseminate information:

1.5.6.1 Public Health Notifications:

THEY ISSUE OFFICIAL public health notifications or press releases to inform the general public about the outbreak, its impact, and the actions being taken to address it. These notifications may be shared through traditional media channels, such as newspapers, television, and radio, as well as through online platforms and social media.

1.5.6.2 Public Briefings and Updates:

PUBLIC HEALTH OFFICIALS conduct regular briefings and updates to provide accurate and up-to-date information to the affected population, healthcare providers, and other stakeholders. These briefings may include details about the investigation findings, updates on the number of cases and their distribution, and any changes in control measures or recommendations.

1.5.6.3 Health Education Campaigns:

PUBLIC HEALTH OFFICIALS design and implement targeted health education campaigns to raise awareness about the disease, its symptoms, modes of transmission, and preventive measures. These campaigns may involve distributing informational materials, conducting community meetings or workshops, and leveraging digital platforms to disseminate educational content.

1.5.6.4 Collaboration with Healthcare Providers:

PUBLIC HEALTH OFFICIALS collaborate closely with healthcare providers, sharing relevant information, guidelines, and protocols to ensure a consistent approach to diagnosis, treatment, and surveillance. This collaboration enhances the ability to identify and manage cases effectively.

1.5.6.5 Engaging the Community:

PUBLIC HEALTH OFFICIALS actively engage with the affected community, listening to their concerns and addressing any misconceptions. They involve community leaders, organizations, and influential figures in disseminating information and encouraging community participation in outbreak control measures. This engagement fosters a sense of ownership and empowers the community to actively contribute to the prevention and control of the outbreak.

Throughout the communication process, public health officials prioritize accuracy, clarity, and empathy. They use plain language, avoiding technical jargon, to ensure that the information is easily understood by the target audience. They also remain accessible to address questions, provide guidance, and alleviate any fears or anxieties related to the outbreak.

Outbreak investigation is indeed a complex process that requires the collaboration and coordination of multiple stakeholders, including public health officials, healthcare providers, researchers, and the affected community. By working together, sharing information, and pooling resources, these stakeholders can effectively identify and control outbreaks, prevent the spread of communicable diseases, and safeguard public health. Such collaborative efforts are vital in mitigating the impact of outbreaks and reducing the burden of disease on the affected population.

1.6 Case study: Malaria in Ghana

MALARIA IS A SIGNIFICANT public health problem in Ghana, posing a major burden on the population's health and well-being. The disease accounts for a substantial proportion of morbidity and mortality in the country, particularly among vulnerable populations such as children and pregnant women. Let's explore a brief case study of malaria in Ghana to understand the impact and efforts made to address this public health challenge.

Ghana, located in West Africa, is endemic for malaria, with transmission occurring throughout the year, although the intensity varies across different regions. The disease is primarily caused by the Plasmodium falciparum parasite, known for its severe form of malaria.

1. ***Disease Burden***: Malaria poses a significant burden on the Ghanaian population. According to the World Health Organization (WHO), Ghana accounted for a considerable number of malaria cases and deaths globally.

The prevalence of the disease varies across the country, with higher rates reported in rural areas and regions with favorable breeding sites for mosquitoes.

2. ***Impact on Vulnerable Populations***: Children under the age of five and pregnant women are particularly vulnerable to malaria in Ghana. The disease can lead to severe illness and complications in these populations, contributing to high morbidity and mortality rates. Malaria-related anemia, low birth weight, and increased risk of maternal and infant mortality are some of the consequences faced by pregnant women.

3. ***Prevention and Control Efforts***: Ghana has implemented various strategies to combat malaria and reduce its impact on the population:

   a. ***Insecticide-Treated Bed Nets***: The distribution of long-lasting insecticidal nets (LLINs) is a key preventive measure. Through mass distribution campaigns and routine distribution at health facilities, Ghana has made substantial progress in increasing bed net coverage, particularly among pregnant women and children.

   b. ***Indoor Residual Spraying (IRS)***: The use of insecticides to spray the inner walls of houses helps control malaria-transmitting mosquitoes. IRS has been implemented in targeted areas with high malaria transmission intensity, further reducing the risk of infection.

   c. ***Diagnosis and Treatment***: Access to prompt and accurate malaria diagnosis is essential for effective case management. Ghana has scaled up the use of rapid diagnostic tests (RDTs) and improved access to artemisinin-based combination therapy (ACT) for the treatment of confirmed cases.

d. ***Intermittent Preventive Treatment in Pregnancy (IPTp)***: Pregnant women receive IPTp doses during antenatal care visits to prevent malaria and associated complications.

e. ***Health Education and Behavior Change***: Health promotion campaigns are conducted to raise awareness about malaria prevention, symptoms, and the importance of seeking early treatment. These campaigns emphasize the use of bed nets, proper sanitation, and prompt treatment-seeking behavior.

4. ***Partnerships and Collaborations***: The Ghanaian government collaborates with international organizations, such as the WHO, Global Fund, and other development partners, to strengthen malaria control efforts. These collaborations provide technical support, funding, and capacity-building initiatives to enhance the country's malaria control programs.

Despite the ongoing efforts, challenges persist in the fight against malaria in Ghana. These include issues related to healthcare access, the emergence of drug-resistant parasites, vector control in hard-to-reach areas, and the need for sustained funding and resources. However, Ghana's commitment to malaria control and its implementation of evidence-based interventions have contributed to significant progress in reducing the burden of the disease.

The case study of malaria in Ghana highlights the multifaceted approach required to combat a complex disease like malaria. Through a combination of preventive measures, early diagnosis, effective treatment, and community engagement, Ghana aims to reduce the impact of malaria on its population and achieve the national goal of malaria elimination in the long run.

Here is a breakdown of the number of confirmed malaria cases reported by WHO in 2019 for some countries in sub-Saharan Africa:

Table 2: Confirmed Malaria Cases

Country	Number of confirmed malaria cases (2019)
Ghana	5.7 million
Nigeria	27 million
Tanzania	5.6 million
Mozambique	4.4 million
Democratic Republic of the Congo (DRC)	15.3 million
Uganda	12 million

This table shows the number of malaria cases reported by WHO in 2019 for selected countries.

Epidemiology:

Malaria is endemic in Ghana, with transmission occurring year-round in many areas. The disease is caused by the Plasmodium parasite, which is transmitted to humans through the bite of infected Anopheles mosquitoes. According to the World Health Organization (WHO), Ghana reported 5.7 million confirmed cases of malaria in 2019, accounting for 3.1% of all malaria cases in sub-Saharan Africa.

Conclusion:

Malaria is a significant public health problem in Ghana, and efforts to control the disease are ongoing. While progress has been made in distributing ITNs, conducting IRS campaigns, and improving case management, significant challenges remain. Addressing these challenges will require sustained investment in malaria control efforts, as well as a focus on strengthening the overall health system in Ghana.

1.7 Exercises

1. Multiple-choice: What is the most common mode of transmission for malaria? a) Airborne b) Foodborne c) Vector-borne d) Waterborne

Answer: c) Vector-borne

1. True or False: TB is caused by a virus.

Answer: False

1. Fill in the blank: HIV attacks the body's ______________

cells.

Answer: immune system

1. Matching: Match the following diseases with their mode of transmission

   I. Cholera a) Airborne
  II. Yellow fever b) Vector-borne
 III. Measles c) Foodborne
 IV. Malaria d) Waterborne

ANSWERS: I-c II-b III-a IV-b

1. Short answer: What is the basic reproductive number (R0) and why is it important in disease transmission?

Answer: R0 is the number of people that one infected person is likely to infect in a susceptible population. It is important in disease transmission because it helps in predicting the potential for an outbreak and in developing control measures.

1. Multiple-choice: Which of the following is not a key element of outbreak investigation? a) Contact tracing b) Laboratory testing c) Mass vaccination d) Surveillance

Answer: c) Mass vaccination

1. True or False: Ebola can be transmitted through the air.

Answer: False

1. Short answer: What are the three key strategies for

preventing the transmission of communicable diseases?

Answer: Vaccination, sanitation, and hygiene measures.

1. Multiple-choice: What is the International Health Regulations? a) A set of guidelines for ensuring food safety b) A global agreement for the prevention and control of communicable diseases c) A framework for promoting mental health d) A treaty for reducing air pollution

Answer: b) A global agreement for the prevention and control of communicable diseases.

Chapter 2. Disease prevention and control

2.1 Prevention strategies for communicable diseases

Prevention strategies for communicable diseases are essential to reduce the burden of disease and prevent their spread. Here are some common prevention strategies for communicable diseases:

2.1.1 Vaccination:

VACCINATION IS WIDELY recognized as one of the most effective strategies for preventing communicable diseases and reducing their burden on public health. Vaccines work by stimulating the body's immune system to recognize and mount a protective response against specific pathogens, such as bacteria or viruses. This immune response helps to prevent infection or reduce the severity of the disease if an individual is exposed to the pathogen.

Vaccines have played a crucial role in controlling and eradicating numerous infectious diseases throughout history. They have been instrumental in preventing millions of cases, reducing hospitalizations, and saving countless lives. Here are some examples of vaccines and their impact:

2.1.1.1 Measles Vaccine:

THE MEASLES VACCINE is highly effective in preventing measles, a highly contagious viral disease. Before the introduction of the vaccine, measles caused significant morbidity and mortality worldwide, particularly among children. Through widespread vaccination campaigns, measles control programs, and routine immunization, many countries have successfully reduced the incidence of measles and even eliminated it in certain regions.

2.1.1.2 Polio Vaccine:

THE POLIO VACCINE HAS been instrumental in the global effort to eradicate poliomyelitis, a highly infectious viral disease that can cause paralysis and even death. The oral polio vaccine (OPV) and the inactivated polio vaccine (IPV) have played a critical role in reducing the number of polio cases worldwide. Thanks to extensive vaccination campaigns, several regions have been certified polio-free, bringing us closer to global eradication.

2.1.1.3 HPV Vaccine:

THE HUMAN PAPILLOMAVIRUS (HPV) vaccine protects against several strains of HPV that can cause cervical, anal, and other types of cancers, as well as genital warts. By vaccinating adolescents and young adults, the HPV vaccine has the potential to significantly reduce the incidence of these HPV-related diseases, leading to improved public health outcomes.

Vaccination programs typically target specific populations based on disease epidemiology, risk factors, and age groups. Immunization schedules outline the recommended vaccines and their timing, ensuring optimal protection throughout life. Routine childhood immunization programs, in particular, play a crucial role in preventing numerous communicable diseases.

In addition to preventing individual cases, vaccination also contributes to herd immunity, wherein a significant portion of the population is immunized, reducing the overall transmission of the disease. This protection benefits vulnerable individuals who may not be eligible for certain vaccines due to age, underlying health conditions, or other factors.

It's important to note that vaccines undergo rigorous testing and monitoring for safety and effectiveness before they are approved for public use. Regulatory authorities carefully assess their benefits and potential risks. Ongoing surveillance and post-marketing studies further monitor vaccine safety.

Public health campaigns and education efforts are essential to address vaccine hesitancy and ensure high vaccine uptake. By promoting accurate information, addressing concerns, and emphasizing the benefits of vaccination, public health authorities strive to build trust and confidence in immunization programs.

2.1.2 Sanitation:

SANITATION MEASURES play a crucial role in preventing the spread of communicable diseases by ensuring proper waste disposal and access to clean water. Contaminated water and food are common sources of pathogens that cause diseases such as cholera, typhoid, and various gastrointestinal infections. Implementing effective sanitation practices is essential in reducing the risk of transmission and improving public health. Here are some key aspects of sanitation measures and their impact:

2.1.2.1 Proper Waste Disposal:

ADEQUATE WASTE MANAGEMENT systems, including proper collection, transportation, and disposal of waste, are critical for preventing the proliferation of disease-causing organisms. Improper disposal of solid waste can attract pests, including rodents and insects, which can carry pathogens and spread diseases. Additionally, untreated or poorly managed sewage can contaminate water sources, leading to the spread of waterborne diseases. By implementing proper waste disposal methods, such as sanitary landfill facilities and waste treatment systems, the risk of disease transmission can be significantly reduced.

2.1.2.2 Access to Clean Water:

ACCESS TO CLEAN AND safe drinking water is essential for maintaining good hygiene and preventing waterborne diseases. Contaminated water sources can harbor pathogens, including bacteria, viruses, and parasites, that cause diseases like cholera, typhoid fever, hepatitis A, and dysentery. Implementing water treatment processes, such as filtration, disinfection, and chlorination, helps eliminate or reduce the presence of pathogens, making the water safe for consumption. Providing communities with access to clean water sources and promoting safe storage practices, such as using covered containers, further ensures the availability of safe drinking water.

2.1.2.3 Improved Sanitary Facilities:

PROPER SANITATION FACILITIES, including toilets and handwashing stations, are critical for preventing the fecal-oral transmission of diseases. Inadequate sanitation infrastructure, such as the absence of toilets or open defecation practices, can lead to the contamination of the environment and water sources, increasing the risk of disease transmission. Promoting the construction and use of improved sanitation facilities, such as flush toilets, pit latrines, or sanitation systems with proper waste disposal mechanisms, can significantly reduce the spread of communicable diseases.

2.1.2.4 Hygiene Practices:

ALONGSIDE SANITATION measures, promoting good hygiene practices is essential in preventing the spread of communicable diseases. This includes regular handwashing with soap and clean water, especially before handling food and after using the toilet. Hand hygiene helps remove pathogens from the hands and prevents their transfer to the mouth or other surfaces. Educating communities about the importance of hygiene practices and providing access to handwashing facilities can significantly improve public health outcomes.

Efforts to improve sanitation and hygiene practices are vital at both the individual and community levels. Governments, public health authorities, and international organizations work together to develop and implement policies, guidelines, and programs to enhance sanitation infrastructure, provide access to clean water, and promote hygiene education. Community engagement, awareness campaigns, and capacity building initiatives are also crucial to foster behavior change and ensure the sustainable adoption of sanitation and hygiene practices.

2.1.3 Hygiene measures:

PERSONAL HYGIENE MEASURES play a crucial role in preventing the spread of communicable diseases. Simple practices such as regular hand washing, covering the mouth and nose when coughing or sneezing, and avoiding close contact with sick individuals are effective in reducing the transmission of diseases like the flu and COVID-19.

Regular hand washing with soap and water, or using alcohol-based hand sanitizers when soap and water are not available, is an essential hygiene measure. Hand washing helps remove pathogens from the hands, preventing their transfer to the face or other surfaces. The Centers for Disease Control and Prevention (CDC) recommends washing hands for at least 20 seconds, especially before eating, after using the restroom, and after coughing, sneezing, or blowing the nose.

Covering the mouth and nose with a tissue or the elbow when coughing or sneezing is another important hygiene practice. This helps prevent the release of respiratory droplets containing infectious agents into the air, reducing the risk of transmission to others. By following this practice, individuals can minimize the spread of respiratory illnesses, including the flu and COVID-19.

Furthermore, avoiding close contact with sick individuals is crucial to prevent the spread of communicable diseases. When someone is ill, maintaining a safe distance helps minimize the risk of inhaling respiratory droplets that may contain infectious pathogens. This practice is especially important during outbreaks or pandemics when the transmission of diseases can be widespread.

These hygiene measures have been emphasized during the COVID-19 pandemic as effective strategies to reduce the transmission of the virus. The World Health Organization (WHO) and health authorities worldwide have promoted these practices as part of public health guidelines to control the spread of COVID-19.

Real-world examples of the impact of personal hygiene measures can be seen during flu seasons or outbreaks of infectious diseases. In many countries, public health campaigns raise awareness about the importance of hand hygiene, cough etiquette, and maintaining distance from sick individuals. These campaigns have been successful in reducing the transmission of diseases and protecting public health.

2.1.4 Environmental measures:

ENVIRONMENTAL MEASURES play a crucial role in preventing the spread of diseases transmitted by insect vectors, such as malaria and dengue fever. Controlling these vectors can significantly reduce the risk of disease transmission and protect public health.

One of the most notable examples of environmental measures to control disease transmission is the fight against malaria. Malaria is a mosquito-borne disease caused by the Plasmodium parasite. To prevent the transmission of malaria, various environmental interventions have been employed. For instance, mosquito breeding sites are targeted for elimination or treatment to reduce the mosquito population. Stagnant water sources, where mosquitoes lay their eggs, are often treated with larvicides to prevent the emergence of adult mosquitoes. Additionally, insecticide-treated bed nets are widely distributed in malaria-endemic regions to protect individuals from mosquito bites while they sleep.

Similarly, dengue fever, another mosquito-borne disease, can be controlled through environmental measures. Mosquitoes of the Aedes genus are the primary vectors responsible for dengue virus transmission. To combat dengue, efforts are made to reduce mosquito breeding sites in urban areas, such as empty containers, tires, and discarded items that can collect rainwater. Community participation in identifying and eliminating potential breeding sites has proven effective in reducing dengue transmission in some regions.

Beyond mosquito-borne diseases, environmental measures have been implemented to control other insect vectors as well. For instance, controlling flies is essential in preventing the spread of diseases like trachoma, which is a leading cause of blindness in certain regions. Trachoma is transmitted through eye-seeking flies, and improved sanitation, waste management, and fly control programs have been successful in reducing its prevalence.

Real-world examples of the impact of environmental measures on disease prevention can be seen in several countries that have implemented vector control programs. Sri Lanka's efforts to control malaria through mosquito control interventions significantly reduced the number of malaria cases, earning the country a malaria-free certification from the World Health Organization in 2016. Similarly, the city of La Paz in Bolivia successfully reduced the transmission of dengue fever by implementing targeted vector control measures These examples demonstrate how environmental measures, such as vector control, are essential components of public health strategies to prevent the spread of diseases transmitted by insect vectors.

2.1.5 Screening and testing:

SCREENING AND TESTING play a crucial role in the early detection and prevention of communicable diseases. These strategies help identify individuals who may be infected with a specific disease, allowing for timely intervention, treatment, and control measures. Here are some examples of screening and testing for communicable diseases:

2.1.5.1 Tuberculosis (TB) screening:

TUBERCULOSIS IS AN infectious disease caused by the bacterium Mycobacterium tuberculosis. Screening for TB involves conducting tests such as the tuberculin skin test (TST) or interferon-gamma release assays (IGRAs). These tests help identify individuals who have been exposed to TB bacteria or have latent TB infection. If the screening test is positive, further diagnostic tests, such as chest X-rays and sputum tests, are performed to confirm active TB disease.

2.1.5.2 HIV testing:

HIV (HUMAN IMMUNODEFICIENCY Virus) is the virus that causes AIDS (Acquired Immunodeficiency Syndrome). HIV testing is crucial for early detection, initiation of treatment, and prevention of transmission. Various types of HIV tests are available, including rapid tests, enzyme immunoassays (EIAs), and nucleic acid tests (NATs). HIV testing can be performed using blood, oral fluid, or urine samples, and can provide results within minutes or a few days, depending on the testing method.

2.1.5.3 Hepatitis screening:

HEPATITIS REFERS TO inflammation of the liver, and several viruses can cause hepatitis, including hepatitis A, B, C, D, and E. Screening for hepatitis involves blood tests to detect specific viral markers, such as antibodies or antigens. Hepatitis B and C are particularly important to screen for, as they can lead to chronic liver disease and complications. Early detection through screening allows for appropriate medical management and preventive measures.

2.1.5.4 Sexually transmitted infection (STI) testing:

STI TESTING IS IMPORTANT for identifying and treating infections that are primarily transmitted through sexual contact. Examples of common STIs include chlamydia, gonorrhea, syphilis, and human papillomavirus (HPV) infection. Testing methods vary depending on the specific infection and may involve urine samples, swabs from genital areas, or blood tests. Prompt diagnosis and treatment of STIs are crucial for preventing the spread of infection and reducing long-term complications.

2.1.5.5 COVID-19 testing:

WITH THE EMERGENCE of the COVID-19 pandemic, testing for the SARS-CoV-2 virus, which causes COVID-19, has become widespread. Testing methods include polymerase chain reaction (PCR) tests, which detect the genetic material of the virus, and antigen tests, which detect specific viral proteins. Testing is used for diagnosis, contact tracing, surveillance, and monitoring the spread of the virus. Rapid and accurate testing has been vital in implementing appropriate public health measures to control the pandemic.

It's important to note that screening and testing for communicable diseases should be conducted in accordance with established guidelines and protocols. These tests should be performed by trained healthcare professionals, and appropriate counseling and follow-up should be provided to individuals who undergo testing.

2.1.6 Isolation and quarantine:

ISOLATION AND QUARANTINE are important measures in preventing the spread of communicable diseases. They involve separating individuals who are infected with a contagious disease or those who have been exposed to the disease from the general population. Here are some key points about isolation and quarantine:

2.1.6.1 Isolation:

ISOLATION IS THE SEPARATION of individuals who have a confirmed infection from those who are healthy. It aims to prevent the spread of the disease to others.

Example: Individuals with active tuberculosis (TB) are isolated until they are no longer infectious. They may be isolated in a healthcare facility or at home, depending on the severity of the disease and the availability of appropriate facilities.

2.1.6.2 Quarantine:

QUARANTINE INVOLVES the separation of individuals who have been exposed to a communicable disease but are not yet showing symptoms. It aims to prevent potential transmission during the incubation period of the disease.

Example: During the COVID-19 pandemic, individuals who have been in close contact with someone infected with the virus may be asked to quarantine for a specific period (e.g., 10-14 days) to monitor for symptoms and prevent further transmission.

Key considerations for isolation and quarantine:

1. ***Timing***: Isolation and quarantine should be implemented as early as possible to reduce the risk of transmission.
2. ***Duration***: The duration of isolation or quarantine depends on the specific disease and public health guidelines. It is based on the incubation period and the duration of infectiousness.
3. ***Facilities and support***: Isolation and quarantine require appropriate facilities, supplies, and support services, including medical care, monitoring of symptoms, and provision of basic needs.
4. ***Communication and education***: Clear communication about the reasons for isolation or quarantine, as well as guidelines for compliance, is essential to ensure understanding and cooperation.
5. ***Compliance and enforcement***: It is important for individuals to comply with isolation and quarantine measures voluntarily. However, enforcement measures may be necessary in certain situations to protect public health.
6. ***Mental health support***: Isolated or quarantined individuals may experience psychological distress, and access to mental health support should be provided.

It is crucial to implement isolation and quarantine measures alongside other preventive measures, such as testing, contact tracing, and vaccination, to effectively control the spread of communicable diseases.

Mostly, a combination of prevention strategies is usually the most effective approach for preventing the spread of communicable diseases. By implementing measures such as vaccination, sanitation, and hygiene measures, we can reduce the burden of disease and protect public health.

2.2 The use of antibiotics and antivirals in disease control

ANTIBIOTICS AND ANTIVIRALS are medications used in disease control to treat infections caused by bacteria and viruses, respectively. Here are some key points regarding the use of antibiotics and antivirals in disease control:

2.2.1 Antibiotics:

ANTIBIOTICS ARE DRUGS that target bacteria and are used to treat bacterial infections such as pneumonia, strep throat, and urinary tract infections. They work by killing or slowing the growth of bacteria, allowing the body's immune system to fight off the infection more effectively. It is important to note that antibiotics are not effective against viral infections such as the common cold, flu, or COVID-19.

Antibiotics play a crucial role in modern medicine, helping to treat and control bacterial infections that can cause significant morbidity and mortality. However, their misuse and overuse have contributed to the emergence of antibiotic resistance, a global public health threat. It is important to use antibiotics judiciously to preserve their effectiveness for future generations.

One real-world example highlighting the importance of responsible antibiotic use is the case of Methicillin-resistant Staphylococcus aureus (MRSA) infections. MRSA is a strain of bacteria that is resistant to many commonly used antibiotics, making it challenging to treat. The widespread use of antibiotics, especially in healthcare settings, has contributed to the emergence and spread of MRSA. Implementing infection prevention and control measures, promoting appropriate antibiotic prescribing practices, and improving surveillance systems have been key strategies in combating MRSA infections.

Another example is the management of tuberculosis (TB). TB is a bacterial infection caused by Mycobacterium tuberculosis. The treatment of TB requires a combination of antibiotics, known as anti-tuberculosis drugs, taken for an extended period. However, the emergence of drug-resistant TB, such as multidrug-resistant TB (MDR-TB) and extensively drug-resistant TB (XDR-TB), poses significant challenges to TB control efforts. Effective management of drug-resistant TB involves appropriate laboratory diagnostics, access to specialized drugs, and strict adherence to treatment.

2.2.2 Antivirals:

ANTIVIRAL MEDICATIONS play a critical role in the treatment and management of various viral infections, helping to reduce symptoms, prevent complications, and improve patient outcomes. They are designed to target specific viral processes and inhibit viral replication. Here are a few real-world examples of antiviral use in different viral infections:

2.2.2.1 HIV/AIDS:

ANTIRETROVIRAL THERAPY (ART) is the cornerstone of HIV treatment and involves the use of a combination of antiviral drugs. ART suppresses the replication of the human immunodeficiency virus (HIV), reduces the viral load in the body, and allows the immune system to recover. This has led to significant improvements in the prognosis and quality of life for individuals living with HIV/AIDS.

2.2.2.2 Hepatitis B and C:

ANTIVIRAL DRUGS ARE used in the treatment of chronic hepatitis B and C infections to reduce viral replication, prevent liver damage, and decrease the risk of complications such as cirrhosis and liver cancer. Examples of antiviral drugs used in hepatitis treatment include entecavir and sofosbuvir, among others.

2.2.2.3 Influenza:

ANTIVIRAL MEDICATIONS such as oseltamivir (Tamiflu) and zanamivir are used to treat and manage influenza infections. These drugs work by inhibiting the neuraminidase enzyme, which is essential for viral replication. Early initiation of antiviral treatment can help reduce the severity and duration of influenza symptoms.

2.2.3 Overuse and misuse:

THE OVERUSE AND MISUSE of antibiotics and antivirals can contribute to the development of drug-resistant bacteria and viruses, making infections more difficult to treat. Therefore, it is important to use these medications only when necessary and to follow the prescribed dosage and duration.

2.2.4 Side effects:

OVERUSE AND MISUSE of antibiotics and antivirals pose significant challenges to public health by promoting the emergence and spread of drug-resistant microorganisms. Inappropriate use includes taking antibiotics for viral infections or using them in improper dosages or durations. Similarly, using antivirals in non-indicated cases or deviating from recommended treatment regimens can also contribute to the development of antiviral resistance.

The consequences of overuse and misuse of these medications are far-reaching. It can lead to treatment failures, prolonged illnesses, increased healthcare costs, and, in severe cases, limited or no treatment options for certain infections. Furthermore, the spread of drug-resistant microorganisms can pose a threat to public health, making it difficult to control outbreaks and increasing the risk of severe infections and complications.

To combat this issue, appropriate prescribing practices, public awareness campaigns, and education programs for healthcare professionals and the general public are crucial. Implementing antimicrobial stewardship programs, which promote responsible and evidence-based use of antibiotics and antivirals, can help preserve the effectiveness of these medications and mitigate the development of drug resistance.

Here are some real-world examples of overuse and misuse of antibiotics and antivirals:

2.2.4.1 Overuse of antibiotics in upper respiratory tract

infections:

UPPER RESPIRATORY TRACT infections, such as the common cold and sinusitis, are primarily caused by viruses. However, antibiotics are often prescribed unnecessarily, leading to their overuse. A study conducted in the United States found that antibiotics were prescribed in approximately 67% of adult acute respiratory tract infection visits, even though antibiotics are not effective against viral infections.

2.2.4.2 Misuse of antibiotics in agricultural practices:

IN SOME COUNTRIES, antibiotics are used as growth promoters in livestock and poultry farming. This practice can lead to the spread of antibiotic-resistant bacteria through the food chain. For example, a study conducted in Nigeria found high levels of antibiotic residues in poultry products, indicating the misuse of antibiotics in the poultry industry.

2.2.4.3 Inappropriate use of antivirals in influenza:

ANTIVIRAL MEDICATIONS such as oseltamivir (Tamiflu) are effective in treating influenza when initiated early and in high-risk patients. However, their inappropriate use, such as using them without a confirmed diagnosis or using them as a preventive measure without appropriate indications, can contribute to the development of antiviral resistance. A study conducted in the United States found that a significant proportion of oseltamivir prescriptions during the 2009 H1N1 influenza pandemic did not adhere to treatment guidelines.

2.2.5 Combination therapy:

COMBINATION THERAPY refers to the use of two or more antibiotics or antivirals simultaneously to treat certain infections. This approach aims to enhance treatment efficacy by targeting multiple aspects of the infection, such as different strains of bacteria or different stages of viral replication. While combination therapy can be effective, it is important to carefully consider its benefits and potential risks.

One example of combination therapy is the treatment of tuberculosis (TB). TB is caused by the bacterium Mycobacterium tuberculosis, which can develop resistance to single antibiotics through genetic mutations. To combat drug-resistant TB, a combination of multiple antibiotics is typically prescribed. This approach helps to prevent the emergence of further drug resistance and increases treatment success rates.

Another example is the treatment of HIV/AIDS. Antiretroviral therapy (ART) for HIV typically involves combining different classes of antiretroviral drugs to target the virus at multiple stages of its replication cycle. This combination therapy approach has significantly improved the prognosis and quality of life for individuals living with HIV, reducing mortality rates and suppressing viral replication.

While combination therapy can be beneficial, it is important to be aware of the potential risks and side effects associated with using multiple medications. Some medications may interact with each other, leading to increased toxicity or reduced effectiveness. Additionally, the use of multiple drugs can increase the complexity of treatment regimens and may result in poor adherence to the prescribed therapy.

To ensure the safe and effective use of combination therapy, healthcare professionals must carefully consider the specific infection, the drug resistance patterns, and the individual patient's health status. The benefits of combination therapy should outweigh the potential risks and side effects.

In summary, antibiotics and antivirals are important tools in disease control for treating bacterial and viral infections, respectively. However, their use should be carefully monitored and controlled to prevent the development of drug resistance and minimize side effects.

2.3 The importance of surveillance and early warning systems

SURVEILLANCE AND EARLY warning systems are crucial in disease control and prevention, as they allow for the timely detection and response to disease outbreaks. Here are some key reasons why surveillance and early warning systems are important:

2.3.1 Early detection:

EARLY DETECTION PLAYS a crucial role in disease surveillance and outbreak response. Surveillance systems, coupled with effective early warning systems, enable the timely detection of disease outbreaks, providing public health officials with the opportunity to respond promptly and mitigate the spread of diseases.

One real-world example of early detection is the Global Public Health Intelligence Network (GPHIN), operated by the World Health Organization (WHO). GPHIN is an automated system that collects and analyzes information from various sources, including media reports, social media, and official health reports, to identify and track potential disease outbreaks globally. This early detection system was instrumental in detecting and reporting the outbreak of severe acute respiratory syndrome (SARS) in 2003, allowing for a swift international response to contain the spread of the disease.

Another example is the use of syndromic surveillance systems, which monitor patterns of symptoms or health events to detect disease outbreaks in real-time. In Africa, the Early Warning and Response System (EWARS) has been implemented in several countries to strengthen surveillance and early detection of epidemics, particularly for diseases such as malaria, cholera, and meningitis. EWARS combines data from health facilities, community-based surveillance, and laboratory results to provide early warnings and trigger rapid response interventions.

The early detection of outbreaks not only allows for the implementation of timely response measures but also enables public health officials to allocate resources effectively and mobilize healthcare providers in affected areas. By identifying outbreaks early, interventions can be initiated promptly, including case management, contact tracing, and public health education campaigns, all of which are essential for reducing morbidity and mortality associated with infectious diseases.

2.3.2 Rapid response:

EARLY DETECTION OF disease outbreaks enables rapid response, which can include measures such as isolation and treatment of infected individuals, vaccination campaigns, and implementation of public health measures such as social distancing and mask mandates.

Rapid response is a crucial component of effective disease surveillance and response systems. Once a potential disease outbreak is detected, prompt action is necessary to contain the spread of the disease, mitigate its impact on public health, and save lives. Rapid response strategies encompass a range of interventions aimed at controlling the outbreak and protecting the population.

One notable real-world example of rapid response is the global response to the Ebola outbreak in West Africa, which occurred between 2014 and 2016. The outbreak, primarily affecting Guinea, Liberia, and Sierra Leone, posed a significant threat to public health. In response, national and international organizations swiftly mobilized resources, including healthcare personnel, medical supplies, and funding, to provide immediate support. Rapid response efforts involved establishing treatment centers, implementing infection control measures, conducting contact tracing, and deploying mobile laboratories for timely diagnosis. These measures, combined with public health messaging and community engagement, played a vital role in curbing the spread of the virus and ultimately bringing the outbreak under control.

Another example is the response to the COVID-19 pandemic. When the novel coronavirus emerged in late 2019, countries around the world faced an urgent need for rapid response. Governments and health authorities implemented a range of measures, such as border controls, travel restrictions, testing and contact tracing, and public health campaigns to promote hygiene and social distancing. Additionally, rapid research and development efforts led to the production and distribution of vaccines within a remarkably short timeframe, allowing for mass immunization campaigns to protect populations from the virus.

These examples highlight the importance of swift and coordinated action in response to disease outbreaks. Rapid response measures help to limit the transmission of infectious diseases, minimize the severity of illness, and reduce the burden on healthcare systems. By promptly identifying cases, implementing appropriate control measures, and engaging communities, public health authorities can effectively mitigate the impact of outbreaks and safeguard public health.

2.3.3 Identification of high-risk populations:

SURVEILLANCE SYSTEMS can help identify high-risk populations, such as individuals with weakened immune systems, elderly populations, or individuals living in crowded or unsanitary conditions, and target interventions to these groups.

Identification of high-risk populations is a critical aspect of disease surveillance and response. By identifying specific groups that are more vulnerable to certain diseases, public health authorities can tailor their interventions and prioritize resources where they are most needed. This targeted approach helps to reduce the burden of disease and prevent severe outcomes among high-risk populations.

Examples:

1. One real-world example of identifying high-risk populations is the surveillance and response to tuberculosis (TB) in high-burden countries. TB primarily affects individuals with weakened immune systems, such as those living with HIV/AIDS, malnutrition, or other underlying health conditions. Surveillance systems are used to identify areas with a high prevalence of TB and to target interventions to these populations. For instance, in sub-Saharan Africa, where TB and HIV co-infection

rates are high, integrated surveillance systems have been implemented to detect and manage TB cases among HIV-positive individuals, ensuring timely diagnosis and treatment.

2. Another example is the identification of high-risk populations during disease outbreaks, such as the COVID-19 pandemic. Elderly individuals, people with chronic medical conditions (such as heart disease, diabetes, or respiratory conditions), and residents of nursing homes or long-term care facilities have been identified as high-risk populations for severe illness and complications from COVID-19. Surveillance systems have played a crucial role in monitoring the spread of the virus within these populations and guiding targeted interventions, such as prioritizing vaccination and implementing infection control measures in high-risk

By using surveillance data to identify high-risk populations, public health authorities can implement preventive measures, provide targeted healthcare services, and allocate resources effectively. This approach enhances the overall effectiveness of disease surveillance and response efforts, leading to better health outcomes for vulnerable populations.

2.3.4 Monitoring of disease trends:

SURVEILLANCE SYSTEMS allow public health officials to monitor disease trends over time, enabling the development of more effective prevention and control strategies.

Monitoring disease trends is a crucial function of surveillance systems in public health. By continuously collecting and analyzing data on disease occurrence, surveillance systems provide valuable insights into the patterns and trends of various diseases. This information is essential for understanding the burden of diseases, identifying emerging threats, and evaluating the impact of control measures.

Examples:

1. One real-world example of monitoring disease trends is the surveillance of vaccine-preventable diseases. Through routine surveillance, public health agencies monitor the incidence and distribution of diseases such as measles, polio, and influenza. This data helps identify areas or populations with low vaccination coverage, detect outbreaks or clusters of cases, and assess the effectiveness of immunization programs. Based on these trends, targeted interventions can be implemented, such as intensified vaccination campaigns or public awareness campaigns to increase vaccine uptake

1. Another example is the monitoring of vector-borne diseases like malaria and dengue fever. Surveillance systems track the number of cases, geographic distribution, and seasonality of these diseases. This information helps identify areas of high transmission, detect changes in disease patterns, and assess the effectiveness of vector control measures. For instance, in malaria-endemic regions, surveillance data can guide the distribution of insecticide-treated bed nets and indoor residual spraying in areas with the highest disease burden.

By monitoring disease trends, public health officials can identify shifts in disease patterns, detect outbreaks or epidemics in a timely manner, and develop evidence-based strategies for prevention and control. Surveillance data also play a crucial role in informing public health policies and interventions, ensuring that resources are allocated effectively and targeted to areas of greatest need.

2.3.5 Early warning:

EARLY WARNING SYSTEMS can provide alerts about potential disease outbreaks, allowing for preemptive measures to be taken to prevent or control the spread of disease.

Early warning systems play a critical role in disease surveillance and response, providing timely alerts and signals about potential disease outbreaks. These systems rely on various indicators and data sources to detect early signs of a disease threat, enabling public health authorities to take preemptive measures and mitigate the impact of the outbreak.

Examples

1. One real-world example of an early warning system is the Global Early Warning and Response System (GLEWS), a collaborative effort between the World Health Organization (WHO), the Food and Agriculture Organization of the United Nations (FAO), and the World Organization for Animal Health (OIE). GLEWS monitors and analyzes data on human health, animal health, and food safety to identify potential public health risks, including zoonotic diseases and foodborne illnesses. By integrating information from different sectors, GLEWS enhances early detection and response capabilities, facilitating rapid action to prevent the spread of diseases.

1. Another example is the ProMED-mail system, an

internet-based global reporting system for emerging infectious diseases and outbreaks. ProMED-mail relies on a network of medical and public health professionals who voluntarily report and share information on unusual disease events. The system serves as an early warning mechanism by disseminating timely alerts and updates about outbreaks, enabling the global health community to respond quickly and effectively.

Early warning systems allow public health authorities to mobilize resources, implement control measures, and coordinate response efforts before a disease outbreak reaches a critical level. By providing early alerts, these systems help prevent or minimize the spread of infectious diseases, reduce morbidity and mortality, and enhance preparedness and response capacities at the local, national, and global levels.

2.3.6 International cooperation:

INTERNATIONAL COOPERATION is vital in the field of disease surveillance and early warning systems. Global health threats recognize no borders, and effective prevention and control efforts require collaboration and information sharing between countries. International cooperation in surveillance and early warning systems plays a crucial role in preventing the global spread of infectious diseases and facilitating timely responses to outbreaks.

One example of international cooperation in disease surveillance is the Global Health Security Agenda (GHSA), a partnership of nations, international organizations, and other stakeholders committed to strengthening global health security. The GHSA promotes cooperation in surveillance, laboratory capacity building, and emergency preparedness to detect and respond to infectious diseases. Through collaboration, countries can share epidemiological data, exchange best practices, and coordinate efforts to enhance global health security.

Furthermore, international organizations such as the World Health Organization (WHO), the Centers for Disease Control and Prevention (CDC), and the World Organization for Animal Health (OIE) play pivotal roles in promoting international cooperation and information sharing in disease surveillance. These organizations facilitate the exchange of data, provide technical support, and foster collaboration among countries to enhance surveillance systems and respond to public health emergencies.

International cooperation also extends to the sharing of resources during outbreaks. For instance, during the 2014-2016 Ebola outbreak in West Africa, various countries and international organizations collaborated to provide financial aid, medical supplies, and personnel to support affected countries in their response efforts. This collective action demonstrated the importance of international cooperation in controlling and containing the spread of infectious diseases.

By fostering collaboration and information sharing, international cooperation in disease surveillance and early warning systems strengthens global preparedness and response capacities. It enables countries to leverage collective expertise, resources, and technologies to detect, prevent, and control the spread of infectious diseases on a global scale.

Overall, surveillance and early warning systems are critical tools in the fight against communicable diseases, allowing for early detection, rapid response, and effective prevention and control strategies.

2.4 Case study: Polio eradication in Nigeria

POLIO IS A VIRAL DISEASE that can cause paralysis and death. Nigeria was one of the last countries in the world to still have endemic polio transmission, with high numbers of polio cases reported in the country as recently as 2012. However, through sustained efforts to eradicate the disease, Nigeria was declared polio-free in 2020. Here is an overview of the efforts to eradicate polio in Nigeria:

1. *Vaccination campaigns*: One of the main strategies for eradicating polio in Nigeria was the use of vaccination campaigns. Millions of children were vaccinated against polio every year, with a focus on reaching children in hard-to-reach and conflict-affected areas.

2. *Surveillance and monitoring*: To ensure that polio cases were detected and responded to quickly, a comprehensive surveillance system was put in place, which included active case searching and environmental surveillance.

3. *Community engagement*: Community engagement was a key component of the polio eradication efforts in Nigeria. Community leaders, religious leaders, and traditional healers were engaged to help promote vaccination campaigns and encourage vaccination uptake.

4. *Innovative strategies*: In addition to traditional vaccination campaigns, innovative strategies were also used to reach children in hard-to-reach areas. These included the use of mobile vaccination teams, the involvement of traditional healers, and the use of community-based surveillance.

5. *Political commitment*: The government of Nigeria demonstrated strong political commitment to polio eradication, with the establishment of a Presidential Task

Force on Polio Eradication, and the allocation of significant resources to support the eradication efforts.

Despite challenges such as insecurity and vaccine hesitancy, Nigeria's polio eradication efforts have been successful, with no cases of wild polio reported in the country since 2016. The efforts in Nigeria demonstrate that sustained commitment, community engagement, and innovative strategies can be effective in eradicating communicable diseases, even in challenging settings.

2.5 Exercises

1. What is the basic reproductive number (R0) in disease transmission, and why is it significant?

Solution: The basic reproductive number (R0) is the average number of people that one infected person can transmit a disease to in a susceptible population. It is significant because it can help predict the potential for an outbreak and inform public health response measures.

1. How do transmission patterns differ in different settings, such as community, hospital, and long-term care facilities?

Solution: Transmission patterns differ in different settings due to factors such as the types of contacts, environmental conditions, and infection control practices. For example, in a hospital setting, patients may be more vulnerable to infections due to weakened immune systems, while long-term care facilities may have residents with more chronic conditions.

1. What are some social and behavioral factors that can affect disease transmission?

Solution: Social and behavioral factors such as cultural beliefs, practices, and norms, as well as socioeconomic status, education, and access to healthcare, can affect disease transmission. For example, lack of access to healthcare may lead to delays in diagnosis and treatment, while cultural beliefs around illness may discourage people from seeking medical attention.

1. What is the International Health Regulations (IHR) and why are they important?

Solution: The IHR are a legally binding framework that outlines the responsibilities of countries in preventing, detecting, and responding to public health emergencies of international concern. They are important because they promote global cooperation in disease surveillance and response, and help prevent the spread of communicable diseases across borders.

1. What are some challenges and opportunities in global health security? *Solution:* Challenges in global health security include issues such as lack of funding, political instability, and insufficient healthcare infrastructure. Opportunities include advancements in technology and international collaborations to address emerging infectious diseases.

1. What is the role of governance and leadership in epidemic control?

Solution: Governance and leadership are crucial in epidemic control as they play a critical role in setting policies, allocating resources, and coordinating response efforts. Effective leadership can help build trust and ensure that public health measures are implemented in a timely and effective manner.

1. What are some ethical considerations in disease surveillance and response?

Solution: Ethical considerations in disease surveillance and response include issues such as informed consent, privacy, and confidentiality. It is important to balance individual rights with public health interests, and to ensure that interventions are implemented in a way that is equitable and respectful of cultural beliefs and practices.

1. How can community engagement and mass media be used to promote public health?

Solution: Community engagement and mass media can be used to raise awareness about public health issues, promote healthy behaviors, and encourage participation in public health interventions. They can also help build trust and improve communication between healthcare providers and communities.

1. What are some best practices and lessons learned from the response to recent outbreaks?

Solution: Best practices from recent outbreaks include early detection and rapid response, effective communication, community engagement, and collaboration between local and international partners. Lessons learned include the need for stronger healthcare systems and improved preparedness and response planning.

1. How has climate change and environmental factors affected the emergence of infectious diseases?

Solution: Climate change and environmental factors have played a role in the emergence of infectious diseases by altering the distribution and abundance of vectors and hosts, as well as influencing human behavior and patterns of interaction with the environment. This can lead to the emergence or re-emergence of infectious diseases, and highlights the need for a One Health approach to disease surveillance and response.

Chapter 3. Emerging and re-emerging infectious diseases

3.1 Understanding the drivers of emerging infectious diseases

Emerging infectious diseases (EIDs) are diseases that have recently appeared in a population or have existed but are rapidly increasing in incidence or geographic range. The drivers of EIDs are complex and multifactorial, but here are some key factors that contribute to their emergence:

3.1.1 Environmental changes:

ENVIRONMENTAL CHANGES have a significant impact on disease dynamics and the emergence of infectious diseases. The alteration of natural habitats due to factors such as deforestation, urbanization, and climate change can lead to increased contact between humans, animals, and their pathogens. This closer interaction creates opportunities for the transmission of zoonotic diseases, which pose a significant public health threat.

Deforestation, for example, involves the removal of large areas of forested land for agricultural expansion, infrastructure development, or logging. This process disrupts ecosystems, displaces wildlife, and forces animals into closer proximity to human settlements. As a result, the chances of direct contact between humans and disease-carrying animals, such as rodents, bats, and primates, are heightened. This proximity increases the risk of zoonotic disease transmission, as pathogens can cross species barriers and infect humans.

Urbanization is another significant environmental change that influences disease dynamics. Rapid urban growth leads to increased population density, inadequate sanitation systems, and suboptimal living conditions. These factors create favorable conditions for the transmission of infectious diseases, including waterborne diseases like cholera and vector-borne diseases like dengue fever and malaria. The concentration of people in urban areas also facilitates the rapid spread of contagious diseases.

Climate change is a global environmental challenge that impacts disease patterns. Rising temperatures, altered rainfall patterns, and extreme weather events can affect the geographic distribution of disease vectors, such as mosquitoes and ticks, as well as the transmission dynamics of waterborne and foodborne diseases. Climate change can also impact the survival and reproduction rates of pathogens, potentially leading to changes in disease prevalence and seasonality.

To address the impact of environmental changes on disease transmission, it is crucial to adopt a holistic One Health approach. This approach recognizes the interconnectedness of human, animal, and environmental health and emphasizes the need for interdisciplinary collaboration. Efforts should focus on sustainable land-use practices, urban planning that prioritizes public health, and climate change mitigation and adaptation strategies. By addressing the root causes of environmental changes and promoting ecosystem health, we can mitigate the risks posed by emerging infectious diseases.

3.1.2 Globalization:

GLOBALIZATION, CHARACTERIZED by the increased interconnectedness and integration of societies and economies worldwide, has had a profound impact on disease transmission dynamics. The rapid movement of people, animals, and goods across borders has facilitated the global spread of infectious diseases, presenting new challenges for disease surveillance and response.

One notable example of how globalization influences disease transmission is the rapid spread of infectious diseases through international travel. Air travel allows individuals to traverse long distances in short periods, leading to the swift introduction and dissemination of pathogens across different regions. A prominent case is the global spread of the severe acute respiratory syndrome (SARS) in 2003. Within a matter of weeks, the SARS virus traveled from its origin in southern China to multiple countries around the world, causing a widespread outbreak.

Another example is the global trade of food products. With the expansion of international trade networks, food items are transported across continents, increasing the risk of foodborne diseases. Contaminated food can carry pathogens such as Salmonella, Escherichia coli, or Listeria monocytogenes, causing outbreaks that span multiple countries. The 2011 E. coli outbreak in Europe, linked to contaminated sprouts, affected numerous countries and highlighted the challenges of tracing the source of contaminated food in a globalized food supply chain.

Furthermore, the illegal wildlife trade has become a significant driver of disease transmission. Animals captured or farmed for the exotic pet trade, traditional medicine, or bushmeat consumption can harbor zoonotic pathogens. The trafficking of wildlife increases the likelihood of introducing novel diseases to new regions, as demonstrated by the transmission of the Ebola virus from wildlife to humans through the hunting and consumption of infected bushmeat.

To address the challenges posed by globalization, international collaborations and partnerships are crucial. Organizations such as the World Health Organization (WHO) and the World Organization for Animal Health (OIE) work to strengthen global surveillance systems, facilitate information sharing, and develop coordinated responses to outbreaks. Improved border health surveillance, effective communication networks, and harmonized public health measures are vital for early detection, rapid response, and containment of infectious diseases in a globalized world.

Real-world examples of disease outbreaks and their global spread underscore the need for ongoing efforts to enhance global health security. By recognizing the interconnectedness of nations and prioritizing collaborative approaches, we can strengthen our collective ability to prevent, detect, and respond to infectious diseases in an increasingly interconnected world.

3.1.3 Agricultural practices:

INTENSIVE AGRICULTURE and livestock production practices can increase the risk of disease transmission from animals to humans, particularly through the use of antibiotics and other drugs that can increase the risk of drug-resistant infections.

Agricultural practices, particularly intensive farming and livestock production, play a significant role in disease transmission dynamics and can pose risks to both animal and human health. The intensification of agriculture involves densely packed livestock populations, increased use of antimicrobials, and alterations in land use patterns, which can contribute to the emergence and spread of infectious diseases.

One notable example of the impact of agricultural practices on disease transmission is the emergence and dissemination of antibiotic-resistant bacteria. The routine use of antibiotics in livestock production for growth promotion and disease prevention has led to the development of antimicrobial resistance. Resistant bacteria can be transmitted to humans through direct contact with animals, consumption of contaminated food products, or exposure to contaminated environmental sources. This poses a significant public health concern, as infections caused by drug-resistant bacteria are more difficult to treat and can lead to increased morbidity and mortality.

Livestock-associated zoonotic diseases also represent a significant concern in relation to agricultural practices. Close proximity between animals and humans in intensive farming systems increases the risk of zoonotic disease transmission. Pathogens such as avian influenza, Salmonella, Campylobacter, and E. coli can be transmitted from animals to humans through direct contact, consumption of contaminated animal products, or environmental exposure. These diseases pose a threat to both farm workers and consumers of animal products.

Furthermore, changes in land use patterns associated with agriculture, such as deforestation and encroachment into wildlife habitats, can lead to the increased contact between humans and wildlife, promoting the transmission of zoonotic diseases. For instance, the conversion of forested areas for agricultural purposes can bring humans into closer proximity to reservoirs of zoonotic pathogens, increasing the likelihood of spillover events and the emergence of novel infectious diseases.

Addressing the risks associated with agricultural practices requires a holistic and One Health approach. This approach recognizes the interconnectedness of human, animal, and environmental health and emphasizes collaboration between different sectors.

Implementing sustainable agricultural practices that prioritize animal welfare, reduce the use of antimicrobials, and promote biodiversity conservation can help mitigate the risks of disease transmission. Strengthening surveillance systems, improving biosecurity measures, and promoting public awareness about safe food handling and hygiene practices are essential components of preventing and controlling zoonotic diseases associated with agricultural practices.

Real-world examples, such as the outbreaks of avian influenza in poultry farms and the emergence of multidrug-resistant pathogens in livestock settings, highlight the importance of addressing the risks posed by agricultural practices to protect both animal and human health.

3.1.4 Human behavior:

HUMAN BEHAVIOR PLAYS a significant role in the transmission and emergence of infectious diseases. Various aspects of human behavior, such as travel, trade, and consumption of wildlife, can increase the risk of disease spread and facilitate the emergence of new diseases.

3.1.4.1 Travel:

THE EASE AND FREQUENCY of travel have greatly accelerated in recent decades, leading to the rapid spread of infectious diseases across geographical boundaries. International travel allows pathogens to move quickly from one region to another, potentially introducing diseases to new populations that may have little or no immunity. Notable examples include the global spread of diseases like SARS (Severe Acute Respiratory Syndrome), H1N1 influenza (swine flu), and COVID-19. Air travel, in particular, can facilitate the rapid dissemination of infectious agents within a short period.

3.1.4.2 Trade:

GLOBAL TRADE IN GOODS and products can also contribute to the spread of infectious diseases. Infected animals, contaminated food products, and other goods can serve as vehicles for disease transmission across borders. For instance, the introduction of infected livestock or animal products can introduce diseases like foot-and-mouth disease or avian influenza to new regions. Similarly, contaminated food products can cause outbreaks of foodborne illnesses in multiple countries. Strict regulations and standards are necessary to ensure the safety and biosecurity of traded goods.

3.1.4.3 Consumption of Wildlife:

THE CONSUMPTION OF wildlife, including bushmeat and exotic animals, can pose significant risks for disease transmission. Some zoonotic diseases, such as Ebola, SARS-CoV-1 (the virus causing SARS), and SARS-CoV-2 (the virus causing COVID-19), are believed to have originated from wildlife. Close contact between humans and wildlife in markets, farms, or during hunting and consumption activities increases the likelihood of disease spillover events. Proper regulation, enforcement of wildlife trade policies, and public awareness campaigns are crucial in mitigating the risks associated with wildlife consumption.

3.1.4.4 Urbanization:

THE RAPID GROWTH OF urban areas and population density can create ideal conditions for the transmission of infectious diseases. Overcrowding, inadequate sanitation, and poor hygiene practices can facilitate the spread of pathogens. Urbanization can also bring humans into closer contact with animal reservoirs of diseases, increasing the risk of zoonotic transmission. Effective urban planning, improved sanitation infrastructure, and public health education are essential to reducing disease transmission in urban settings.

Real-world examples of the impact of human behavior on disease transmission include the spread of HIV/AIDS through global travel and migration, the emergence of the H1N1 influenza virus through international travel and trade, and the transmission of zoonotic diseases like Ebola and Nipah virus through the consumption of wildlife.

Understanding and addressing the role of human behavior in disease transmission is vital for developing effective prevention and control strategies. Promoting behavior change through public health education, implementing travel and trade regulations, and promoting sustainable practices can help mitigate the risks associated with human behavior and reduce the emergence and spread of infectious diseases.

3.1.5 Pathogen evolution:

PATHOGEN EVOLUTION is a natural and ongoing process that allows microorganisms to adapt and change over time. This evolution can have significant implications for human health, as pathogens can acquire new traits, such as antibiotic resistance or the ability to infect new hosts, leading to the emergence of new diseases or the resurgence of previously controlled infections.

3.1.5.1 Antibiotic Resistance:

PATHOGENS, PARTICULARLY bacteria, have the ability to develop resistance to antibiotics through genetic changes. Overuse and misuse of antibiotics in human and animal health settings have accelerated the evolution of drug-resistant strains, rendering certain antibiotics ineffective against infections. Methicillin-resistant Staphylococcus aureus (MRSA) and multi-drug-resistant tuberculosis (MDR-TB) are examples of bacterial infections that have become increasingly difficult to treat due to antibiotic resistance.

3.1.5.2 Host Adaptation:

PATHOGENS CAN UNDERGO genetic changes that allow them to infect new hosts or adapt to different environmental conditions. This adaptation can result in the emergence of novel diseases or the spread of existing diseases to new populations. For instance, the avian influenza virus (H5N1) underwent genetic changes that allowed it to infect humans, leading to sporadic cases of severe respiratory illness. Similarly, the coronavirus responsible for the COVID-19 pandemic (SARS-CoV-2) is believed to have originated from an animal source and subsequently adapted to infect humans.

3.1.5.3 Viral Reassortment and Genetic Shift:

VIRUSES, ESPECIALLY RNA viruses, have a high mutation rate, making them prone to genetic changes. This genetic variability can lead to the emergence of new strains or the recombination of genetic material from different viruses, known as reassortment. This process can result in the generation of novel strains with altered virulence or transmissibility. Influenza viruses undergo frequent genetic reassortment, leading to the emergence of new influenza strains with the potential to cause pandemics.

3.1.5.4 Vector Adaptation:

VECTOR-BORNE DISEASES, such as malaria and dengue fever, are transmitted by insects or other arthropods. Pathogens that rely on vectors for transmission can undergo evolutionary changes that enhance their ability to survive and replicate within the vector, increasing the efficiency of disease transmission. This adaptation can result in the expansion of vector habitats, increased vector abundance, and a higher risk of disease transmission to human populations.

Real-world examples of pathogen evolution include the development of antibiotic-resistant strains of bacteria, such as vancomycin-resistant Enterococcus (VRE) and carbapenem-resistant Enterobacteriaceae (CRE). Additionally, the ongoing evolution of the influenza virus, resulting in the emergence of new strains with pandemic potential, highlights the dynamic nature of pathogen evolution.

Understanding pathogen evolution is crucial for public health strategies, as it helps inform surveillance, prevention, and control efforts. Effective monitoring of pathogen evolution, research on mechanisms of resistance, and the development of novel interventions are essential in combating the challenges posed by evolving pathogens.

3.1.6 Health systems and infrastructure:

WEAK HEALTH SYSTEMS and infrastructure can also contribute to the emergence of EIDs, as they may not have the resources or capacity to detect and respond to outbreaks quickly and effectively.

Health systems and infrastructure play a critical role in preventing, detecting, and responding to emerging infectious diseases (EIDs). However, weak health systems and inadequate infrastructure can pose significant challenges in controlling and managing these outbreaks. Several factors associated with health systems and infrastructure can contribute to the emergence and spread of EIDs:

3.1.6.1 Limited Surveillance and Detection Capacity:

WEAK HEALTH SYSTEMS may lack robust surveillance systems and diagnostic capabilities to promptly identify and monitor emerging infectious diseases. This can delay the detection of outbreaks, allowing the disease to spread undetected and potentially reach epidemic proportions before appropriate control measures can be implemented.

3.1.6.2 Inadequate Healthcare Facilities and Personnel:

INSUFFICIENT HEALTHCARE facilities, including hospitals, clinics, and laboratories, can limit the capacity to diagnose and manage EIDs effectively. Additionally, a shortage of healthcare professionals, including doctors, nurses, and laboratory technicians, can further strain the response efforts, leading to delayed diagnosis and treatment.

3.1.6.3 Poor Healthcare Access and Infrastructure:

LIMITED ACCESS TO HEALTHCARE services, particularly in remote or underserved areas, can hinder timely access to medical care and disease prevention measures. Inadequate transportation systems, including roads and infrastructure, can further impede the delivery of healthcare resources, including medical supplies, vaccines, and personnel, to affected areas.

3.1.6.4 Inadequate Infection Prevention and Control Measures:

WEAK HEALTH SYSTEMS may lack adequate infection prevention and control measures, including proper hand hygiene, personal protective equipment, and isolation facilities. This can contribute to the spread of infectious diseases within healthcare settings and among healthcare workers, amplifying the outbreak.

3.1.6.5 Limited Health Financing and Resources:

INSUFFICIENT FUNDING for public health and healthcare systems can hinder preparedness and response efforts for emerging infectious diseases. This includes the availability of financial resources to invest in surveillance, laboratory infrastructure, workforce training, and the procurement of necessary medical supplies and equipment.

Real-world examples of the impact of weak health systems and infrastructure on the emergence and spread of EIDs can be seen in various outbreaks, such as the Ebola virus disease outbreak in West Africa in 2014-2016. The limited healthcare infrastructure, inadequate infection control measures, and weak surveillance systems in affected countries contributed to the rapid spread and high mortality rates associated with the outbreak.

To address these challenges, strengthening health systems and infrastructure is crucial. This includes improving surveillance and early warning systems, enhancing laboratory capacity, training healthcare workers, establishing robust healthcare delivery systems, ensuring access to essential medicines and vaccines, and strengthening emergency preparedness and response mechanisms.

Understanding the drivers of EIDs is critical for developing effective prevention and control strategies. Addressing the underlying factors that contribute to the emergence of EIDs, such as environmental changes, agricultural practices, and human behavior, can help prevent the emergence of new diseases and reduce the impact of existing ones.

3.2 The role of climate change and environmental factors

CLIMATE CHANGE AND environmental factors play a significant role in the emergence and transmission of infectious diseases. Here are some ways in which they impact disease transmission:

3.2.1 Altering the distribution of disease vectors:

ALTERING THE DISTRIBUTION of disease vectors is a significant consequence of climate change and environmental changes. These changes can disrupt the natural ecological balance and impact the habitats of disease-transmitting vectors, such as mosquitoes and ticks. As a result, the geographical range and abundance of these vectors can shift, leading to changes in disease transmission patterns and increased risk to human populations.

Climate change, characterized by rising temperatures, altered precipitation patterns, and changing weather conditions, can create more favorable environments for disease vectors. For instance, increased temperatures can accelerate the breeding cycles of mosquitoes, allowing them to reproduce more rapidly and expand their range into previously non-endemic areas. Similarly, altered rainfall patterns can create stagnant water bodies, providing ideal breeding sites for mosquitoes.

Real-world examples demonstrate the impact of altering disease vector distribution due to climate change and environmental factors. In regions where malaria was previously non-endemic, such as high-altitude areas, increased temperatures and changing rainfall patterns have created conditions suitable for malaria-carrying mosquitoes to survive and multiply. Consequently, these areas have experienced an emergence or re-emergence of malaria cases.

Likewise, Lyme disease, primarily transmitted by ticks, has seen an expansion of its geographical range in regions where climate conditions have become more favorable for tick populations. This expansion has been observed in various parts of North America and Europe, resulting in an increased incidence of Lyme disease in areas where it was previously uncommon.

To mitigate the impacts of altering disease vector distribution, proactive measures are essential. This includes:

1. **Strengthening vector surveillance**: Monitoring and tracking changes in the distribution and abundance of disease vectors through surveillance systems can help identify areas at risk and guide targeted interventions.
2. **Implementing vector control strategies**: Employing effective vector control measures, such as insecticide-treated bed nets, indoor residual spraying, and

environmental management techniques, can help reduce vector populations and prevent disease transmission.

3. **Promoting community engagement and education**: Raising awareness among communities about the risks of vector-borne diseases and providing education on personal protective measures, such as using insect repellents and wearing protective clothing, can help individuals protect themselves from vector bites.

4. **Supporting research and innovation:** Investing in research to better understand the impact of climate change on vector distribution and developing innovative tools and strategies for vector control can aid in effectively combating vector-borne diseases.

3.2.2 Changing host-pathogen dynamics:

CHANGING HOST-PATHOGEN dynamics is a significant consequence of climate change and environmental changes. These changes can disrupt the delicate balance between hosts and pathogens, influencing their physiology, behavior, and interactions. As a result, new diseases can emerge or existing ones can spread to new areas, posing challenges to public health.

Climate change and environmental factors can impact host populations in several ways. Increased temperatures, altered precipitation patterns, and changes in ecological systems can influence the distribution, migration, and breeding patterns of animals and plants. For instance, rising temperatures can affect the phenology and behavior of migratory birds, altering their migration routes and potentially exposing them to new pathogens. Changes in vegetation patterns and availability of resources can also affect the distribution and behavior of host species.

These alterations in host populations can directly influence the dynamics of pathogens. Pathogens may adapt to new host species, expand their range, or increase their replication rates in response to changes in host physiology and behavior. Environmental changes can also create more favorable conditions for the survival and transmission of pathogens. For example, increased rainfall can lead to the proliferation of water bodies, providing breeding sites for disease-transmitting mosquitoes.

One real-world example of changing host-pathogen dynamics is the Zika virus outbreak. The Zika virus, primarily transmitted by Aedes mosquitoes, gained international attention in recent years due to its association with neurological disorders such as microcephaly. Environmental changes, including urbanization, deforestation, and climate change, have created conditions conducive to the spread of Zika virus. The expansion of mosquito habitats, increased human-mosquito contact, and the presence of susceptible populations have contributed to the rapid dissemination of the virus in various regions.

To address the challenges posed by changing host-pathogen dynamics, comprehensive strategies are necessary:

1. **Enhanced surveillance**: Surveillance systems should be strengthened to monitor changes in host populations and the emergence of new diseases. Early detection and prompt response are crucial in containing outbreaks and preventing further spread.

2. **Integrated approach**: Collaboration between public health, environmental, and veterinary sectors is vital to understanding the complex interactions between hosts, pathogens, and the environment. This interdisciplinary approach can facilitate effective disease prevention and

control strategies.

3. **Risk assessment and management**: Conducting risk assessments to identify vulnerable populations and areas susceptible to emerging diseases can guide targeted interventions. Implementing appropriate control measures, such as vector control programs, can help mitigate the impact of changing host-pathogen dynamics.

4. **Research and innovation**: Continued research on the ecological, environmental, and molecular aspects of host-pathogen interactions is essential for better understanding and predicting disease dynamics. Investment in innovative technologies and approaches can aid in developing effective prevention and control strategies.

3.2.3 Impacting food and water security:

CLIMATE CHANGE AND environmental changes have significant implications for food and water security, which in turn can impact human health and increase the risk of infectious diseases. These changes can disrupt agricultural systems, alter the availability and quality of water resources, and affect food production and distribution. As a result, communities may face challenges in accessing safe and nutritious food and clean water, leading to malnutrition and compromised immune systems.

Here are some key points to consider regarding the impact of climate change and environmental changes on food and water security:

3.2.3.1 Agricultural systems:

CLIMATE CHANGE CAN disrupt agricultural practices by altering rainfall patterns, temperature regimes, and the prevalence of extreme weather events such as droughts and floods. These changes can negatively affect crop yields, livestock productivity, and overall agricultural production. Reduced agricultural output can lead to food shortages, price volatility, and increased reliance on imported food, potentially exacerbating food insecurity.

3.2.3.2 Water resources:

CLIMATE CHANGE CAN influence the availability and quality of water resources, including surface water and groundwater. Changes in precipitation patterns can lead to water scarcity or excessive rainfall, affecting water availability for agricultural irrigation, domestic use, and sanitation. Additionally, rising temperatures can exacerbate water stress, leading to increased competition for limited water resources. Water scarcity and poor water quality can contribute to malnutrition and the spread of waterborne diseases.

3.2.3.3 Malnutrition and weakened immune systems:

LIMITED ACCESS TO DIVERSE and nutritious food can result in malnutrition, including both undernutrition and overnutrition. Undernutrition weakens the immune system, making individuals more susceptible to infectious diseases. Conversely, overnutrition and unhealthy dietary patterns can increase the risk of non-communicable diseases, such as diabetes and cardiovascular diseases, which can further compromise immune function.

3.2.3.4 Altered disease patterns:

CHANGES IN ENVIRONMENTAL conditions can impact the distribution and prevalence of infectious diseases. For example, water scarcity and changes in water storage practices can promote the breeding of disease vectors, such as mosquitoes, leading to an increased risk of vector-borne diseases like malaria and dengue fever. Furthermore, shifts in agricultural practices and land use can bring humans into closer contact with wildlife, increasing the potential for zoonotic disease transmission.

To address the impact of climate change and environmental changes on food and water security, it is crucial to:

1. **Promote sustainable agriculture**: Implementing climate-smart agricultural practices, such as conservation agriculture, agroforestry, and water-efficient irrigation, can help adapt to changing environmental conditions and enhance food production.

2. **Strengthen water resource management**: Implementing integrated water resource management strategies, including water conservation measures, wastewater treatment and reuse, and improved water governance, can help ensure equitable access to safe and clean water for agricultural, domestic, and industrial purposes.

3. **Enhance nutrition and health interventions**: Implementing comprehensive strategies to improve nutrition, including promoting diverse and locally sourced food, fortifying staple foods, and addressing underlying determinants of malnutrition, can help strengthen immune systems and reduce the risk of infectious diseases.

4. **Strengthen disease surveillance and response**:

Enhancing disease surveillance systems and response mechanisms can help monitor changes in disease patterns, detect outbreaks early, and implement appropriate control measures to prevent the spread of infectious diseases.

3.2.4 Displacing populations:

CLIMATE CHANGE AND environmental changes can result in the displacement of populations, forcing people to migrate from their homes due to the adverse effects of these changes. Displacement can occur as a result of various factors, including sea-level rise, coastal erosion, drought, flooding, and desertification. These environmental challenges can have significant implications for public health, leading to increased vulnerability to disease transmission and the spread of infectious diseases.

Here are some real-world examples and references illustrating the link between displacement and the risk of disease transmission:

3.2.4.1 Displacement due to sea-level rise:

RISING SEA LEVELS POSE a threat to low-lying coastal regions and islands, forcing communities to relocate. This displacement can lead to overcrowding in temporary settlements or urban areas, where inadequate sanitation, poor access to clean water, and limited healthcare services increase the risk of infectious diseases. For instance, in the aftermath of Hurricane Katrina in 2005, the displacement of populations in New Orleans resulted in an increased incidence of waterborne diseases such as gastrointestinal infections.

3.2.4.2 Displacement due to drought and desertification:

DROUGHTS AND DESERTIFICATION can lead to the displacement of rural communities, as arable land becomes unsuitable for agriculture and water resources become scarce. Displaced populations may be forced to live in overcrowded and unsanitary conditions, increasing the risk of infectious diseases such as respiratory infections, diarrheal diseases, and vector-borne diseases. The Sahel region in Africa has experienced significant population displacement due to desertification, with subsequent health challenges.

3.2.4.3 Displacement due to natural disasters:

NATURAL DISASTERS, such as hurricanes, floods, and earthquakes, can result in large-scale population displacement. Displaced individuals often face inadequate shelter, limited access to clean water and sanitation facilities, and reduced healthcare services, increasing their vulnerability to infectious diseases. Following the earthquake in Haiti in 2010, the displacement of populations led to overcrowded living conditions and the spread of communicable diseases such as cholera.

3.2.4.4 Displacement due to climate-related conflicts:

CLIMATE CHANGE IMPACTS can exacerbate existing conflicts and contribute to the displacement of populations. Displaced individuals may face overcrowding in camps or host communities, limited access to healthcare, and compromised sanitation, increasing the risk of infectious diseases. The ongoing conflict in Syria, combined with drought and water scarcity, has led to population displacement and heightened health risks.

These examples highlight the relationship between displacement, climate change, and the increased risk of disease transmission. It underscores the importance of addressing the health needs of displaced populations, providing adequate healthcare services, improving living conditions, and implementing measures to prevent the spread of infectious diseases in these vulnerable settings.

3.2.5 Amplifying extreme weather events:

EXTREME WEATHER EVENTS can have significant impacts on public health, and climate change is amplifying the frequency and intensity of such events. Floods, droughts, and heatwaves are examples of extreme weather events that can create favorable conditions for the transmission of diseases.

Floods, for instance, can contaminate water sources, leading to the spread of waterborne diseases like cholera, dysentery, and hepatitis A. Standing water left after a flood can also provide breeding grounds for mosquitoes, increasing the risk of diseases such as malaria and dengue fever.

Droughts, on the other hand, can lead to water scarcity and compromised hygiene practices, contributing to the spread of waterborne diseases. Additionally, droughts can affect agricultural productivity, leading to food shortages and malnutrition, which weaken immune systems and increase vulnerability to diseases.

Heatwaves, characterized by prolonged periods of excessive heat, can have direct health impacts such as heatstroke, dehydration, and cardiovascular issues. Heatwaves can also exacerbate air pollution and the formation of harmful algal blooms, leading to respiratory problems and the spread of harmful toxins.

Real-world examples of the impact of extreme weather events on disease transmission include the flooding in Bangladesh in 2004, which resulted in a cholera outbreak affecting thousands of people (Lipp et al., 2008), and the heatwave in Europe in 2003, which caused an estimated excess mortality of tens of thousands of individuals.

Addressing climate change and environmental factors is critical for preventing and controlling infectious diseases. Mitigating the impact of climate change, protecting natural habitats, and promoting sustainable practices can help reduce the emergence and transmission of infectious diseases.

3.3 The need for preparedness and response plans

THE NEED FOR PREPAREDNESS and response plans is crucial in the face of emerging infectious diseases and outbreaks of communicable diseases. Here are some reasons why preparedness and response plans are essential:

3.3.1 Early detection and response:

EARLY DETECTION AND response to disease outbreaks are essential for effectively controlling and mitigating the spread of infectious diseases. Preparedness plans play a vital role in facilitating early detection and rapid response efforts, enabling public health authorities to intervene promptly and implement appropriate measures to limit the impact of outbreaks.

Early detection involves the timely identification of disease cases or clusters through surveillance systems and early warning systems. These systems utilize various data sources, such as hospital records, laboratory reports, and syndromic surveillance, to detect unusual patterns or increases in disease incidence. For example, in the case of an influenza outbreak, monitoring the number of influenza-like illness (ILI) cases reported by healthcare facilities can provide early indications of an impending outbreak.

Once a potential outbreak is identified, response plans are activated to initiate a coordinated and efficient response. This may involve activating emergency operations centers, mobilizing response teams, and implementing control measures. Outbreak investigation protocols are followed to determine the source, transmission pathways, and risk factors associated with the outbreak. This information guides the implementation of targeted interventions to prevent further transmission.

Real-world examples of early detection and response include the response to the Ebola outbreak in West Africa in 2014-2016. Early detection through enhanced surveillance systems and rapid response efforts, including contact tracing, isolation of cases, and safe burials, helped contain the outbreak and prevent its further spread.

Another example is the global response to the COVID-19 pandemic. Early detection of the novel coronavirus and prompt implementation of public health measures, such as testing, contact tracing, quarantine, and social distancing, have been critical in controlling the spread of the virus and saving lives.

3.3.2 Coordination and communication:

COORDINATION AND COMMUNICATION are crucial components of preparedness plans in responding to disease outbreaks. These aspects play a vital role in ensuring effective collaboration and cooperation between various stakeholders involved in the response efforts.

Coordination involves bringing together different entities, such as government agencies, healthcare institutions, non-governmental organizations, and community leaders, to work collectively towards a common goal. This includes establishing clear roles and responsibilities, coordinating resources and logistics, and fostering partnerships to leverage expertise and capacities.

Effective communication is essential in providing accurate and timely information to the public, healthcare providers, and decision-makers. Transparent and reliable communication helps to build trust, facilitate compliance with preventive measures, and dispel rumors or misinformation. Communication channels may include public health announcements, press releases, social media, community engagement activities, and regular updates to relevant stakeholders.

Real-world examples demonstrate the importance of coordination and communication in outbreak response. During the H1N1 influenza pandemic in 2009, countries and international health organizations collaborated closely to share information, coordinate surveillance activities, and develop response strategies (CDC, 2019). This facilitated a coordinated global effort in monitoring the pandemic and implementing control measures.

In the context of the COVID-19 pandemic, effective coordination and communication have been crucial in sharing best practices, coordinating research efforts, and disseminating public health guidance. Countries and international organizations have worked together to exchange information, coordinate travel restrictions, and develop unified messaging to promote public health measures.

3.3.3 Resource mobilization:

RESOURCE MOBILIZATION is a crucial aspect of preparedness plans in managing and responding to public health emergencies. These plans are designed to facilitate the efficient and timely allocation of essential resources, including medical supplies, personnel, and funding, to effectively address the needs of affected populations.

During a public health emergency, such as a disease outbreak or a natural disaster, the demand for resources can quickly surpass the available supply. Adequate resource mobilization ensures that the necessary resources are in place to support response efforts and mitigate the impact of the emergency.

Real-world examples demonstrate the importance of resource mobilization in effectively responding to public health emergencies. The COVID-19 pandemic highlighted the significance of preparedness plans and resource mobilization on a global scale. Countries with robust preparedness plans and effective resource mobilization strategies were better equipped to respond to the rapidly evolving situation. They were able to swiftly allocate medical supplies, deploy healthcare personnel to affected areas, and secure funding for testing, treatment, and research initiatives.

For instance, countries like South Korea and New Zealand, which had well-developed preparedness plans and effective resource mobilization mechanisms, were able to implement widespread testing, contact tracing, and isolation measures early on in the pandemic. This proactive approach contributed to their success in containing the spread of the virus and minimizing its impact on public health and the economy.

Furthermore, resource mobilization extends beyond national responses. International organizations, such as the World Health Organization (WHO) and various humanitarian agencies, play a crucial role in mobilizing resources during global health emergencies. These organizations coordinate efforts to secure funding, procure medical supplies, and deploy healthcare professionals to support affected regions.

In addition to emergencies, resource mobilization is essential for long-term public health programs and initiatives. For example, efforts to control and eliminate diseases like polio and malaria require sustained resource mobilization to ensure the availability of vaccines, diagnostic tools, treatment medications, and skilled personnel.

Overall, resource mobilization through preparedness plans is vital for effective emergency response and public health interventions. By facilitating the timely allocation of resources, preparedness plans help ensure that response efforts are adequately supported and that resources are directed to the areas where they are most needed.

3.3.4 Capacity building:

CAPACITY BUILDING IS a vital component of preparedness plans in response to disease outbreaks. It involves enhancing the skills, knowledge, and resources of healthcare workers and public health officials, as well as strengthening the infrastructure and capabilities of healthcare systems.

Preparedness plans recognize the importance of equipping healthcare workers with the necessary skills and knowledge to effectively detect, diagnose, and manage outbreaks. This includes training programs on surveillance methods, outbreak investigation techniques, infection prevention and control measures, and the proper use of personal protective equipment. By investing in training and education, healthcare workers become better prepared to respond to outbreaks and provide quality care to affected individuals.

In addition to training, preparedness plans also focus on the establishment and enhancement of laboratory and diagnostic capacities. This includes ensuring the availability of reliable laboratory services for timely and accurate diagnosis of infectious diseases. Diagnostic facilities play a crucial role in early detection, monitoring disease trends, and facilitating targeted interventions.

Real-world examples demonstrate the importance of capacity building in outbreak response. During the Ebola outbreak in West Africa in 2014-2016, capacity building efforts were prioritized to strengthen the healthcare system's ability to detect, diagnose, and manage Ebola cases. This involved training healthcare workers, establishing Ebola treatment centers, and improving laboratory capacities for Ebola testing (WHO, 2016).

In the context of the COVID-19 pandemic, capacity building initiatives have focused on training healthcare workers in infection prevention and control, expanding testing capabilities, and establishing specialized COVID-19 treatment facilities. These efforts have aimed to enhance the healthcare system's ability to respond effectively to the surge in cases and provide optimal care to patients.

3.3.5 Prevention and control:

PREVENTION AND CONTROL strategies play a crucial role in preparedness plans for disease outbreaks. These strategies aim to minimize the occurrence and spread of infectious diseases, ultimately reducing the impact on public health. Preparedness plans encompass a range of preventive measures and control strategies that address various aspects of disease transmission.

Vaccination programs are a key component of prevention and control efforts. Vaccines help to protect individuals and communities by stimulating the immune system to produce a specific response against a particular pathogen. Through widespread vaccination, the incidence of vaccine-preventable diseases can be significantly reduced, contributing to disease control and prevention.

Sanitation measures are essential in preventing the transmission of infectious diseases. Access to clean water, proper sanitation facilities, and hygiene practices are vital in reducing the spread of waterborne and foodborne diseases. Adequate sanitation infrastructure, including safe disposal of waste and promotion of hand hygiene, can help minimize the risk of disease transmission.

Education campaigns are another important aspect of prevention and control strategies. These campaigns aim to raise awareness among the population about the risks associated with infectious diseases and promote behavior changes that can help prevent transmission. Education campaigns may focus on topics such as proper handwashing techniques, safe food handling practices, and the importance of vaccination.

Real-world examples demonstrate the effectiveness of prevention and control strategies. For instance, the global immunization campaigns for diseases such as polio, measles, and hepatitis have significantly reduced the incidence of these diseases worldwide.

In the context of the COVID-19 pandemic, prevention and control measures have included widespread mask usage, physical distancing guidelines, and public health messaging to promote hand hygiene and respiratory etiquette. These measures have been crucial in slowing the transmission of the virus and reducing the impact of the pandemic.

Preparedness and response plans are essential for effective prevention and control of infectious diseases. They enable early detection and response, coordination and communication, resource mobilization, capacity building, and prevention and control strategies.

3.4 Case study: Zika outbreak in Brazil

IN 2015, AN OUTBREAK of Zika virus occurred in Brazil and quickly spread to other parts of South and Central America, the Caribbean, and eventually the United States. Here is a brief overview of the outbreak and its impact:

The Zika virus is primarily transmitted by Aedes mosquitoes, which also transmit dengue and chikungunya viruses. Symptoms of Zika infection are typically mild and include fever, rash, joint pain, and conjunctivitis. However, the virus can also cause severe neurological complications, such as Guillain-Barré syndrome, and has been linked to birth defects in infants born to mothers infected during pregnancy.

The outbreak began in northeastern Brazil in early 2015 and quickly spread to other parts of the country. By the end of the year, there were an estimated 1.5 million cases in Brazil alone. The outbreak also affected other parts of South and Central America, as well as the Caribbean. The World Health Organization declared the outbreak a public health emergency of international concern in February 2016.

The outbreak had a significant impact on public health, as well as on tourism and the economy in affected areas. The Brazilian government launched a massive public awareness campaign to educate people about the risks of Zika virus and to encourage measures to prevent mosquito bites and reduce mosquito breeding sites. The government also deployed thousands of soldiers to help with mosquito control efforts.

Research efforts focused on developing a vaccine against the virus, as well as on understanding the link between Zika infection during pregnancy and birth defects, such as microcephaly. In 2016, the first Zika vaccine trials were conducted, and in 2018, the FDA approved the first Zika vaccine for emergency use.

The Zika outbreak highlighted the importance of preparedness and response plans for emerging infectious diseases, as well as the need for global collaboration and research efforts to address these diseases.

3.5 Exercises

1. What are the different transmission patterns of communicable diseases and how do they differ between settings?

   Solution: The different transmission patterns include person-to-person transmission, vector-borne transmission, and environmental transmission. The patterns differ between settings depending on factors such as population density, climate, and social and cultural practices.

1. What is the role of social and behavioral factors in disease

transmission and how can they be addressed?

Solution: Social and behavioral factors such as poor hygiene practices, inadequate sanitation, and lack of access to healthcare can contribute to disease transmission. They can be addressed through education and awareness campaigns, improved infrastructure and resources, and community engagement.

1. What were the key factors that contributed to the Zika outbreak in Brazil? *Solution:* Key factors included the presence of the Aedes mosquito, which is a vector for the virus, and a lack of immunity in the population. The outbreak was also exacerbated by social and environmental factors such as poor sanitation and urbanization.

1. What is the role of surveillance in public health decision-making and how can it be improved?

Solution: Surveillance plays a critical role in detecting and monitoring disease outbreaks and informing public health decision-making. It can be improved through the use of new technologies and data analysis methods, as well as increased collaboration and coordination between stakeholders.

1. How did the Ebola outbreak in Sierra Leone highlight the importance of governance and leadership in epidemic control?

Solution: The Ebola outbreak in Sierra Leone highlighted the critical role of governance and leadership in epidemic control. The country's weak healthcare infrastructure and lack of preparedness were major contributing factors to the spread of the virus. Effective leadership and coordinated response efforts were necessary to contain the outbreak and prevent further transmission.

1. What were the ethical considerations involved in the response to the COVID-19 pandemic and how were they addressed?

Solution: Ethical considerations in the response to the COVID-19 pandemic included issues such as access to healthcare and resources, privacy and data protection, and the balancing of individual rights and public health interests. They were addressed through the development of guidelines and protocols, as well as ongoing communication and engagement with stakeholders.

1. What are the key challenges and opportunities in global health security, and how can they be addressed?

Solution: Key challenges include inadequate resources and infrastructure, limited access to healthcare and resources in low-income countries, and the threat of emerging infectious diseases. Opportunities include the use of new technologies and data analysis methods, as well as increased collaboration and coordination between stakeholders. They can be addressed through improved funding and resources, increased global cooperation, and strengthened health systems.

1. How did the measles outbreak in Ukraine highlight the

importance of vaccination in disease prevention?

Solution: The measles outbreak in Ukraine highlighted the critical importance of vaccination in disease prevention. The outbreak was largely due to low vaccination rates and a lack of herd immunity in the population. Effective vaccination campaigns were necessary to contain the outbreak and prevent further transmission.

1. What is the role of the International Health Regulations in global disease surveillance and response, and how can they be improved?

Solution: The International Health Regulations provide a framework for global disease surveillance and response, and outline the responsibilities of countries and international organizations in this regard. They can be improved through increased funding and resources, strengthened reporting and data collection systems, and enhanced collaboration and coordination between stakeholders.

Chapter 4. Public health surveillance systems

4.1 Overview of surveillance systems in Africa and Europe

Surveillance systems in Africa and Europe are essential tools for monitoring and controlling the spread of communicable diseases. Here is an overview of surveillance systems in both regions:

4.1.1 Africa:

IN AFRICA, THE SURVEILLANCE systems for communicable diseases have historically faced challenges, including limited resources, inadequate infrastructure, and a lack of trained personnel. These factors have made it challenging to detect and respond to outbreaks in a timely manner. However, there have been significant efforts in recent years to strengthen surveillance systems across the continent.

The World Health Organization (WHO) has been at the forefront of these efforts, working closely with African countries to establish integrated disease surveillance and response (IDSR) systems. The IDSR framework aims to enhance the capacity of countries to monitor and control priority communicable diseases. These diseases include malaria, tuberculosis, HIV/AIDS, and viral hemorrhagic fevers, which pose significant health threats in the region.

Through the IDSR system, countries collect, analyze, and report data on disease occurrences in a standardized manner. This enables the early detection of outbreaks and the implementation of timely response measures. For example, in countries like Ghana, Kenya, and Tanzania, the implementation of IDSR has led to improvements in disease surveillance and response capabilities, resulting in more effective control of diseases like malaria and tuberculosis.

Moreover, African countries have developed national action plans for health security, which prioritize strengthening surveillance systems and building capacity for outbreak response. These plans align with international frameworks, such as the *International Health Regulations (IHR),* which emphasize the importance of effective surveillance and response to prevent the spread of infectious diseases across borders.

One example of a national action plan is Nigeria's National Action Plan for Health Security. This plan focuses on enhancing the country's surveillance capacity, strengthening laboratory networks, and improving the coordination of disease control programs. The plan also emphasizes the integration of surveillance systems for different diseases, including malaria, to facilitate a more comprehensive and coordinated approach to disease control.

Ghana has developed a comprehensive National Action Plan for Health Security (NAPHS) to strengthen its capacity for disease surveillance and outbreak response. The plan focuses on the implementation of the International Health Regulations (IHR) and aims to enhance the country's overall health security.

The key components of Ghana's NAPHS include:

1. *Surveillance and Early Warning Systems*: The plan

emphasizes the establishment and strengthening of surveillance systems to enhance the early detection and timely reporting of diseases. This includes improving the capacity for laboratory diagnostics and expanding the use of digital technologies for real-time data collection and analysis.

2. *Laboratory Capacity*: The NAPHS highlights the need to enhance laboratory capacity across the country. This involves strengthening laboratory infrastructure, improving the quality assurance of laboratory services, and promoting collaboration and information sharing between laboratories.

3. *Emergency Preparedness and Response*: The plan emphasizes the importance of developing and implementing emergency response mechanisms. This includes enhancing the coordination and communication among different stakeholders involved in outbreak response, establishing rapid response teams, and conducting simulation exercises and drills to test the preparedness of the health system.

4. *Health System Strengthening*: The NAPHS recognizes the need for overall health system strengthening to support effective disease surveillance and response. This includes improving human resource capacity, ensuring sustainable financing for health security, and promoting research and innovation in disease surveillance and control.

4.1.2 National Action Plan for Health Security in Liberia:

LIBERIA HAS ALSO DEVELOPED a National Action Plan for Health Security (NAPHS) to enhance its capacity for disease surveillance and response. The plan aligns with international frameworks such as the International Health Regulations (IHR) and focuses on strengthening the country's overall health security.

The key elements of Liberia's NAPHS include:

1. **Disease Surveillance and Response**: The plan emphasizes the establishment of a robust disease surveillance system to monitor the occurrence and spread of diseases. This involves strengthening the capacity for data collection, analysis, and reporting, as well as improving the integration of surveillance systems for different diseases.

2. *Laboratory Strengthening*: Liberia's NAPHS prioritizes the strengthening of laboratory services to support disease diagnosis and surveillance. This includes improving laboratory infrastructure, enhancing quality assurance and quality control measures, and promoting the training and retention of laboratory personnel.

3. **Health Emergency Preparedness and Response**: The plan focuses on enhancing the country's preparedness and response capabilities for public health emergencies. This includes developing emergency response plans, establishing emergency operations centers, and conducting regular drills and exercises to test the readiness of the health system.

4. *Workforce Development*: Liberia's NAPHS highlights the importance of building the capacity of healthcare workers and public health professionals in disease surveillance and response. This involves providing training and continuing education opportunities, promoting cross-sectoral collaboration, and strengthening the coordination and communication

among different stakeholders.

4.1.3 Europe:

SURVEILLANCE SYSTEMS in Europe are generally more robust than those in Africa, benefiting from well-established public health infrastructure and coordinated efforts at the regional level. The European Centre for Disease Prevention and Control (ECDC) plays a crucial role in coordinating surveillance and response efforts across the European Union (EU) and the European Economic Area (EEA). The ECDC works closely with national public health institutes and other partners to ensure the timely and accurate collection of data on communicable diseases, facilitating effective disease control and response.

One of the key surveillance systems operated by the ECDC is the European Surveillance System (TESSy). TESSy serves as a central repository for data on a wide range of communicable diseases, including vaccine-preventable diseases, HIV/AIDS, sexually transmitted infections, and others. The system allows for the standardized collection, analysis, and sharing of surveillance data among participating countries, enabling the detection and monitoring of disease trends at the European level.

In addition to TESSy, the ECDC operates several other surveillance systems and networks focused on specific diseases or risk factors. For example, the European Influenza Surveillance Network monitors the circulation and impact of influenza viruses in Europe, providing timely information for seasonal influenza vaccine composition and public health interventions. The European Antimicrobial Resistance Surveillance Network (EARS-Net) tracks antimicrobial resistance patterns across Europe, aiding in the development of effective antibiotic stewardship strategies.

Despite the overall robustness of surveillance systems in Europe, there are still challenges to be addressed. These challenges include variations in data quality and reporting practices among countries, differences in the availability of resources and capacity for surveillance, and the need for improved integration and interoperability of surveillance systems across borders. The ECDC works closely with member states to address these challenges and strengthen surveillance systems further.

In conclusion, while there are differences in the strength and capacity of surveillance systems between Africa and Europe, both regions recognize the crucial role of surveillance in disease control. Efforts are underway in Africa to strengthen surveillance systems and improve their capacity for early detection and response. In Europe, the ECDC plays a pivotal role in coordinating surveillance and response efforts, operating systems like TESSy and collaborating with national public health institutes. By working together and addressing the challenges, both regions aim to enhance their surveillance capabilities and effectively monitor and control communicable diseases.

4.2 The role of surveillance in public health decision-making

SURVEILLANCE PLAYS a critical role in public health decision-making by providing timely and accurate information about the occurrence and spread of diseases. Here are some of the key ways in which surveillance supports public health decision-making:

4.2.1 Detecting outbreaks:

SURVEILLANCE SYSTEMS play a crucial role in detecting outbreaks of communicable diseases, enabling public health officials to respond quickly and effectively. By continuously monitoring data from various sources, including healthcare facilities, laboratories, and community reports, surveillance systems can identify unusual patterns or increases in disease incidence, indicating the presence of an outbreak. Early detection of outbreaks is vital as it allows for timely intervention to control the spread of diseases and minimize their impact on public health.

One example of an effective surveillance system for outbreak detection is the Global Public Health Intelligence Network (GPHIN), operated by the World Health Organization (WHO). GPHIN uses a combination of automated data collection, data mining, and natural language processing techniques to monitor global news sources, social media, and other online platforms in real-time. The system analyzes these sources for signals of potential disease outbreaks, allowing for early detection and rapid response.

Another notable surveillance system is ProMED-mail (Program for Monitoring Emerging Diseases), an internet-based platform where health professionals and disease experts report and discuss unusual or emerging disease events. ProMED-mail serves as an early warning system, providing valuable insights into outbreaks and emerging diseases from around the world. The system has been instrumental in detecting and reporting outbreaks, including the severe acute respiratory syndrome (SARS) outbreak in 2003 and the Ebola outbreak in West Africa in 2014.

Surveillance systems also facilitate cross-border detection of outbreaks, playing a critical role in preventing the spread of diseases between countries. International collaborations and information sharing platforms, such as the Global Outbreak Alert and Response Network (GOARN), enhance the global surveillance efforts. GOARN, coordinated by WHO, brings together various partners and organizations to strengthen global surveillance and response capacities. This network enables rapid communication and collaboration during outbreaks, ensuring that relevant information is shared promptly, and coordinated response measures are implemented across borders.

4.2.2 Monitoring disease trends:

SURVEILLANCE SYSTEMS play a crucial role in monitoring disease trends over time, providing valuable insights into the patterns and dynamics of various diseases. By continuously collecting and analyzing data on disease incidence, prevalence, and other relevant factors, surveillance systems enable public health officials to identify patterns, trends, and changes in disease occurrence. This information is essential for understanding the burden of diseases, assessing their impact on populations, and developing effective strategies for prevention, control, and treatment.

One of the primary benefits of monitoring disease trends is the ability to identify populations at high risk for certain diseases. Surveillance data can reveal disparities in disease occurrence among different demographic groups, geographic regions, or socioeconomic backgrounds. For instance, surveillance data may highlight higher rates of a specific infectious disease among vulnerable populations, such as individuals with weakened immune systems, the elderly, or those living in crowded or unsanitary conditions. This information allows public health officials to target interventions and allocate resources to these high-risk populations, tailoring prevention and treatment strategies to address their specific needs. By focusing efforts on these at-risk groups, surveillance systems contribute to more effective and efficient public health interventions.

In addition to identifying high-risk populations, monitoring disease trends helps public health officials to detect changes in disease patterns and take appropriate actions. Surveillance systems enable the early detection of outbreaks or unusual spikes in disease incidence. By comparing current disease data with historical trends and thresholds, public health officials can identify deviations or sudden increases in disease occurrence, indicating a potential outbreak or a change in disease transmission dynamics. This early warning allows for timely response measures, such as enhanced surveillance, targeted interventions, public health messaging, and resource allocation, to control the outbreak and prevent further spread. Furthermore, monitoring disease trends allows for the evaluation of the effectiveness of interventions and the assessment of progress towards disease control and elimination goals.

Real-world examples demonstrate the significance of monitoring disease trends in shaping public health responses. The Centers for Disease Control and Prevention (CDC) in the United States operates the National Notifiable Diseases Surveillance System (NNDSS), which monitors and tracks the occurrence of nationally notifiable infectious diseases. This system collects data from healthcare providers, laboratories, and public health agencies across the country, providing essential information on disease trends, geographic distribution, and population groups affected. The data collected through the NNDSS helps guide public health interventions, inform policy decisions, and allocate resources to prevent and control the spread of infectious diseases.

Another example is the Global Polio Surveillance System (GPSS), a comprehensive network of laboratories, health facilities, and surveillance officers dedicated to monitoring the transmission of poliovirus worldwide. The GPSS enables the timely detection of polio cases, tracks the circulation of wild and vaccine-derived polioviruses, and supports vaccination campaigns and outbreak response activities. Through its robust surveillance system, the GPSS has contributed to the significant reduction of polio cases globally and brings us closer to the goal of eradicating polio.

4.2.3 Evaluating interventions:

SURVEILLANCE DATA PLAYS a crucial role in evaluating the effectiveness of public health interventions. By analyzing the data collected before and after the implementation of interventions, public health officials can assess the impact of these measures on disease incidence, prevalence, and transmission patterns. This evaluation helps determine the success of interventions, identify areas for improvement, and inform future public health strategies.

One important application of surveillance data in evaluating interventions is assessing the effectiveness of vaccination campaigns. Vaccination is a key strategy for preventing the spread of infectious diseases, and surveillance systems provide valuable information on vaccine coverage and disease incidence. By comparing vaccination rates and disease data, public health officials can evaluate the impact of vaccination campaigns on reducing disease burden and transmission. For example, surveillance data on vaccine-preventable diseases like measles or polio can indicate whether vaccination efforts have led to a decrease in the number of cases and the interruption of transmission chains.

Surveillance data is also valuable for evaluating control measures for vector-borne diseases. Vector-borne diseases, such as malaria, dengue fever, or Zika virus, require targeted interventions to control the vectors (mosquitoes, ticks) and prevent disease transmission. Surveillance systems collect data on disease incidence, vector populations, and vector control measures. By analyzing this data, public health officials can assess the effectiveness of vector control interventions, such as insecticide-treated bed nets, indoor residual spraying, or community-based vector control programs. This evaluation helps determine the impact of these interventions on reducing vector populations and disease transmission rates.

Real-world examples demonstrate the use of surveillance data in evaluating public health interventions. In the case of polio eradication efforts, surveillance data is used to assess the impact of vaccination campaigns and detect any remaining cases. The Global Polio Eradication Initiative closely monitors polio cases and the effectiveness of vaccination efforts through surveillance systems, allowing for the evaluation of intervention strategies and adjustment of tactics to achieve eradication goals.

Another example is the evaluation of malaria control measures. In many malaria-endemic countries, surveillance systems collect data on malaria cases, vector populations, and the implementation of control interventions, such as distribution of insecticide-treated bed nets and indoor residual spraying. By analyzing these data, public health authorities can evaluate the impact of these interventions on reducing malaria incidence and transmission rates. This information helps guide decision-making and optimize the allocation of resources for future control efforts.

4.2.4 Planning resource allocation:

SURVEILLANCE DATA PLAYS a crucial role in planning resource allocation for public health interventions. By analyzing surveillance data, public health officials can identify areas with high disease burden, populations at risk, and specific needs for interventions. This information enables them to allocate resources effectively and efficiently to maximize the impact of their interventions.

One key aspect of resource allocation is the distribution of vaccines. Surveillance data provides insights into disease incidence and prevalence, helping to identify regions or populations that require prioritized vaccination efforts. For example, in the case of a vaccine-preventable disease outbreak, surveillance data can reveal areas with high case counts or low vaccination coverage, indicating the need for increased vaccine supply and targeted vaccination campaigns in those regions. By utilizing surveillance data, public health officials can ensure that vaccines are distributed where they are most needed, minimizing the spread of disease and protecting vulnerable populations.

Surveillance data also informs the allocation of drugs and other medical supplies. For infectious diseases that require treatment, such as tuberculosis or HIV/AIDS, surveillance systems provide information on disease prevalence, drug resistance patterns, and treatment outcomes. This data helps determine the quantity and distribution of drugs needed to effectively manage and control these diseases. It ensures that medical supplies are available in sufficient quantities in regions with higher disease burden and may require additional support.

Additionally, surveillance data aids in identifying emerging threats and allocating resources for early response. Surveillance systems can detect and monitor outbreaks or the emergence of new infectious diseases. By analyzing these data, public health officials can quickly identify hotspots, assess the magnitude of the outbreak, and allocate resources for timely response and containment measures. This includes deploying medical personnel, establishing treatment centers, procuring diagnostic tests, and providing necessary supplies to affected areas.

Real-world examples illustrate the importance of surveillance data in resource allocation. During the COVID-19 pandemic, surveillance data on case counts, hospitalizations, and deaths played a crucial role in guiding resource allocation decisions. Governments and health agencies used this data to determine the distribution of personal protective equipment (PPE), ventilators, testing kits, and vaccines to regions experiencing higher transmission rates and healthcare burden. This approach ensured that resources were directed to areas with the greatest need, facilitating effective response and control of the pandemic.

In conclusion, surveillance data is essential for planning resource allocation in public health interventions. By analyzing this data, public health officials can identify areas with high disease burden, populations at risk, and specific needs for interventions. This information guides the distribution of vaccines, drugs, and other medical supplies, ensuring that resources are allocated where they are most needed. By utilizing surveillance data for resource allocation, public health authorities can maximize the impact of their interventions and effectively address the challenges posed by infectious diseases.

4.2.5 Informing policy decisions:

SURVEILLANCE DATA PLAYS a vital role in informing policy decisions related to disease prevention and control. By providing accurate and up-to-date information on disease burden, transmission patterns, and emerging threats, surveillance data guides policymakers in formulating evidence-based policies and strategies to mitigate the impact of infectious diseases.

One area where surveillance data informs policy decisions is in addressing antibiotic resistance. Antibiotic-resistant bacteria pose a significant threat to public health, making it crucial to implement appropriate policies to combat this problem. Surveillance systems collect data on the prevalence and trends of antibiotic-resistant bacteria, helping policymakers understand the scope of the issue and make informed decisions. This data can guide the development of policies and guidelines for appropriate antibiotic use, infection control measures, and antimicrobial stewardship programs. It can also identify areas or populations with higher rates of resistance, allowing policymakers to target interventions and resources to those specific areas.

For example, based on surveillance data showing a high prevalence of antibiotic-resistant strains of tuberculosis, policymakers may implement policies to ensure appropriate use of antibiotics for tuberculosis treatment, promote infection control practices in healthcare settings, and strengthen laboratory capacity for drug susceptibility testing. These policies aim to prevent the further emergence and spread of drug-resistant strains and improve treatment outcomes for patients.

Surveillance data also informs policy decisions related to disease prevention and control strategies. For example, in the case of vaccine-preventable diseases, surveillance data on disease incidence, vaccination coverage, and vaccine effectiveness can guide policymakers in formulating vaccination policies. This includes decisions on vaccine schedules, target populations, and the introduction of new vaccines. Surveillance data can also help evaluate the impact of vaccination programs and guide adjustments to immunization strategies to achieve desired outcomes.

Furthermore, surveillance data can inform policies related to public health interventions, such as vector control measures for diseases like malaria or dengue fever. By analyzing surveillance data on vector abundance, disease transmission rates, and the effectiveness of control strategies, policymakers can make informed decisions on the allocation of resources for vector control, including the distribution of insecticide-treated bed nets, indoor residual spraying, and environmental management.

Real-world examples highlight the role of surveillance data in informing policy decisions. The Global Antimicrobial Resistance Surveillance System (GLASS), coordinated by the World Health Organization, collects and analyzes data on antimicrobial resistance from participating countries. This data helps inform global policies and strategies to combat antibiotic resistance. Additionally, the Global Polio Surveillance Network, established by the World Health Organization, provides surveillance data on polio cases worldwide, enabling policymakers to make informed decisions on immunization strategies to achieve polio eradication.

Surveillance data plays a critical role in informing policy decisions related to disease prevention and control. It provides policymakers with essential information on disease burden, transmission patterns, and emerging threats, enabling evidence based policy formulation. Surveillance data guides policies related to antibiotic use, vaccination strategies, vector control measures, and other interventions to mitigate the impact of infectious diseases. By utilizing surveillance data to inform policy decisions, policymakers can effectively allocate resources and implement measures to protect public health.

In summary, surveillance is a critical tool for public health decision-making, providing valuable information that can help to prevent and control the spread of communicable diseases.

4.3 The challenges and opportunities of digital surveillance

DIGITAL SURVEILLANCE, also known as electronic surveillance, refers to the use of technology such as mobile phones, social media, and other digital platforms to track and monitor the spread of communicable diseases. While digital surveillance offers many opportunities for improving disease surveillance and response, it also presents several challenges. Here are some of the challenges and opportunities of digital surveillance:

4.3.1 Challenges:

1. *Data privacy*: The use of digital surveillance raises concerns about data privacy and the potential misuse of personal information.
2. *Access to technology*: Digital surveillance requires access to technology, such as mobile phones and computers, which may not be available to all populations, particularly in low-income settings.
3. *Data accuracy*: The accuracy of digital surveillance data may be affected by factors such as incomplete reporting and inaccurate self-reporting.
4. *Technical challenges*: The use of digital surveillance requires technical expertise and infrastructure, which may be lacking in some settings.

4.3.2 Opportunities:

REAL-TIME DATA COLLECTION is a significant opportunity offered by digital surveillance systems. Traditional surveillance methods often rely on manual data collection and reporting, which can be time-consuming and delay the detection of outbreaks. With digital surveillance, data can be collected and transmitted in real-time, allowing for the immediate identification of disease outbreaks and timely response. For example, mobile-based reporting systems have been implemented in various countries to enable healthcare workers to report cases of infectious diseases directly from the field, providing real-time information to public health authorities.

Digital surveillance also facilitates rapid communication between public health officials and the public. Through various digital platforms such as websites, social media, and mobile applications, important health messages, updates, and guidelines can be disseminated quickly to a wide audience. This enables public health agencies to communicate preventive measures, promote health-seeking behaviors, and provide timely information during disease outbreaks. For instance, during the COVID-19 pandemic, digital surveillance systems have been utilized to share information about symptoms, testing locations, and vaccination campaigns.

The use of digital surveillance can also expand coverage and reach a larger population. Traditional surveillance methods may be limited by factors such as geographical barriers, inadequate healthcare infrastructure, or underreporting. Digital surveillance, on the other hand, has the potential to capture a broader range of cases by leveraging technologies such as mobile phones, internet connectivity, and telemedicine. This can help to identify cases that would have otherwise gone unreported, leading to a more comprehensive understanding of disease burden and transmission patterns.

Another opportunity offered by digital surveillance is the ability to analyze data using advanced techniques. With the increasing availability of big data and the advancements in data analytics, digital surveillance data can be processed and analyzed using machine learning algorithms, artificial intelligence, and other computational methods. These techniques can identify patterns, correlations, and trends in disease transmission, allowing for more accurate and timely decision-making. For example, predictive models can be developed to forecast disease outbreaks based on historical data, helping public health officials allocate resources and implement targeted interventions.

Real-world examples demonstrate the opportunities of digital surveillance in public health. The Global Public Health Intelligence Network (GPHIN), operated by the Public Health Agency of Canada, is a digital surveillance system that monitors global media sources in multiple languages to detect early signs of disease outbreaks. It has been successful in detecting various outbreaks, including the emergence of the severe acute respiratory syndrome (SARS) in 2003. In addition, the use of mobile-based reporting systems in countries like India and Kenya has enabled real-time disease surveillance and response, improving the detection and control of infectious diseases.

Overall, while digital surveillance presents several challenges, it also offers many opportunities for improving disease surveillance and response, particularly in the context of emerging infectious diseases and pandemics. To realize the potential of digital surveillance, it is essential to address the challenges and ensure that privacy and ethical considerations are taken into account.

4.4 Case Studies of Surveillance of Communicable diseases in Africa

4.4.1 COVID-19 pandemic in Kenya

THE COVID-19 PANDEMIC, caused by the novel coronavirus SARS-CoV-2, has had a significant impact on Kenya since the first case was reported on March 13, 2020. Here is a brief overview of the COVID-19 situation in Kenya:

Epidemiology:

As of April 22, 2023, Kenya has recorded over 240,000 confirmed cases of COVID-19 and over 4,700 deaths. The country experienced a surge in cases in the second half of 2020, peaking in November, before declining in early 2021. However, the number of cases has been rising again since September 2021.

Response: The Kenyan government implemented a range of measures to control the spread of COVID-19, including lockdowns, curfews, and restrictions on public gatherings. The government also launched a mass testing campaign, increased hospital capacity, and provided economic support to affected populations. Kenya received vaccines through the COVAX initiative and also purchased additional doses, and as of April 2023, over 10 million doses of vaccine have been administered.

Challenges: Kenya faced several challenges in its response to the COVID-19 pandemic. These included a shortage of medical supplies, particularly personal protective equipment (PPE), and a lack of resources to support affected populations, particularly those in informal settlements. The pandemic also highlighted existing social and economic inequalities in the country.

Lessons learned: The COVID-19 pandemic has highlighted the need for investment in health systems and the importance of strong public health infrastructure. It has also demonstrated the importance of community engagement and the need for equitable access to healthcare and economic support. The pandemic has also spurred innovation, with the development of new technologies and approaches to disease surveillance and response.

Overall, the COVID-19 pandemic has had a significant impact on Kenya and has highlighted both the challenges and opportunities in responding to emerging infectious diseases.

4.4.2 COVID-19 Pandemic in South Africa Epidemiology:

SOUTH AFRICA HAS BEEN heavily impacted by the COVID-19 pandemic. As of April 22, 2023, the country has recorded over 5 million confirmed cases of COVID-19 and over 95,000 deaths. The country experienced multiple waves of infections, with the first wave occurring in 2020 and subsequent waves in 2021 and 2022.

Response: The South African government implemented various measures to control the spread of COVID-19, including lockdowns, travel restrictions, and widespread testing. The government also initiated a comprehensive vaccination campaign and has administered millions of vaccine doses to its population.

Challenges: South Africa faced challenges in its COVID-19 response, including strained healthcare systems, shortages of medical supplies, and vaccine distribution challenges. The country also experienced socioeconomic impacts, particularly affecting vulnerable populations and the economy.

Lessons learned: The COVID-19 pandemic in South Africa highlighted the importance of a strong and resilient healthcare system, effective communication strategies, and equitable access to healthcare and vaccines. It emphasized the need for robust surveillance systems and the importance of international collaboration in responding to global health crises.

4.4.3 COVID-19 Pandemic in Nigeria
Epidemiology:

NIGERIA HAS BEEN SIGNIFICANTLY affected by the COVID-19 pandemic. As of April 22, 2023, the country has recorded over 2.5 million confirmed cases of COVID-19 and over 45,000 deaths. Nigeria experienced multiple waves of infections, with the highest number of cases reported between 2020 and 2021.

Response: The Nigerian government implemented measures to control the spread of COVID-19, including the enforcement of lockdowns, travel restrictions, and the establishment of isolation and treatment centers. The government also launched a national vaccination campaign and has administered millions of vaccine doses.

Challenges: Nigeria faced challenges in its COVID-19 response, including limited healthcare infrastructure, vaccine hesitancy, and misinformation. The country also dealt with socioeconomic impacts, including disruptions to businesses and livelihoods.

Lessons learned: The COVID-19 pandemic in Nigeria highlighted the importance of strengthening healthcare systems, improving testing and contact tracing capacity, and enhancing public health education. It emphasized the need for collaboration between the government, healthcare providers, and communities to effectively respond to a public health crisis.

4.4.4 COVID-19 Pandemic in Ethiopia Epidemiology:

ETHIOPIA HAS BEEN SIGNIFICANTLY impacted by the COVID-19 pandemic. As of April 22, 2023, the country has recorded over 400,000 confirmed cases of COVID-19 and over 6,500 deaths. Ethiopia experienced multiple waves of infections, with the highest number of cases reported in 2021.

Response: The Ethiopian government implemented measures to control the spread of COVID-19, including the enforcement of lockdowns, travel restrictions, and the establishment of quarantine and treatment centers. The government also launched a vaccination campaign and has administered a significant number of vaccine doses.

Challenges: Ethiopia faced challenges in its COVID-19 response, including limited healthcare infrastructure, testing capacity, and access to healthcare in remote areas. The country also dealt with socioeconomic impacts, including disruptions to education and livelihoods.

Lessons learned: The COVID-19 pandemic in Ethiopia highlighted the importance of strengthening healthcare systems, improving laboratory capacity for testing, and enhancing coordination between the government and regional health authorities. It emphasized the need for community engagement, public health education, and equitable vaccine distribution to effectively control the spread of the virus.

4.4.5 COVID-19 Pandemic in Egypt Epidemiology:

EGYPT HAS BEEN SIGNIFICANTLY affected by the COVID-19 pandemic. As of April 22, 2023, the country has recorded over 1.5 million confirmed cases of COVID-19 and over 50,000 deaths. Egypt experienced multiple waves of infections, with the highest number of cases reported between 2020 and 2021.

Response: The Egyptian government implemented various measures to control the spread of COVID-19, including curfews, travel restrictions, and the closure of public spaces. The government also initiated a national vaccination campaign and has administered millions of vaccine doses to its population.

Challenges: Egypt faced challenges in its COVID-19 response, including the strain on healthcare facilities, shortage of medical supplies, and adherence to preventive measures. The country also dealt with socioeconomic impacts, particularly affecting tourism and the economy.

Lessons learned: The COVID-19 pandemic in Egypt highlighted the importance of effective risk communication, public health awareness, and collaboration between the government, healthcare professionals, and the public. It emphasized the need for investment in healthcare infrastructure and the development of local manufacturing capabilities for medical supplies.

4.4.6 COVID-19 Pandemic in Senegal
Epidemiology:

SENEGAL HAS BEEN SIGNIFICANTLY impacted by the COVID-19 pandemic. As of April 22, 2023, the country has recorded over 100,000 confirmed cases of COVID-19 and over 2,000 deaths. Senegal experienced multiple waves of infections, with varying intensity throughout different periods.

Response: The Senegalese government implemented measures to control the spread of COVID-19, including curfews, travel restrictions, and the establishment of testing and treatment centers. The government also launched a vaccination campaign and has administered vaccine doses to a significant portion of its population.

Challenges: Senegal faced challenges in its COVID-19 response, including limited healthcare resources, access to testing in remote areas, and vaccine distribution to vulnerable populations. The country also dealt with socioeconomic impacts, particularly affecting informal workers and small businesses.

Lessons learned: The COVID-19 pandemic in Senegal highlighted the importance of community engagement, public health education, and the involvement of local leaders in disseminating accurate information. It emphasized the need for research and innovation in diagnostics and treatment, as well as the strengthening of health systems to respond effectively to future health crises.

4.4.7 COVID-19 Pandemic in Morocco
Epidemiology:

MOROCCO HAS BEEN SIGNIFICANTLY affected by the COVID-19 pandemic. As of April 22, 2023, the country has recorded over 800,000 confirmed cases of COVID-19 and over 10,000 deaths. Morocco experienced multiple waves of infections, with varying intensity throughout different periods.

Response: The Moroccan government implemented measures to control the spread of COVID-19, including curfews, travel restrictions, and the establishment of field hospitals. The government also launched a national vaccination campaign and has administered millions of vaccine doses to its population.

Challenges: Morocco faced challenges in its COVID-19 response, including strain on healthcare facilities, vaccine hesitancy, and socioeconomic impacts on vulnerable populations. The country also dealt with the disruption of tourism and the economy.

Lessons learned: The COVID-19 pandemic in Morocco highlighted the importance of proactive and coordinated decision-making, effective risk communication, and the involvement of local communities in implementing preventive measures. It emphasized the need for international cooperation and solidarity to address global health emergencies effectively.

4.4.8 Ebola Outbreak in Democratic Republic of the Congo (DRC) Epidemiology:

THE DEMOCRATIC REPUBLIC of the Congo has experienced multiple Ebola outbreaks. One notable outbreak occurred between 2018 and 2020, with over 3,400 cases and approximately 2,200 deaths reported. The outbreak affected several provinces in the country, including North Kivu, Ituri, and Equateur.

Response: The response to the Ebola outbreak in DRC involved a multi-sectoral approach, including surveillance, contact tracing, isolation of cases, and vaccination campaigns. International organizations, such as the World Health Organization (WHO), worked closely with the DRC government and local communities to control the spread of the virus.

Challenges: The response to the Ebola outbreak faced various challenges, including insecurity and armed conflict in affected areas, resistance from some communities, and the remote and hard-to-reach nature of certain regions. The outbreak response required extensive coordination among local and international partners.

Lessons learned: The Ebola outbreak in DRC highlighted the importance of community engagement, trust-building, and cultural sensitivity in disease control efforts. It underscored the need for robust surveillance systems, effective coordination between national and international stakeholders, and investment in healthcare infrastructure to respond promptly to outbreaks.

4.4.9 Malaria Control in Tanzania Epidemiology:

MALARIA IS ENDEMIC in Tanzania, with high transmission rates across the country. It remains a leading cause of illness and death, particularly among young children and pregnant women. In 2020, Tanzania reported over 10 million confirmed malaria cases and thousands of deaths.

Response: The Tanzanian government, in collaboration with international partners, has implemented comprehensive malaria control strategies, including vector control measures (such as bed nets and indoor residual spraying), prompt diagnosis, and effective treatment with antimalarial drugs. The government has also prioritized community education and mobilization to promote preventive measures.

Challenges: Tanzania faces challenges in malaria control, including limited access to healthcare in remote areas, inadequate funding for prevention and treatment programs, and the emergence of drug-resistant malaria strains. The country also experiences seasonal variations in transmission intensity, requiring targeted interventions.

Lessons learned: The malaria control efforts in Tanzania emphasize the importance of a multi-faceted approach, including vector control, diagnosis, treatment, and community involvement. It underscores the need for sustained investment in malaria programs, research for new tools and strategies, and close collaboration between the government, healthcare providers, and communities.

4.4.10 Yellow Fever Outbreak in Nigeria Epidemiology:

NIGERIA HAS EXPERIENCED multiple yellow fever outbreaks in recent years. One significant outbreak occurred in 2017, with over 3,000 suspected cases and hundreds of deaths reported. The outbreak affected several states across the country.

Response: The Nigerian government, with support from the WHO and other partners, launched a large-scale yellow fever vaccination campaign to control the outbreak. The campaign targeted high-risk areas and involved widespread vaccination coverage, particularly among children and vulnerable populations. **Challenges:** The response to the yellow fever outbreak faced challenges, including limited vaccine supply, logistical difficulties in reaching remote and underserved areas, and vaccine hesitancy among some communities. The outbreak response required coordination among multiple stakeholders and the mobilization of resources.

Lessons learned: The yellow fever outbreak in Nigeria highlighted the importance of proactive surveillance, early detection, and rapid response to prevent the spread of the disease. It emphasized the need for sustainable vaccination programs, strengthening of laboratory capacity for diagnosis, and addressing vaccine hesitancy through community engagement and health education.

4.4.11 Cholera Outbreak in Zambia Epidemiology:

ZAMBIA HAS FACED RECURRENT cholera outbreaks, with the most recent major outbreak occurring in 2017-2018. During that period, over 5,900 cases and approximately 114 deaths were reported. Cholera transmission is often associated with poor sanitation and limited access to safe drinking water. **Response**: The Zambian government, in collaboration with international partners, implemented a comprehensive response to the cholera outbreak. This included enhancing water and sanitation infrastructure, conducting hygiene promotion campaigns, improving case management, and strengthening surveillance and early warning systems.

Challenges: The response to the cholera outbreak in Zambia faced challenges such as inadequate sanitation facilities in densely populated areas, limited access to clean water sources, and the need for sustained behavior change to promote proper hygiene practices. Coordinating efforts across different sectors and ensuring the availability of resources were crucial challenges as well.

Lessons learned: The cholera outbreak in Zambia highlighted the importance of addressing underlying factors such as inadequate sanitation and water infrastructure to prevent future outbreaks. It underscored the need for integrated approaches that combine health interventions with improvements in water, sanitation, and hygiene (WASH) infrastructure. Additionally, community engagement and behavior change programs were recognized as essential components of cholera control efforts.

4.4.12 HIV/AIDS Epidemic in South Africa
Epidemiology:

SOUTH AFRICA HAS ONE of the highest burdens of HIV/AIDS globally. The country has experienced a significant HIV epidemic, with an estimated 7.7 million people living with HIV in 2020. The epidemic disproportionately affects certain populations, such as young women and key populations including sex workers and men who have sex with men.

Response: The South African government, along with civil society organizations and international partners, has implemented a comprehensive response to the HIV/AIDS epidemic. This includes widespread access to antiretroviral therapy (ART), prevention programs, HIV testing and counseling services, and efforts to reduce mother-to-child transmission of HIV.

Challenges: The response to the HIV/AIDS epidemic in South Africa faced challenges such as ensuring universal access to HIV testing and treatment, reducing stigma and discrimination, addressing health disparities, and reaching key populations with tailored prevention and care services. The country also had to address the social and economic factors driving the epidemic, including poverty and gender inequality.

Lessons learned: The HIV/AIDS epidemic in South Africa highlighted the importance of political commitment, strong leadership, and collaboration among various sectors and stakeholders. It emphasized the need for a comprehensive approach that combines prevention, treatment, and care services with efforts to address social determinants of health and reduce stigma. The country's experience also emphasized the significance of community engagement and meaningful involvement of affected populations in shaping the response.

These case studies provide insights into the challenges, responses, and lessons learned from different disease outbreaks and epidemics in Southern and Central African countries. Each case study highlights the importance of coordinated efforts, community engagement, and the integration of various interventions to effectively control and mitigate the impact of diseases.

4.5 Exercises

1. What is the purpose of disease surveillance systems?

Solution: Disease surveillance systems are used to collect, analyze, and interpret data on the occurrence of diseases in populations to help identify outbreaks and guide public health interventions.

1. What is the difference between active and passive surveillance?

Solution: Active surveillance involves actively seeking out cases of a disease, while passive surveillance relies on healthcare providers and laboratories reporting cases to public health authorities.

1. What are some challenges associated with disease surveillance in low-resource settings?

Solution: Some challenges include limited resources for surveillance, inadequate laboratory capacity, and poor infrastructure for data collection and reporting.

1. What are some of the components of an effective outbreak response plan? *Solution*: An effective outbreak

response plan should include a system for early detection and reporting of cases, rapid investigation of cases and outbreaks, development and implementation of control measures, and communication with the public and other stakeholders.

1. What is the role of contact tracing in outbreak response?

Solution: Contact tracing involves identifying and monitoring individuals who have had close contact with a person infected with a disease in order to prevent further transmission.

1. How can social and behavioral factors impact disease transmission and response efforts?

Solution: Social and behavioral factors such as stigma, distrust of healthcare providers, and cultural practices can impact disease transmission and response efforts by affecting willingness to seek care, comply with control measures, and participate in surveillance activities.

1. What is the International Health Regulations (IHR) and why are they important?

Solution: The IHR are a legally binding agreement between countries that establish the rights and obligations of countries to report public health events, including disease outbreaks, to the international community. They are important for promoting global health security and preventing the spread of infectious diseases.

1. What is the role of the World Health Organization (WHO) in disease surveillance and response?

Solution: The WHO plays a key role in disease surveillance and response by providing technical guidance and support to member countries, coordinating global efforts to prevent and control outbreaks, and facilitating the sharing of information and resources.

1. What are some ethical considerations in disease surveillance and response?

Solution: Ethical considerations in disease surveillance and response include protecting the privacy and confidentiality of individuals, ensuring equitable access to healthcare services, and balancing individual rights with public health interests.

1. What are some potential challenges in achieving global cooperation for disease surveillance and response?

Solution: Potential challenges include differences in political systems and priorities, limited resources for surveillance and response, and concerns about sovereignty and national security.

Chapter 5. Disease surveillance and response in Europe

5.1 Comparative analysis of disease surveillance systems in Europe

Europe has a diverse range of disease surveillance systems, reflecting the differences in health systems, legal frameworks, and cultural contexts across the continent. Here are some examples of disease surveillance systems in Europe:

5.1.1 European Centre for Disease Prevention and Control (ECDC):

THE EUROPEAN CENTRE for Disease Prevention and Control (ECDC) plays a vital role in the prevention and control of communicable diseases in Europe. As an agency of the European Union (EU), the ECDC provides technical expertise, surveillance, and support to member states in their efforts to combat infectious diseases.

One of the primary functions of the ECDC is the collection and analysis of data on infectious disease outbreaks in Europe. The agency collaborates with national authorities and surveillance systems across the EU to gather information on the occurrence and spread of communicable diseases. By monitoring and analyzing this data, the ECDC can identify trends, detect emerging threats, and assess the impact of infectious diseases on public health.

In addition to data collection, the ECDC conducts risk assessments to evaluate the threat posed by different infectious diseases. These assessments consider factors such as the transmissibility of the disease, severity of illness, potential for outbreaks, and effectiveness of control measures. Based on these assessments, the ECDC provides evidence-based guidance and recommendations to member states on disease prevention, surveillance, and response strategies.

Real-world examples demonstrate the significant role of the ECDC in effectively responding to infectious disease outbreaks in Europe. During the COVID-19 pandemic, the ECDC has been at the forefront of coordinating and disseminating information to member states. The agency has provided regular updates on the epidemiological situation, risk assessments, and guidance on testing, contact tracing, quarantine measures, and vaccination strategies. This collaborative approach has helped member states align their response efforts and implement effective public health measures to control the spread of the virus.

Furthermore, the ECDC actively supports member states in strengthening their surveillance systems, laboratory capacities, and preparedness plans for infectious diseases. Through training programs, technical assistance, and knowledge sharing, the ECDC promotes a standardized and coordinated approach to disease surveillance and response across Europe.

The ECDC's role in providing timely and accurate information, technical expertise, and guidance to member states has been instrumental in enhancing Europe's ability to prevent, detect, and respond to communicable diseases. By facilitating collaboration and cooperation among countries, the ECDC contributes to a more effective and efficient response to outbreaks and the protection of public health in Europe.

5.1.2 Health Protection Surveillance Centre

(HPSC) in Ireland:

THE HEALTH PROTECTION Surveillance Centre (HPSC) plays a crucial role in the surveillance and control of infectious diseases in Ireland. Established in 1998, the HPSC operates under the auspices of the Health Service Executive (HSE) and the Department of Health. Its primary objective is to protect public health by providing timely and accurate information on infectious diseases and supporting healthcare professionals in their efforts to prevent and control outbreaks.

The HPSC operates a comprehensive national surveillance system for notifiable diseases, which includes both mandatory reporting and voluntary reporting by healthcare providers and laboratories across the country. Notifiable diseases are those that are required by law to be reported to public health authorities due to their potential impact on public health. The HPSC works closely with these reporting entities to ensure timely and accurate data collection, analysis, and reporting of infectious diseases.

One of the key functions of the HPSC is to collect, collate, and analyze surveillance data to monitor the incidence and prevalence of infectious diseases in Ireland. This data provides insights into disease trends, geographical distribution, and population-specific risk factors, helping public health officials and policymakers make informed decisions regarding prevention and control measures.

In addition to surveillance, the HPSC plays a vital role in providing expert advice and support to healthcare professionals, government agencies, and the public on infectious disease prevention and control. The center produces guidelines, protocols, and recommendations for disease-specific management and control measures, which are regularly updated based on emerging evidence and best practices. The HPSC also collaborates with international partners and participates in global networks to stay informed about emerging infectious disease threats and contribute to international efforts in disease surveillance and response.

The HPSC's expertise extends beyond infectious diseases to include public health emergencies and health protection issues. The center actively participates in emergency preparedness and response activities, providing guidance and coordination during public health crises such as pandemics or large-scale outbreaks. It works closely with other national and international stakeholders, including the European Centre for Disease Prevention and Control (ECDC) and the World Health Organization (WHO), to ensure a coordinated and effective response to public health threats.

5.1.3 Robert Koch Institute (RKI) in Germany:

THE ROBERT KOCH INSTITUTE (RKI) is a renowned federal institution in Germany that plays a pivotal role in disease surveillance, prevention, and control. Established in 1891, the RKI is named after the eminent physician and microbiologist, Robert Koch, who made groundbreaking contributions to the field of infectious diseases.

The primary objective of the RKI is to safeguard public health by monitoring and analyzing infectious diseases in Germany. The institute operates a comprehensive national surveillance system for infectious diseases, which involves mandatory reporting by healthcare providers and laboratories across the country. This surveillance system ensures timely collection and analysis of data on disease incidence, prevalence, and trends, enabling the RKI to identify potential outbreaks and take appropriate actions.

One of the key functions of the RKI is to conduct risk assessments and provide evidence-based recommendations on disease prevention and control measures. The institute's expert scientists and epidemiologists continuously evaluate the epidemiological situation, conduct research, and generate guidelines to inform healthcare professionals, policymakers, and the public on best practices for disease prevention, diagnosis, and treatment. These recommendations help guide public health interventions, vaccination strategies, and the implementation of control measures.

The RKI is actively involved in scientific research and collaboration with national and international partners. Its scientists conduct studies and investigations to enhance the understanding of infectious diseases, including their transmission dynamics, risk factors, and impact on public health. The institute also collaborates with other national and international institutions, such as the World Health Organization (WHO) and the European Centre for Disease Prevention and Control (ECDC), to exchange information, share expertise, and contribute to global efforts in disease surveillance and control.

In addition to its surveillance and research activities, the RKI plays a critical role in crisis management during public health emergencies. The institute provides rapid risk assessments, develops response plans, and coordinates the national response to outbreaks or other health emergencies. It collaborates closely with regional health authorities, laboratories, and healthcare providers to ensure a coordinated and effective response, including the deployment of diagnostic tests, provision of medical supplies, and implementation of control measures.

Furthermore, the RKI plays an important role in health communication and public education. The institute regularly disseminates information to the public and healthcare professionals through various channels, including its website, press releases, and public awareness campaigns. It aims to raise awareness about infectious diseases, promote healthy behaviors, and address any misconceptions or concerns among the population.

The work of the RKI is essential in maintaining and enhancing the health security of the German population. By conducting disease surveillance, providing evidence-based recommendations, conducting research, and coordinating crisis response, the institute contributes significantly to the prevention, control, and management of infectious diseases in Germany.

5.1.4 National Institute of Public Health and the Environment (RIVM) in the Netherlands:

THE NATIONAL INSTITUTE for Public Health and the Environment (RIVM) is the leading authority in the Netherlands for disease surveillance, prevention, and control. Established in 1909, the RIVM plays a crucial role in safeguarding public health and promoting a healthy living environment.

One of the primary functions of the RIVM is to operate a comprehensive national surveillance system for infectious diseases. The institute collaborates with healthcare providers, laboratories, and other stakeholders to ensure the timely and accurate reporting of infectious disease cases. This surveillance system enables the RIVM to monitor disease trends, identify potential outbreaks, and assess the effectiveness of control measures. By collecting and analyzing data on disease incidence, prevalence, and other epidemiological factors, the RIVM provides valuable insights into the dynamics of infectious diseases in the Netherlands.

In addition to surveillance, the RIVM conducts research on various aspects of infectious diseases. Its team of scientists and experts explore topics such as disease transmission, risk factors, and the impact of interventions. Through epidemiological studies, laboratory investigations, and modeling, the RIVM generates evidence-based knowledge to inform public health policies and interventions. This research also contributes to the global understanding of infectious diseases and supports international collaborations.

The RIVM plays a vital role in providing advice and guidance on disease prevention and control. It develops evidence-based guidelines and recommendations for healthcare professionals, policymakers, and the general public. These guidelines cover a wide range of topics, including vaccination strategies, infection prevention measures, and outbreak management. The RIVM's expertise and guidance help ensure that healthcare providers and the public have access to accurate and up-to-date information on disease prevention, diagnosis, and treatment.

Furthermore, the RIVM actively participates in national and international collaborations to address global health challenges. It collaborates with other public health agencies, research institutions, and international organizations to share knowledge, exchange best practices, and strengthen global disease surveillance and response systems. Through these collaborations, the RIVM contributes to the collective effort of preventing and controlling infectious diseases worldwide.

The RIVM also plays a key role in crisis management during public health emergencies. It provides rapid risk assessments, supports outbreak investigations, and coordinates the national response to disease outbreaks or other health threats. The institute works closely with regional health authorities, healthcare providers, and other stakeholders to ensure a coordinated and effective response, including the dissemination of timely and accurate information to the public.

Additionally, the RIVM engages in health promotion and public awareness activities. It educates the public on infectious diseases, promotes healthy behaviors, and raises awareness about emerging health risks. Through its communication channels, such as its website, social media platforms, and public campaigns, the RIVM strives to empower individuals and communities to take proactive measures for disease prevention and control.

The work of the RIVM is crucial in protecting and promoting public health in the Netherlands. By operating a robust surveillance system, conducting research, providing expert advice, and coordinating response efforts, the RIVM contributes to the prevention, control, and management of infectious diseases in the country.

5.1.5 Comparative analysis:

THE DISEASE SURVEILLANCE systems in Europe vary in terms of their organization, scope, and methods. However, they share some common features, such as the use of mandatory reporting, risk assessments, and guidance on disease prevention and control. The ECDC plays a key role in coordinating and supporting disease surveillance across Europe, while national institutions such as the HPSC, RKI, and RIVM provide country-specific expertise and guidance.

In terms of challenges, some disease surveillance systems in Europe face issues such as underreporting, limited resources, and the need for greater collaboration and data sharing across borders. The

COVID-19 pandemic has highlighted both the strengths and weaknesses of disease surveillance systems in Europe, and has spurred innovation in areas such as digital surveillance and vaccine development. Overall, the comparative analysis of disease surveillance systems in Europe highlights the importance of strong public health infrastructure, collaboration, and innovation in preventing and controlling infectious diseases.

5.2 The role of the European Centre for Disease Prevention and Control

THE EUROPEAN CENTRE for Disease Prevention and Control (ECDC) is an EU agency that plays a key role in supporting disease surveillance and prevention across Europe. The main role of the ECDC is to provide technical expertise, guidance, and support to EU member states in their efforts to prevent and control infectious diseases. Some of the specific functions of the ECDC include:

1. *Surveillance and monitoring*: The ECDC collects and analyzes data on infectious disease outbreaks in Europe, and provides regular updates on the spread of diseases such as COVID-19, influenza, and tuberculosis.

2. *Risk assessment and communication*: The ECDC provides risk assessments and guidance to member states on the prevention and control of infectious diseases. This includes developing protocols for outbreak investigation, contact tracing, and quarantine measures.

3. *Response coordination*: In the event of a disease outbreak or public health emergency, the ECDC works closely with member states to coordinate their response efforts. This includes providing technical support, coordinating the distribution of medical supplies and equipment, and

assisting with the deployment of public health experts and emergency responders.

4. ***Capacity building***: The ECDC provides training and technical assistance to member states to enhance their capacity for disease surveillance, prevention, and control. This includes supporting the development of national public health strategies and emergency response plans.

Overall, the role of the ECDC is to support EU member states in their efforts to prevent and control infectious diseases, and to promote cooperation and collaboration among public health authorities across Europe. The ECDC plays a vital role in enhancing the preparedness and response capacity of Europe to emerging infectious diseases and other public health threats.

5.3 Best practices and lessons learned from the response to recent outbreaks

THE RESPONSE TO RECENT outbreaks has provided valuable insights into best practices and lessons learned in outbreak response. Here are some key takeaways:

5.3.1 Early detection and rapid response are critical:

EARLY DETECTION AND rapid response are crucial components in containing and mitigating the spread of infectious diseases. By identifying outbreaks early on and implementing prompt response measures, public health authorities can effectively limit the transmission of the disease and protect communities. Various real-world examples highlight the significance of early detection and rapid response in controlling infectious disease outbreaks.

During the 2014-2016 Ebola outbreak in West Africa, early detection and rapid response played a critical role in containing the spread of the virus. In Guinea, Sierra Leone, and Liberia, where the outbreak was most severe, efforts were made to improve surveillance systems, enhance laboratory capacities, and establish emergency response mechanisms. By quickly detecting cases, isolating infected individuals, and conducting contact tracing, public health officials were able to identify and quarantine individuals who may have been exposed to the virus, effectively breaking the chain of transmission and preventing further spread of Ebola.

Another example is the response to the COVID-19 pandemic. Early detection of the novel coronavirus and the implementation of rapid response measures have been essential in curbing the spread of the disease. Countries that adopted proactive testing strategies, contact tracing, and quarantine measures for confirmed cases and their contacts have demonstrated better control over the virus. For instance, South Korea's successful response to COVID-19 was largely attributed to its extensive testing, contact tracing, and strict quarantine measures.

In addition to these examples, the importance of early detection and rapid response has been highlighted in outbreaks of other infectious diseases such as SARS (Severe Acute Respiratory Syndrome) and MERS (Middle East Respiratory Syndrome). Prompt identification of cases, implementation of infection control measures, and isolation of individuals with symptoms or positive test results have been key strategies in limiting the spread of these diseases.

5.3.2 Communication and community engagement are essential:

COMMUNICATION AND COMMUNITY engagement play a crucial role in outbreak response efforts. Effective communication strategies that provide clear and accurate information to the public can help build trust, dispel misinformation, and ensure widespread adherence to recommended prevention measures. Engaging with local communities and stakeholders fosters collaboration and empowers individuals to take an active role in mitigating the spread of infectious diseases. Numerous real-world examples highlight the significance of communication and community engagement in outbreak response.

During the COVID-19 pandemic, countries that prioritized transparent and consistent communication with their populations experienced better outcomes in terms of public compliance and understanding of preventive measures. New Zealand's Prime Minister, Jacinda Ardern, gained international recognition for her clear and empathetic communication style, which helped build trust and unity among the public during the crisis (Bergman, 2020). The effective communication strategies employed in New Zealand contributed to the country's successful management of the pandemic.

Community engagement was a vital component of the response to the Ebola outbreak in West Africa. In Liberia, for instance, community leaders and organizations played a critical role in disseminating accurate information, dispelling rumors, and mobilizing community support for control measures. This community-led approach helped in gaining the trust of the local population, which resulted in increased compliance with preventive measures and reduced transmission.

Engaging with communities also proved instrumental in combating the Zika virus outbreak in Brazil. The government, along with health authorities, collaborated with community leaders, non-governmental organizations, and local residents to raise awareness about the virus, promote vector control measures, and provide support to affected individuals and families. This community-centered approach facilitated a more comprehensive and effective response to the outbreak.

5.3.3 Collaboration and coordination are key:

COLLABORATION AND COORDINATION among various stakeholders are crucial for an effective outbreak response. By working together, public health authorities, healthcare providers, community leaders, and international organizations can pool their resources, expertise, and knowledge to develop coordinated strategies, share information, and implement effective interventions. Real-world examples highlight the importance of collaboration and coordination in outbreak response efforts.

The response to the COVID-19 pandemic has demonstrated the significance of collaboration at the global level. The World Health Organization (WHO) has played a central role in coordinating the global response and facilitating collaboration among countries. Through its International Health Regulations (IHR), the WHO has provided a platform for countries to exchange information, coordinate response efforts, and support each other in managing the pandemic. Collaborative initiatives such as the Access to COVID-19 Tools Accelerator (ACT-A) and its COVAX facility have brought together multiple stakeholders to ensure equitable access to COVID-19 diagnostics, treatments, and vaccines globally. These collaborative efforts have been essential in addressing the challenges posed by the pandemic.

Another example of collaboration and coordination can be seen in the response to the Ebola outbreak in West Africa. Multiple organizations, including the WHO, national health ministries, non-governmental organizations, and international partners, collaborated to control the outbreak and provide healthcare services to affected communities. This collaborative approach involved sharing expertise, coordinating response activities, and providing technical assistance to affected countries. The successful containment of the Ebola outbreak in Nigeria was largely attributed to the coordinated efforts of various stakeholders, including government agencies, healthcare providers, and international partners.

Collaboration and coordination are not limited to global or national levels but also extend to local communities. Local public health agencies, healthcare facilities, community organizations, and first responders often work together during outbreaks to ensure a coordinated response. For instance, during the H1N1 influenza pandemic, local health departments collaborated with schools, workplaces, and community organizations to disseminate information, provide vaccinations, and implement preventive measures.

These examples highlight the importance of collaboration and coordination in outbreak response. By working together, stakeholders can leverage their collective strengths, optimize resource allocation, and ensure a more effective and efficient response to outbreaks.

5.3.4 Preparedness is essential:

PREPAREDNESS IS INDEED crucial in effectively responding to outbreaks, and there have been several real-world examples highlighting the significance of preparedness measures. Here are a few examples:

5.3.4.1 Global Influenza Surveillance and Response System (GISRS):

GISRS IS A GLOBAL NETWORK of laboratories and health organizations that monitor and respond to seasonal and pandemic influenza threats. The system collects and analyzes influenza viruses, conducts risk assessments, and provides recommendations for vaccine strain selection. The surveillance and preparedness activities of GISRS have been instrumental in monitoring and responding to influenza outbreaks worldwide.

5.3.4.2 West Africa Ebola Outbreak (2014-2016):

THE EBOLA OUTBREAK in West Africa emphasized the importance of preparedness in responding to emerging infectious diseases. Following the outbreak, countries in the region, along with international partners, strengthened their preparedness capacities by developing national emergency response plans, establishing surveillance systems, enhancing laboratory capacity, and conducting simulation exercises. These preparedness efforts helped mitigate the impact of subsequent Ebola outbreaks in the region.

5.3.4.3 Strategic National Stockpile (SNS) - United States:

THE SNS IS A NATIONAL repository of critical medical supplies and pharmaceuticals maintained by the U.S. Centers for Disease Control and Prevention (CDC). The stockpile enables a rapid response to public health emergencies by ensuring the availability of essential medical resources. During outbreaks such as the H1N1 influenza pandemic and Hurricane Katrina, the SNS played a vital role in delivering medical supplies and equipment to affected areas.

5.3.4.4 Exercise Cygnus - United Kingdom:

EXERCISE CYGNUS WAS a pandemic preparedness exercise conducted in the United Kingdom in 2016. It simulated a severe influenza pandemic to assess the country's readiness and identify areas for improvement. The findings from the exercise highlighted the importance of preparedness planning, coordination, and resource allocation. The lessons learned from Exercise Cygnus informed subsequent pandemic response strategies.

These examples underscore the significance of preparedness in outbreak response. By stockpiling essential resources, developing response plans, and conducting simulation exercises, countries and organizations can enhance their readiness to effectively mitigate the impact of outbreaks.

5.3.5 Investment in public health infrastructure is crucial:

INVESTMENT IN PUBLIC health infrastructure is indeed crucial for effective outbreak response. Here are some real-world examples that highlight the significance of investing in public health infrastructure:

5.3.5.1 Global Polio Eradication Initiative:

THE GLOBAL POLIO ERADICATION Initiative is a partnership of organizations, including the World Health

Organization (WHO), UNICEF, Rotary International, and the U.S. Centers for Disease Control and Prevention (CDC), working towards eradicating polio worldwide. The initiative focuses on strengthening disease surveillance systems, establishing laboratory networks, and improving immunization programs. Investments in public health infrastructure have been key to the success of the initiative, leading to a significant reduction in polio cases globally.

5.3.5.2 Strengthening Health Systems - Liberia:

FOLLOWING THE DEVASTATING Ebola outbreak in 2014-2016, Liberia made substantial investments in strengthening its health system. This included improving disease surveillance systems, enhancing laboratory capacity, and training healthcare workers. These investments helped build a resilient health system that is better equipped to detect and respond to future outbreaks.

5.3.5.3 Integrated Disease Surveillance and Response - Africa:

THE INTEGRATED DISEASE Surveillance and Response (IDSR) strategy, implemented in many African countries, focuses on enhancing disease surveillance, laboratory capacity, and emergency response systems. This approach has been instrumental in improving early detection and response to outbreaks, including diseases such as Ebola, cholera, and meningitis.

5.3.5.4 Global Health Security Agenda (GHSA):

THE GHSA IS A COLLABORATIVE effort among multiple countries and organizations to strengthen global health security. It aims to prevent, detect, and respond to infectious disease threats through investments in public health infrastructure, including disease surveillance, laboratory networks, and healthcare systems. The GHSA has supported countries in improving their readiness to respond to outbreaks and enhancing their overall health security.

These examples demonstrate that investment in public health infrastructure is critical for building resilient healthcare systems and effectively responding to outbreaks. By strengthening disease surveillance, laboratory networks, and healthcare systems, countries can enhance their capacity to detect, monitor, and respond to emerging infectious diseases.

5.3.6 Health equity and social determinants of health must be addressed:

HEALTH EQUITY AND SOCIAL determinants of health play a critical role in outbreak response. Addressing underlying health disparities and ensuring access to healthcare services for all populations can help prevent the spread of infectious diseases.

Overall, recent outbreaks have highlighted the importance of a coordinated, collaborative, and prepared approach to outbreak response. By implementing best practices and lessons learned from past outbreaks, we can better protect public health and prevent the spread of infectious diseases.

5.4 Case study: Measles outbreak in Ukraine

IN RECENT YEARS, UKRAINE has experienced a large outbreak of measles, with over 56,000 cases reported between January 2018 and June 2019. Measles is a highly contagious viral disease that can cause severe health complications, particularly in children. The outbreak in Ukraine was attributed to a combination of factors, including low vaccination coverage, weak disease surveillance systems, and limited access to healthcare services in some areas.

The Ukrainian government and international organizations responded to the outbreak by implementing a range of measures to increase vaccination coverage and improve disease surveillance. These measures included:

5.4.1.1 Strengthening disease surveillance systems:

THE UKRAINIAN MINISTRY of Health worked with international organizations to improve disease surveillance systems and increase the number of reported cases. This helped to identify the extent of the outbreak and target response efforts.

5.4.1.2 Conducting vaccination campaigns:

THE UKRAINIAN GOVERNMENT and international organizations conducted vaccination campaigns to increase coverage rates and prevent further spread of the disease. The campaigns targeted vulnerable populations such as children and healthcare workers.

5.4.1.3 Improving access to healthcare services:

THE UKRAINIAN GOVERNMENT and international organizations worked to improve access to healthcare services in areas where there were shortages of medical personnel or facilities. This included providing mobile medical clinics and increasing the number of medical professionals in affected areas.

5.4.1.4 Increasing public awareness:

THE UKRAINIAN GOVERNMENT and international organizations worked to increase public awareness about the importance of vaccination and disease prevention measures. This included providing information about the risks of measles and the benefits of vaccination.

Overall, the response to the measles outbreak in Ukraine highlights the importance of a coordinated and comprehensive approach to outbreak response. By strengthening disease surveillance systems, increasing vaccination coverage, improving access to healthcare services, and increasing public awareness, it is possible to prevent and control the spread of infectious diseases like measles.

5.5 Exercises

1. What is the basic reproductive number (R0) in disease transmission?

   Solution: The basic reproductive number (R0) is the average number of new infections that one infected person will generate in a completely susceptible population.

1. What are some factors that can affect the transmission of communicable diseases?

   Solution: Factors that can affect the transmission of communicable diseases include population density, sanitation, hygiene, and social and behavioral factors.

1. How can mass media be used to promote public health?

Solution: Mass media can be used to promote public health by disseminating information on disease prevention and control measures, and by encouraging behaviors that promote health.

1. What is the International Health Regulations (IHR)?

Solution: The International Health Regulations (IHR) is a legally binding instrument of international law that aims to prevent, protect against, control, and provide a public health response to the international spread of disease.

1. What is the role of the Africa Centers for Disease Control and Prevention (Africa CDC) in disease surveillance and response?

Solution: The Africa CDC plays a key role in disease surveillance and response in Africa by providing technical and operational support to member states, coordinating regional and continental responses, and strengthening health systems.

1. What are some challenges and opportunities in global health security? *Solution*: Some challenges in global health security include the emergence of new infectious diseases, inadequate public health infrastructure, and the potential for bioterrorism. Some opportunities include advances in technology and communication, increased international cooperation, and the potential for innovative financing mechanisms.

1. What are some ethical considerations in disease surveillance and response?

Solution: Ethical considerations in disease surveillance and response include balancing individual rights and public health interests, ensuring privacy and confidentiality of personal health information, and providing equitable access to resources and services.

1. What is the role of governance and leadership in epidemic control?

Solution: Governance and leadership play a critical role in epidemic control by setting priorities, establishing policies and guidelines, allocating resources, and ensuring accountability and transparency in decision-making.

1. How can global cooperation improve disease surveillance and response? *Solution*: Global cooperation can improve disease surveillance and response by facilitating the sharing of information, resources, and expertise, promoting best practices, and coordinating responses to outbreaks and epidemics.

1. What are some best practices and lessons learned from recent outbreaks? *Solution:* Best practices and lessons learned from recent outbreaks include the importance of early detection and response, the need for strong public health systems and infrastructure, the role of community engagement and social mobilization, and the potential benefits of technology and innovation in disease surveillance and response.

Chapter 6. Disease surveillance and response in Africa

6.1 Comparative analysis of disease surveillance systems in Africa

Disease surveillance systems in Africa vary widely depending on the country and region. Some countries have well-established systems that can effectively detect and respond to disease outbreaks, while others have weaker systems that struggle to provide timely and accurate information.

One of the major challenges facing disease surveillance systems in Africa is limited resources and infrastructure. Many countries lack the necessary funding, technology, and trained personnel to effectively monitor and respond to disease outbreaks. This can lead to delays in detecting outbreaks, which can then spread rapidly and become more difficult to control.

However, there have been some successful disease surveillance programs in Africa. For example, the Global Polio Eradication Initiative has worked with African countries to develop and implement polio surveillance systems. These systems have been instrumental in identifying and responding to outbreaks of polio, leading to a significant reduction in the number of cases in recent years.

Another example is the Integrated Disease Surveillance and Response (IDSR) system, which has been implemented in many African countries to improve surveillance and response to priority diseases, including measles, cholera, and meningitis. The IDSR system is based on a standardized framework that includes case definitions, reporting mechanisms, and response protocols, which can help to ensure consistent and effective surveillance across different countries.

Despite these successes, there is still much work to be done to improve disease surveillance in Africa. This includes increasing funding and resources for surveillance systems, strengthening collaboration between countries and international organizations, and investing in training and capacity-building for surveillance staff. By doing so, it is possible to build more robust and effective disease surveillance systems that can help to prevent and control outbreaks of infectious diseases in Africa.

6.2 The role of the Africa Centers for Disease Control and Prevention

THE AFRICA CENTERS for Disease Control and Prevention (Africa CDC) is a specialized technical institution of the African Union (AU) that is responsible for supporting African Union Member States in their efforts to prevent, detect, and respond to infectious disease outbreaks and other public health emergencies. The Africa CDC was established in 2016 in response to the Ebola outbreak in West Africa, which highlighted the need for a more coordinated and effective response to public health emergencies in Africa.

The Africa CDC has several key roles in supporting disease surveillance and response in Africa. These include:

6.2.1.1 Coordinating and harmonizing disease surveillance and response efforts across the continent:

THE AFRICA CDC WORKS to ensure that surveillance and response activities are aligned with international standards and best practices. It provides technical assistance to African Union Member States in the development and implementation of national disease surveillance and response plans.

6.2.1.2 Strengthening laboratory networks:

THE AFRICA CDC IS WORKING to establish a continent-wide network of public health laboratories that can rapidly detect and respond to disease outbreaks. This includes supporting the development of laboratory capacity, promoting the sharing of laboratory data, and providing training and technical support to laboratory staff.

6.2.1.3 Developing and disseminating public health information:

THE AFRICA CDC WORKS to disseminate accurate and timely information about disease outbreaks and public health emergencies to stakeholders across the continent. This includes developing and disseminating public health advisories, providing training on risk communication, and establishing partnerships with media outlets to promote accurate reporting.

6.2.1.4 Mobilizing resources for disease surveillance and response:

THE AFRICA CDC WORKS to mobilize resources from African Union Member States, international partners, and other stakeholders to support disease surveillance and response efforts across the continent. This includes supporting the development of funding proposals, advocating for increased funding for public health, and providing technical assistance to ensure that resources are used effectively.

Overall, the Africa CDC plays a critical role in strengthening disease surveillance and response in Africa, and in supporting African Union Member States in their efforts to prevent, detect, and respond to public health emergencies. By working collaboratively with partners across the continent and around the world, the Africa CDC is helping to build a more resilient and effective public health system in Africa.

6.3 Best practices and lessons learned from the response to recent outbreaks

THE RESPONSE TO RECENT outbreaks, such as Ebola in West Africa, Zika in the Americas, and COVID-19 globally, has provided important lessons on best practices for disease surveillance and response. Some of these best practices include:

6.3.1 Early detection and reporting:

EARLY DETECTION AND reporting of outbreaks plays a crucial role in preventing the rapid spread of diseases and implementing timely control measures. Robust disease surveillance systems are essential for promptly identifying and reporting potential cases to public health authorities. These systems enable the collection, analysis, and interpretation of data on disease incidence and prevalence, allowing for early detection and response.

One real-world example of early detection and reporting is the Global Public Health Intelligence Network (GPHIN), developed by the Public Health Agency of Canada. GPHIN is an automated system that uses artificial intelligence algorithms to monitor news reports and online sources for disease outbreaks and other public health events. The system detected the outbreak of severe acute respiratory syndrome (SARS) in 2003 before it was officially recognized, allowing for rapid response and containment efforts.

Another example is the ProMED-mail system, a global electronic reporting system for emerging infectious diseases and outbreaks. ProMED-mail relies on a network of dedicated volunteers who monitor and report on disease events worldwide. The system has been instrumental in detecting and reporting outbreaks such as Ebola, Zika virus, and Middle East respiratory syndrome (MERS).

In Africa, the Integrated Disease Surveillance and Response (IDSR) framework, developed by the World Health Organization (WHO), aims to strengthen disease surveillance and response capacities. Many African countries have implemented the IDSR system, which includes the establishment of surveillance units at various levels of the health system, training of surveillance officers, and the use of standard case definitions and reporting protocols. For instance, Uganda's IDSR program has improved the country's capacity for early detection and reporting of diseases, leading to more effective response and control efforts.

6.3.2 Rapid response:

IN THE CONTEXT OF THE Integrated Disease Surveillance and Response (IDSR) system in Africa, a rapid response is a critical component of outbreak control. Once an outbreak is detected through the surveillance system, immediate action is required to prevent further spread of the disease and mitigate its impact.

Rapid response involves the mobilization of resources, both human and logistical, to effectively address the outbreak. Public health teams, including epidemiologists, surveillance officers, and healthcare professionals, are deployed to the affected areas to conduct investigations, collect samples, and provide medical care. They work closely with local health authorities and communities to implement control measures and interventions.

Effective control measures may include quarantine and isolation of cases, contact tracing to identify and monitor individuals who have come into contact with confirmed cases, provision of appropriate treatment and care, and implementation of preventive measures such as vaccination campaigns, distribution of insecticide-treated bed nets, or water and sanitation interventions, depending on the nature of the disease.

The IDSR system in Africa emphasizes the need for timely response by setting specific time frames for investigation, reporting, and response to outbreaks. This ensures that actions are taken swiftly to contain the outbreak and prevent further transmission. Rapid response is crucial in preventing the escalation of outbreaks into larger epidemics or pandemics and reducing the impact on affected populations.

6.3.3 Coordination and collaboration:

COORDINATION AND COLLABORATION are fundamental aspects of effective disease surveillance and prevention efforts. In the context of public health, coordination refers to the harmonization and integration of activities among various entities involved in disease surveillance and response, while collaboration entails active cooperation and partnership between these entities. By working together, public health authorities, healthcare providers, and other stakeholders can leverage their collective expertise, resources, and capabilities to achieve common goals in disease surveillance and control.

Coordinating and collaborating with public health authorities is essential for establishing a strong framework for disease surveillance and response. Public health authorities, such as national health ministries or agencies, provide overall leadership and guidance in the implementation of surveillance programs and response strategies. They set policies, regulations, and guidelines to ensure consistency and standardization in disease reporting, data collection, and response protocols. Public health authorities also play a crucial role in coordinating activities across different regions or jurisdictions within a country to ensure a unified and efficient approach to disease surveillance.

Effective coordination and collaboration between public health authorities and healthcare providers are vital for timely and accurate disease reporting. Healthcare providers, including hospitals, clinics, and laboratories, are often the first point of contact for individuals seeking medical care. They play a critical role in recognizing and reporting suspected cases of communicable diseases to public health authorities. Close collaboration between public health authorities and healthcare providers helps to establish robust reporting systems, facilitate the exchange of information, and ensure that data on disease incidence and prevalence are collected and shared in a timely manner. This collaboration also enables public health authorities to provide guidance and support to healthcare providers in implementing control measures and managing disease outbreaks.

Collaboration with other stakeholders, such as academic institutions, research organizations, non-governmental organizations (NGOs), and international agencies, is also essential for comprehensive disease surveillance and response. Academic institutions and research organizations contribute to the development of innovative surveillance methods, data analysis techniques, and predictive modeling to enhance disease detection and forecasting capabilities. NGOs often play a significant role in community engagement, awareness campaigns, and support services for affected populations. International agencies, such as the World Health Organization (WHO), facilitate global collaborations, provide technical expertise, and promote knowledge exchange and capacity building in disease surveillance and response.

Through coordination and collaboration, stakeholders can pool their resources, expertise, and knowledge to address the complex challenges of disease surveillance and prevention. They can share best practices, lessons learned, and technological advancements to strengthen surveillance systems, enhance data quality and analysis, and improve response strategies. Coordinated efforts can also help optimize resource allocation, avoid duplication of efforts, and ensure a cohesive and efficient response to disease outbreaks and other health threats.

Moreover, coordination and collaboration are particularly crucial in the context of cross-border and international disease surveillance. Infectious diseases know no boundaries, and cooperation between countries is vital for early detection, timely information sharing, and joint response efforts. Regional and global networks, such as the European Centre for Disease Prevention and Control (ECDC), the African Union's Africa Centres for Disease Control and Prevention (Africa CDC), and the Global Outbreak Alert and Response Network (GOARN), facilitate coordination and collaboration among countries, enabling rapid response and effective control of infectious diseases on a broader scale.

6.3.4 Risk communication:

EFFECTIVE RISK COMMUNICATION is essential to ensuring that the public is informed about the outbreak and the measures being taken to control its spread. This includes clear and timely communication of risk, guidance on preventative measures, and engagement with affected communities.

In the context of the Integrated Disease Surveillance and Response (IDSR) system in Africa, risk communication plays a critical role in outbreak response. It is a vital component that helps to inform and empower the public and affected communities during disease outbreaks. Effective risk communication ensures that accurate and timely information is disseminated to the public, enabling them to make informed decisions and take appropriate preventive measures.

6.3.4.1 Timely Information Dissemination:

IDSR EMPHASIZES THE importance of timely information dissemination to the public and relevant stakeholders. During an outbreak, health authorities must quickly communicate the risks associated with the disease, its transmission modes, symptoms, and preventive measures to be taken. This information is crucial in helping individuals and communities understand the outbreak's severity and take necessary precautions.

For example, during the COVID-19 pandemic, countries in Africa used various communication channels, including radio, television, and social media, to share information about the virus, preventive measures, and updates on the outbreak's status.

6.3.4.2 Community Engagement:

IDSR RECOGNIZES THE importance of engaging with communities during outbreaks. It encourages the involvement of local leaders, community health workers, and other community-based organizations in the risk communication process. Engaging with communities helps to build trust, address concerns, and encourage compliance with control measures.

In West Africa, during the Ebola outbreak, community engagement was vital in gaining the trust of affected populations. By involving community leaders and traditional healers in the response efforts, health authorities could better explain the disease and the need for safe burial practices, leading to greater acceptance of preventive measures.

6.3.4.3 Tailored Messaging:

EFFECTIVE RISK COMMUNICATION under IDSR considers the diverse cultural, linguistic, and socio-economic backgrounds of the target audience. Messages need to be tailored to be easily understood and accepted by different groups within the population. Using culturally appropriate communication strategies can enhance the effectiveness of risk communication efforts.

For instance, during the outbreak of meningitis in the "Meningitis Belt" of Africa, health authorities tailored their risk communication messages to resonate with nomadic communities, who were particularly vulnerable. By using local languages and engaging with community leaders, they were able to promote vaccination and preventive behaviors.

6.3.4.4 Addressing Misinformation:

DURING OUTBREAKS, MISINFORMATION and rumors can spread quickly, leading to confusion and fear in the community. The IDSR system recognizes the importance of addressing misinformation promptly and providing accurate information to counter rumors. This requires continuous monitoring of public perceptions and concerns to address misconceptions effectively.

In Ethiopia, during the cholera outbreak, health authorities worked closely with local media to dispel myths and address rumors related to the disease. By providing accurate information through trusted sources, they could prevent unnecessary panic and promote appropriate responses.

In conclusion, risk communication is a vital aspect of the IDSR system in Africa. By effectively communicating risks, preventive measures, and response actions, health authorities can engage and empower the public to play an active role in outbreak control. Timely, clear, and culturally appropriate communication helps to build trust and encourage compliance, ultimately contributing to more effective outbreak response efforts.

6.3.5 Capacity building:

BUILDING CAPACITY FOR disease surveillance and response is indeed crucial in ensuring effective outbreak response and preparedness. It involves various key components that contribute to a robust and well-functioning system. Here are some examples of capacity-building efforts in disease surveillance and response:

6.3.5.1 Strengthening Laboratory Capacity:

LABORATORY CAPACITY is essential for timely and accurate diagnosis of diseases, which is crucial for effective outbreak response. Building and strengthening laboratory systems involves upgrading infrastructure, procuring necessary equipment and supplies, and training laboratory personnel in diagnostic techniques and quality assurance. For instance, the African Society for Laboratory Medicine (ASLM) works towards strengthening laboratory systems across Africa through training programs, accreditation initiatives, and quality improvement activities.

6.3.5.2 Training Healthcare Workers:

TRAINING HEALTHCARE workers, including physicians, nurses, and community health workers, is vital to enhance their skills and knowledge in disease surveillance and response. Training programs focus on areas such as case detection, data collection and reporting, outbreak investigation, infection prevention and control, and emergency response protocols. These programs can be conducted through workshops, simulation exercises, and online training platforms. The Field Epidemiology Training Programs (FETPs), such as the African Field Epidemiology Network (AFENET), provide field-based training for epidemiologists and other public health professionals, equipping them with the skills necessary for outbreak investigation and response.

6.3.5.3 Developing Emergency Response Plans:

DEVELOPING COMPREHENSIVE emergency response plans ensures that countries have a clear roadmap for managing outbreaks. These plans outline the roles and responsibilities of different stakeholders, delineate lines of communication and coordination, and establish mechanisms for resource mobilization and deployment. Emergency response plans are often developed in collaboration with national and international partners and are regularly reviewed and updated to incorporate lessons learned from previous outbreaks. For example, the Nigeria Centre for Disease Control (NCDC) has developed the National Action Plan for Health Security, which serves as a blueprint for strengthening the country's capacity to prevent, detect, and respond to public health threats.

6.3.5.4 Enhancing Surveillance Systems:

CAPACITY-BUILDING EFFORTS also focus on enhancing disease surveillance systems by implementing integrated and interoperable surveillance platforms. This includes the use of digital technologies, such as mobile applications and electronic reporting systems, to facilitate real-time data collection, analysis, and reporting. Strengthening surveillance systems also involves establishing mechanisms for data sharing and collaboration between different sectors and organizations involved in disease surveillance. The East African Integrated Disease Surveillance Network (EAIDSNet) is an example of a regional network that promotes collaboration and information sharing among countries in East Africa to enhance disease surveillance and response.

These capacity-building efforts are essential to ensure that countries have the necessary infrastructure, knowledge, and resources to effectively detect, monitor, and respond to outbreaks. By investing in laboratory capacity, training healthcare workers, and developing emergency response plans, countries can strengthen their overall preparedness and response capabilities, reducing the impact of outbreaks and protecting public health.

6.3.6 Sustainable financing:

SUSTAINABLE FINANCING is indeed crucial for maintaining the capacity and resilience of public health systems in responding to outbreaks. It involves developing funding mechanisms and structures that can effectively support outbreak response and ensure ongoing preparedness. Here are some examples of sustainable financing approaches in the context of outbreak response:

6.3.6.1 Emergency Response Funds:

ESTABLISHING EMERGENCY response funds allows countries to quickly mobilize financial resources during outbreaks. These funds are specifically dedicated to responding to public health emergencies and can be accessed rapidly to support activities such as disease surveillance, laboratory testing, case management, and public health interventions. Emergency response funds can be set up at national or regional levels, and contributions can come from various sources, including government allocations, international donors, and public-private partnerships. For instance, the African Union established the Africa CDC COVID-19 Response Fund to support member states in responding to the COVID-19 pandemic.

6.3.6.2 Public Health Emergency Preparedness and Response Budgeting:

INTEGRATING PUBLIC health emergency preparedness and response into national budgets is an effective approach to ensure sustained funding. This involves allocating specific budget lines for outbreak response activities, such as disease surveillance, laboratory systems, human resources, and logistics. By including these budget lines, countries demonstrate a commitment to investing in public health preparedness and can better plan and allocate resources to respond to outbreaks in a timely manner. For example, the World Bank's Pandemic Emergency Financing Facility provides countries with financial support during disease outbreaks by linking disbursements to pre-determined triggers based on epidemiological and operational criteria.

6.3.6.3 Health Insurance and Social Protection Schemes:

INTEGRATING OUTBREAK response and public health interventions into health insurance and social protection schemes can provide sustainable financing for outbreak-related activities. By incorporating coverage for preventive measures, diagnostic tests, and treatment of communicable diseases, these schemes can ensure access to healthcare services during outbreaks. This approach helps to distribute the financial burden and increase financial protection for individuals and communities, particularly vulnerable populations. For instance, the National Health Insurance Scheme in Ghana covers a range of services, including preventive care and treatment for communicable diseases.

6.3.6.4 International Partnerships and Donor Support:

INTERNATIONAL PARTNERSHIPS and donor support play a vital role in providing financial resources for outbreak response. Collaboration with international organizations, development agencies, and philanthropic foundations can help countries access funding for capacity-building initiatives, infrastructure development, and implementation of public health interventions. Donor support can also contribute to sustainable financing by assisting countries in strengthening their health systems and building resilience to future outbreaks. For example, the Global Fund to Fight AIDS, Tuberculosis, and Malaria provides financial support to countries for disease control programs, including surveillance and response activities.

By implementing sustainable financing mechanisms, countries can ensure the availability of financial resources for outbreak response and maintain long-term investments in public health systems. This enables them to effectively respond to outbreaks, strengthen their preparedness, and protect the health of their populations.

Generally, the response to recent outbreaks has demonstrated the importance of strong disease surveillance and response systems, as well as effective coordination and collaboration between stakeholders. By implementing these best practices and building strong public health systems, countries can be better prepared to respond to future outbreaks and prevent the spread of disease.

6.4 Case study: Lassa fever outbreak in Nigeria

IN 2018, NIGERIA EXPERIENCED an outbreak of Lassa fever, a viral hemorrhagic fever that is endemic in West Africa. The outbreak began in January 2018 and by the end of the year, over 600 cases had been reported, with a case fatality rate of 23.6%.

The outbreak was initially reported in Ebonyi state, but cases were also reported in other states including Ondo, Edo, and Delta. The Nigerian government responded quickly to the outbreak, with the establishment of a national Lassa fever emergency operations center to coordinate the response.

The response included active case finding, contact tracing, and isolation and treatment of cases. Healthcare workers were trained in infection prevention and control measures, and health facilities were provided with personal protective equipment and other necessary supplies.

The Nigerian Centre for Disease Control (NCDC) worked closely with state health authorities and international partners to support the response. The NCDC also developed a public health advisory to inform the public about the outbreak and provide guidance on prevention and control measures.

One of the challenges of the response was the limited availability of diagnostic tools, which made it difficult to confirm cases and determine the extent of the outbreak. To address this, the NCDC collaborated with international partners to provide laboratory support, including the deployment of a mobile laboratory to Ondo state.

Overall, the response to the Lassa fever outbreak in Nigeria demonstrated the importance of early detection, rapid response, and effective coordination between stakeholders. The establishment of the national emergency operations center and the collaboration between the NCDC, state health authorities, and international partners were key to the success of the response. However, the limited availability of diagnostic tools highlights the need for continued investment in laboratory capacity to strengthen disease surveillance and response in Nigeria and other countries in the region.

6.5 Exercises

1. What are some potential ethical concerns with using digital surveillance technologies in disease surveillance?

Solution: Potential ethical concerns include privacy violations, data security, and the potential for discrimination or stigmatization of certain groups.

1. How can cultural and religious beliefs impact disease response efforts in a community?

Solution: Cultural and religious beliefs may impact willingness to participate in disease response efforts or comply with public health measures such as vaccination or quarantine.

1. In the context of communicable diseases, what is the difference between isolation and quarantine?

Solution: Isolation refers to separating individuals who are already sick with a contagious disease from healthy individuals. Quarantine refers to separating individuals who have been exposed to a contagious disease but may not be showing symptoms yet.

1. What ethical principles should guide the allocation of scarce medical resources during a disease outbreak?

Solution: Ethical principles such as beneficence, non-maleficence, justice, and respect for autonomy should guide the allocation of scarce medical resources during a disease outbreak.

1. What are some potential conflicts between individual rights and public health interests in disease response efforts?

Solution: Conflicts can arise when public health measures such as quarantine or mandatory vaccination are perceived as infringing on individual rights such as freedom of movement or autonomy.

1. What is the principle of reciprocity in public health ethics?

Solution: The principle of reciprocity holds that those who bear the burdens of public health interventions should also benefit from the interventions.

1. How might power imbalances between countries impact global disease surveillance and response efforts?

Solution: Power imbalances can result in unequal distribution of resources and unequal representation in decision-making, which can impact the effectiveness of global disease surveillance and response efforts.

1. What are some potential challenges with conducting clinical trials during a disease outbreak?

Solution: Challenges can include ethical considerations around informed consent, limited resources and infrastructure, and logistical challenges in accessing affected populations.

1. What is the role of transparency in disease surveillance and response? *Solution*: Transparency is important for building trust in public health interventions, promoting accountability, and ensuring equitable distribution of resources.
2. In the context of communicable diseases, what is the difference between a public health emergency of international concern (PHEIC) and a pandemic? *Solution*: A PHEIC is a situation that is serious, unexpected, and has potential for international spread, while a pandemic refers to a global outbreak of a disease.

Chapter 7. Integrated Disease Surveillance and Response (IDSR)

7.1 Definition of Integrated Disease Surveillance and Response (IDSR)

Intgrated Disease Surveillance and Response (IDSR) is a comprehensive approach to disease surveillance and response that integrates different disease surveillance systems and response activities into a unified and coordinated system. IDSR aims to improve early detection and rapid response to outbreaks of communicable diseases, and to strengthen overall public health surveillance and response systems. It involves the collection, analysis, interpretation, dissemination, and use of health data, as well as the development and implementation of response plans to control and prevent the spread of diseases. The IDSR system also involves collaboration between various stakeholders including health workers, laboratories, public health officials, and communities.

7.2 Importance of IDSR in Africa

IDSR IS CRUCIAL IN Africa due to the high burden of communicable diseases in the continent, including outbreaks of emerging and re-emerging diseases. The implementation of IDSR helps to strengthen the capacity of African countries to detect and respond to these diseases, including the ones that have the potential to cause widespread epidemics or pandemics. Some of the specific reasons why IDSR is important in Africa include:

7.2.1 Early detection of disease outbreaks:

IDSR SYSTEMS ARE DESIGNED to detect outbreaks early through timely reporting, investigation, and response. This is crucial in Africa, where many outbreaks go undetected until they have already spread widely.

7.2.2 Rapid response to outbreaks:

IDSR FACILITATES THE rapid mobilization of resources and response teams to control and prevent the spread of disease outbreaks. This is important in Africa where outbreaks can quickly overwhelm health systems and lead to high morbidity and mortality rates.

7.2.3 Improved disease surveillance:

IDSR HELPS TO IMPROVE overall public health surveillance systems by integrating different surveillance systems into a unified system. This results in more accurate and timely data on disease trends and outbreaks.

7.2.4 Strengthened laboratory services:

IDSR REQUIRES THE DEVELOPMENT of laboratory services that are able to diagnose and confirm diseases. This strengthens laboratory systems in Africa, which are often weak and poorly resourced.

7.2.5 Better coordination and collaboration:

IDSR PROMOTES COLLABORATION between different stakeholders including health workers, public health officials, laboratories, and communities. This helps to ensure a more coordinated and effective response to outbreaks and other public health emergencies.

Overall, IDSR is important in Africa as it helps to build the capacity of countries to detect, respond, and prevent communicable disease outbreaks, ultimately leading to improved public health outcomes.

7.3 Historical background of IDSR implementation in Africa

THE HISTORY OF IDSR implementation in Africa dates back to the early 1990s, when the World Health Organization (WHO) recognized the need for a comprehensive approach to disease surveillance and response on the continent. At the time, many African countries had separate surveillance systems for different diseases, resulting in duplication of efforts, inefficiencies, and missed opportunities for early detection of outbreaks.

In 1998, the WHO, in collaboration with the African Regional Office (AFRO) and other partners, developed the IDSR strategy as a framework for strengthening disease surveillance and response in Africa. The strategy aimed to integrate existing surveillance systems for different diseases into a single, harmonized system that would enable timely detection and response to outbreaks.

The initial implementation of IDSR was limited to a few pilot countries, but it gradually expanded to other countries on the continent. In 2000, the WHO and partners launched the Regional IDSR Enhancement Initiative (RISE), which aimed to provide technical support and resources to countries for the implementation of IDSR.

Over the years, several milestones have been achieved in the implementation of IDSR in Africa. In 2002, the African Union adopted a resolution on IDSR, calling on member states to implement the strategy. In 2005, the WHO revised the IDSR strategy to include non-communicable diseases, zoonotic diseases, and other public health emergencies.

Despite the progress made in IDSR implementation, there have been challenges, including inadequate resources, weak health systems, and limited political commitment in some countries. However, efforts continue to be made to address these challenges and strengthen the implementation of IDSR in Africa.

7.4 Recap of Definition and classification of communicable diseases

AS DISCUSSED IN CHAPTER one, communicable diseases are illnesses caused by infectious agents such as bacteria, viruses, fungi, and parasites that can be transmitted directly or indirectly from one person to another, from an animal to a person, or from an environmental source to a person.

Communicable diseases can be classified based on the type of agent that causes the disease, the mode of transmission, the severity of illness, and the population affected. Here are some common classifications:

7.4.1 Bacterial infections:

THESE DISEASES ARE caused by the presence and proliferation of bacteria, which are microscopic organisms that can have harmful effects on the human body. Bacterial infections can be transmitted through various means, including contaminated food, water, air, as well as direct contact with infected individuals or animals. Some notable examples of bacterial infections include tuberculosis, cholera, and streptococcal infections.

Tuberculosis (TB) is a highly contagious bacterial infection caused by Mycobacterium tuberculosis. It primarily affects the lungs but can also spread to other parts of the body. TB is usually transmitted through the inhalation of airborne droplets containing the bacteria, which are released when an infected individual coughs or sneezes. Although TB can be a serious and potentially life-threatening disease, it is treatable with appropriate antibiotics.

Cholera is an acute diarrheal illness caused by the bacterium Vibrio cholerae. It is usually spread through the ingestion of contaminated food or water. Cholera outbreaks often occur in areas with inadequate sanitation and limited access to clean drinking water. The infection can lead to severe dehydration and, if left untreated, can be fatal. Prompt rehydration and administration of antibiotics are key in managing cholera cases.

Streptococcal infections are caused by various bacteria belonging to the Streptococcus genus, particularly Streptococcus pyogenes. These infections can range from mild, such as strep throat, to more severe conditions like scarlet fever or invasive streptococcal disease. Streptococcal bacteria are commonly transmitted through respiratory droplets from infected individuals or through direct contact with infected skin or wounds. Prompt treatment with antibiotics is crucial to prevent complications and further spread of the infection.

It's important to note that there are numerous other bacterial infections that can affect humans, each with its own mode of transmission, symptoms, and treatments. Proper hygiene practices, such as regular handwashing, safe food handling, and vaccination, can help reduce the risk of bacterial infections and their spread.

7.4.2 Viral infections:

THESE DISEASES ARE caused by viruses, which are tiny infectious agents that can invade and replicate within living cells. Viral infections can be transmitted through various means, including direct contact with infected body fluids, contaminated surfaces, or through droplets in the air. Here are some examples of viral infections: influenza, HIV/AIDS, and COVID-19.

Influenza, commonly known as the flu, is a highly contagious respiratory illness caused by the influenza virus. It is primarily transmitted through respiratory droplets when an infected person coughs, sneezes, or talks. Influenza viruses can also survive on surfaces, and touching these surfaces and then touching the face can lead to infection. The flu typically presents with symptoms such as fever, cough, sore throat, body aches, and fatigue. Vaccination is available each year to help prevent influenza and its complications.

HIV/AIDS (Human Immunodeficiency Virus/Acquired Immunodeficiency Syndrome) is a viral infection that attacks the immune system, specifically CD4 cells, which are crucial in fighting infections. HIV is most commonly transmitted through unprotected sexual intercourse, sharing needles or syringes contaminated with the virus, or from an infected mother to her child during childbirth or breastfeeding. If left untreated, HIV can progress to AIDS, a condition in which the immune system becomes severely compromised. Antiretroviral therapy (ART) can help control the virus and prevent the progression to AIDS.

COVID-19, caused by the novel coronavirus SARS-CoV-2, emerged as a global pandemic in 2019. The virus spreads mainly through respiratory droplets generated when an infected person coughs, sneezes, talks, or breathes heavily. Close contact with an infected individual or touching surfaces contaminated with the virus and then touching the face can also lead to transmission. COVID-19 can range from mild to severe respiratory illness and may cause complications, particularly in vulnerable populations. Vaccination, along with preventive measures such as mask-wearing, hand hygiene, and physical distancing, is crucial in controlling the spread of the virus.

It's important to note that viral infections can vary in their severity, transmission routes, and available treatments. Vaccinations, when available, play a critical role in preventing certain viral infections. Following public health guidelines and practicing good hygiene can help reduce the risk of viral transmission and protect both individuals and communities.

7.4.3 Fungal infections:

THESE DISEASES ARE caused by fungi, which are multicellular or single-celled organisms that can exist as molds, yeasts, or mushrooms. Fungal infections, also known as mycoses, can be transmitted through various means, including contact with contaminated soil or surfaces, inhalation of fungal spores, or direct contact with infected animals or people. Here are some examples of fungal infections: ringworm, candidiasis, and aspergillosis.

Ringworm, despite its name, is not caused by a worm but by various types of fungi known as dermatophytes. It manifests as a skin infection characterized by a red, ring-shaped rash that is often itchy. Ringworm can be transmitted through direct contact with infected humans or animals, as well as contact with contaminated surfaces such as towels, clothing, or sports equipment. Good hygiene practices, such as regular handwashing and avoiding sharing personal items, can help prevent the spread of ringworm. Antifungal medications are typically used for treatment.

Candidiasis, also called yeast infection, is caused by Candida, a type of yeast that normally resides in the body but can overgrow under certain conditions. It can affect various parts of the body, including the skin, mouth, throat, and genital area. Candidiasis can be transmitted through direct contact with infected individuals, sexual intercourse, or through the use of contaminated items such as towels or oral hygiene products. Treatment typically involves antifungal medications, both topical and oral, depending on the severity and location of the infection.

Aspergillosis is a group of infections caused by the fungus Aspergillus, which is commonly found in the environment. Inhalation of Aspergillus spores is the primary route of transmission. While most people are not affected by exposure to Aspergillus, individuals with weakened immune systems or pre-existing lung conditions are at higher risk of developing aspergillosis. The infection can present in various forms, ranging from allergic reactions to invasive lung infections. Treatment options include antifungal medications and, in severe cases, surgical intervention.

It's important to note that there are numerous other fungal infections that can affect humans, each with its own unique characteristics and modes of transmission. Maintaining good personal hygiene, avoiding direct contact with infected individuals or animals, and taking precautions in environments where fungal growth is likely (such as damp or moldy areas) can help reduce the risk of fungal infections. Seeking medical attention for proper diagnosis and treatment is essential in managing fungal infections effectively.

7.4.4 Parasitic infections:

THESE DISEASES ARE caused by parasites, which are organisms that live in or on another organism (known as the host) and derive nutrients at the expense of the host. Parasitic infections can be transmitted through various means, including consumption of contaminated food or water, direct contact with infected animals, or insect bites. Here are some examples of parasitic infections: malaria, schistosomiasis, and lice infestations.

Malaria is a life-threatening disease caused by the Plasmodium parasite, which is transmitted to humans through the bite of infected female Anopheles mosquitoes. The parasites multiply within the host's liver and then infect red blood cells, leading to symptoms such as fever, chills, fatigue, and flu-like symptoms. Malaria is prevalent in tropical and subtropical regions. Prevention measures include using insecticide-treated bed nets, indoor residual spraying, and taking antimalarial medications.

Schistosomiasis, also known as bilharzia, is caused by parasitic worms called schistosomes. The larvae of these worms are released by freshwater snails and penetrate the skin of individuals in contact with contaminated water. Schistosomiasis is common in areas with poor sanitation and unsafe water sources. The infection can affect various organs, leading to symptoms such as abdominal pain, diarrhea, and blood in urine or stool. Preventive measures include avoiding contact with contaminated water and receiving treatment with antiparasitic medications.

Lice infestations occur when parasitic insects, such as head lice, body lice, or pubic lice (also known as crabs), infest the hair or body of humans. These parasites are typically spread through direct contact with an infested person or by sharing personal items such as combs, hats, or clothing. Lice infestations can cause intense itching and discomfort. Treatment involves using special shampoos, lotions, or medications designed to kill the lice and their eggs, along with thorough cleaning of infested items.

It's important to note that there are numerous other parasitic infections that can affect humans, each with its own specific transmission mechanisms, symptoms, and treatment options. Preventive measures such as practicing good hygiene, avoiding exposure to contaminated sources, and using appropriate protective measures (such as insect repellents or bed nets) can help reduce the risk of parasitic infections. Seeking medical advice and treatment from healthcare professionals is essential for effectively managing and controlling parasitic infections.

7.4.5 Sexually transmitted infections:

THESE INFECTIONS ARE transmitted through sexual contact with infected individuals and are commonly referred to as sexually transmitted infections (STIs) or sexually transmitted diseases (STDs). They are caused by various bacteria, viruses, or parasites and can be passed on through vaginal, anal, or oral sex. Here are some examples of sexually transmitted infections: gonorrhea, syphilis, and herpes.

Gonorrhea is a bacterial infection caused by Neisseria gonorrhoeae. It can affect the urethra, cervix, rectum, throat, or eyes. The infection is transmitted through unprotected sexual intercourse with an infected person. Symptoms may include painful urination, discharge, and pelvic pain. However, some individuals may not experience any noticeable symptoms. Gonorrhea can lead to serious complications if left untreated, such as pelvic inflammatory disease (PID) in women and epididymitis in men. Antibiotics are commonly used for treatment.

Syphilis is a bacterial infection caused by the spirochete bacterium Treponema pallidum. It progresses in stages if left untreated. Syphilis is transmitted through direct contact with syphilis sores, which can occur on the genitals, anus, lips, or mouth. In the early stages, a painless sore (chancre) appears. If left untreated, it can progress to a rash, flu-like symptoms, and eventually lead to serious complications affecting the heart, brain, and other organs. Syphilis can be treated with antibiotics, especially in the early stages.

Herpes is a viral infection caused by the herpes simplex virus (HSV). There are two types of HSV: HSV-1 and HSV-2. HSV-1 is commonly associated with oral herpes (cold sores), while HSV-2 is typically linked to genital herpes. Herpes is transmitted through direct skin-to-skin contact during oral, genital, or anal sex. The infection can cause painful blisters or sores in the affected areas, along with flu-like symptoms during initial outbreaks. While there is no cure for herpes, antiviral medications can help manage symptoms and reduce the frequency of outbreaks.

It's crucial to practice safe sex by using barrier methods such as condoms, getting tested regularly for STIs, and discussing sexual health with partners. Early detection and treatment of STIs are vital to prevent complications and reduce the risk of further transmission. Seeking medical advice, undergoing appropriate testing, and following the prescribed treatment are essential steps in managing sexually transmitted infections effectively.

7.4.6 Vector-borne infections:

THESE INFECTIONS ARE transmitted by vectors, which are organisms such as mosquitoes, ticks, and fleas that can carry and transmit disease-causing pathogens. Vector-borne diseases are a significant global health concern and can have severe consequences. Here are some examples of vector-borne infections: malaria, Lyme disease, and dengue fever.

Malaria is a life-threatening disease caused by the Plasmodium parasite, which is primarily transmitted through the bites of infected female Anopheles mosquitoes. These mosquitoes act as vectors, carrying the parasite and transferring it to humans when they bite. Malaria is prevalent in tropical and subtropical regions and can cause symptoms such as high fever, chills, flu-like symptoms, and, in severe cases, organ failure. Prevention strategies include vector control measures such as insecticide-treated bed nets, indoor residual spraying, and antimalarial medications.

Lyme disease is caused by the bacterium Borrelia burgdorferi and is transmitted to humans through the bite of infected black-legged ticks, commonly known as deer ticks. Ticks acquire the bacterium by feeding on infected animals, such as mice or deer. Lyme disease can lead to a range of symptoms, including a characteristic skin rash, fatigue, joint pain, and neurological problems if left untreated. Prevention includes avoiding tick-infested areas, wearing protective clothing, using tick repellents, and conducting thorough tick checks after potential exposure.

Dengue fever is a viral infection caused by the dengue virus, which is primarily transmitted by Aedes mosquitoes. These mosquitoes can breed in stagnant water and are often found in urban areas. Dengue fever can cause a wide range of symptoms, from mild flu-like illness to severe dengue, also known as dengue hemorrhagic fever. Symptoms may include high fever, severe headache, joint and muscle pain, rash, and bleeding complications. Prevention measures focus on mosquito control, such as eliminating breeding sites, using insect repellents, and wearing protective clothing.

In addition to their mode of transmission, communicable diseases can be classified based on the severity of illness they cause and the populations they affect. Some diseases may cause mild symptoms, while others can be severe, leading to complications and even death. Certain infectious diseases disproportionately affect specific populations, such as children, the elderly, or individuals with weakened immune systems. Understanding these classifications is crucial for developing targeted prevention and control strategies, including vaccination campaigns, public health education, and access to healthcare resources.

Efforts to prevent and control communicable diseases involve a multi-faceted approach, including surveillance, early detection, proper diagnosis, treatment, and preventive measures. By understanding the modes of transmission, severity, and affected populations, public health authorities and healthcare providers can implement effective strategies to mitigate the impact of communicable diseases and protect the health of communities.

7.5 The role of epidemiology in understanding disease transmission and control

EPIDEMIOLOGY PLAYS a critical role in understanding disease transmission and control by providing scientific methods for investigating the patterns, causes, and effects of communicable diseases within populations. Epidemiology helps to:

7.5.1 Identify the agent responsible for the disease:

EPIDEMIOLOGISTS USE laboratory testing and other methods to identify the agent responsible for a particular disease. This information is crucial in developing effective control measures.

7.5.2 Determine the mode of transmission:

EPIDEMIOLOGISTS USE surveillance data and outbreak investigations to determine how a disease is transmitted from person to person or from animals to humans. This information is important in developing strategies to interrupt the transmission chain.

7.5.3 Identify the populations at risk:

EPIDEMIOLOGISTS ANALYZE data to identify populations at increased risk for disease transmission, such as people living in crowded conditions or those with weakened immune systems. This information helps to target interventions to those who need them most.

7.5.4 Monitor disease trends:

EPIDEMIOLOGISTS MONITOR disease trends over time to identify changes in disease patterns and to detect outbreaks early. This information helps public health officials to implement control measures quickly.

7.5.5 Evaluate interventions:

EPIDEMIOLOGISTS EVALUATE the effectiveness of interventions, such as vaccination programs or quarantine measures, to determine their impact on disease transmission. This information is important in refining strategies for controlling the spread of communicable diseases.

Overall, epidemiology provides critical information to inform public health policy and decision-making, and plays an important role in preventing and controlling communicable diseases.

7.6 Overview of epidemic surveillance and response systems

EPIDEMIC SURVEILLANCE and response systems are designed to detect, track, and respond to outbreaks of communicable diseases. These systems are crucial in preventing and controlling the spread of infectious diseases, particularly in areas where the risk of epidemics is high. Here's an overview of epidemic surveillance and response systems:

7.6.1 Surveillance:

THE FIRST STEP IN AN epidemic surveillance and response system is surveillance. Surveillance plays a critical role in public health by systematically collecting, analyzing, and interpreting data related to the occurrence and distribution of communicable diseases. This information is vital for identifying outbreaks, monitoring disease trends, and implementing appropriate control and prevention measures. Here's a further explanation of the process:

7.6.1.1 Data Collection:

SURVEILLANCE BEGINS with the collection of relevant data. This includes information on diagnosed cases of communicable diseases, such as the number of cases, demographic characteristics of affected individuals, geographical locations, and time of occurrence. Data collection can involve multiple sources, including healthcare facilities, laboratories, public health agencies, and other reporting systems.

7.6.1.2 Data Analysis:

ONCE COLLECTED, THE data undergoes analysis to identify patterns, trends, and potential outbreaks. Epidemiologists and public health professionals analyze the data to detect unusual or unexpected occurrences, such as a sudden increase in the number of cases or a geographic clustering of infections. Statistical techniques and mathematical models may be employed to aid in data analysis and to generate meaningful insights.

7.6.1.3 Interpretation:

THE ANALYZED DATA IS then interpreted to understand the implications and significance of the findings. This involves assessing the magnitude and severity of the disease occurrence, identifying high-risk populations or geographical areas, and evaluating the potential impact on public health. The interpretation helps guide public health responses and interventions.

7.6.1.4 Outbreak Detection:

SURVEILLANCE SYSTEMS are designed to promptly detect outbreaks of communicable diseases. By continuously monitoring disease patterns, surveillance can identify clusters of cases that exceed expected levels, indicating a potential outbreak. Early detection allows for immediate response and implementation of control measures to mitigate the spread of the disease.

1. ***Monitoring Disease Trends***: Surveillance systems provide valuable information on the long-term trends and changes in the occurrence and distribution of communicable

diseases. By monitoring disease trends over time, public health authorities can identify shifts in patterns, emergence of new pathogens, changes in transmission dynamics, and effectiveness of control measures. This information helps in planning and implementing targeted prevention and control strategies.

Effective surveillance systems are crucial for timely detection, response, and management of communicable diseases. They provide a basis for evidence-based decision-making, resource allocation, and coordination of public health efforts. Surveillance data also facilitates communication and collaboration among different stakeholders, including local, national, and international health agencies, enabling a coordinated response to outbreaks and the implementation of appropriate preventive measures.

7.6.2 Early warning:

EARLY WARNING SYSTEMS are crucial components of public health infrastructure, designed to detect outbreaks at their earliest stages before they become widespread and pose significant threats to public health. These systems utilize a variety of methods and approaches, such as laboratory testing, clinical surveillance, and disease reporting, to identify potential outbreaks. Here's a detailed explanation of the components and methods involved in early warning systems:

7.6.2.1 Laboratory Testing:

LABORATORY TESTING plays a vital role in the early detection of outbreaks. It involves the analysis of clinical specimens, such as blood, urine, or respiratory samples, to identify the presence of pathogens responsible for communicable diseases.

By conducting tests on samples from patients displaying symptoms, laboratories can quickly detect the causative agents of the disease and confirm suspected cases. Advanced diagnostic techniques, including molecular testing and genetic sequencing, enable rapid and accurate identification of pathogens, facilitating early warning and response.

7.6.2.2 Clinical Surveillance:

CLINICAL SURVEILLANCE involves the monitoring of patients seeking healthcare for symptoms that may indicate a potential outbreak. Healthcare providers, including doctors, nurses, and other medical professionals, play a critical role in recognizing and reporting unusual patterns of diseases or symptoms. By maintaining a high index of suspicion and promptly reporting suspicious cases to public health authorities, healthcare providers contribute to the early detection of outbreaks. Clinical surveillance can involve regular monitoring of patients, sentinel surveillance systems, or syndromic surveillance, which tracks symptoms rather than confirmed diagnoses.

7.6.2.3 Disease Reporting:

DISEASE REPORTING IS an essential component of early warning systems. It involves the timely reporting of diagnosed cases or suspected outbreaks to public health authorities. Healthcare providers, laboratories, and other healthcare facilities are typically mandated to report specific communicable diseases to local or national health departments. The reporting systems facilitate the collection and analysis of data, enabling public health officials to identify clusters of cases and potential outbreaks. Efficient reporting mechanisms, both manual and electronic, promote early detection and response to emerging threats.

7.6.2.4 Data Analysis and Integration:

EARLY WARNING SYSTEMS rely on the analysis and integration of data from various sources. This includes epidemiological data, laboratory results, clinical surveillance data, and disease reporting. By integrating these datasets, public health officials can identify trends, patterns, and anomalies that may indicate the emergence of an outbreak. Advanced data analytics, including statistical modeling and data visualization techniques, facilitate the identification of clusters, hotspots, or changes in disease patterns that require immediate attention.

7.6.2.5 Alert Systems and Communication:

ONCE POTENTIAL OUTBREAKS are identified, early warning systems use alert systems to rapidly notify public health authorities and relevant stakeholders. These alert systems may involve automated notifications, email alerts, or mobile-based systems, ensuring that critical information reaches decision-makers in a timely manner. Effective communication channels and protocols allow for the swift dissemination of information, enabling rapid response, resource mobilization, and coordination among different agencies and sectors involved in outbreak management.

Early warning systems play a vital role in preventing and controlling outbreaks by providing timely information for effective response. By detecting outbreaks at their early stages, public health authorities can implement targeted interventions, such as contact tracing, quarantine measures, public health campaigns, or vaccination programs, to minimize the spread of the disease and mitigate its impact on public health. These systems are continuously improved and refined through ongoing evaluation, research, and technological advancements to enhance their sensitivity and effectiveness in detecting and responding to emerging threats.

7.6.3 Outbreak investigation:

WHEN AN OUTBREAK IS detected, a comprehensive outbreak investigation is conducted to gather crucial information about the source of the outbreak, the mode of transmission, and the populations at risk. This investigation aims to identify the underlying causes and factors contributing to the outbreak, enabling public health officials to develop and implement targeted interventions to control and mitigate its impact. Here's a detailed explanation of the process involved in outbreak investigations:

7.6.3.1 Case Identification and Confirmation:

THE FIRST STEP IN AN outbreak investigation is to identify and confirm cases related to the outbreak. This involves reviewing reported cases, conducting interviews with affected individuals, and analyzing clinical and laboratory data to establish a clear case definition. By determining the scope and magnitude of the outbreak, investigators can focus their efforts on understanding the dynamics of the disease and its spread.

7.6.3.2 Source Identification:

THE INVESTIGATION SEEKS to identify the source of the outbreak, which could be a specific food or water source, a contaminated environment, an infected individual, or other potential reservoirs. Investigators gather information on the activities, exposures, and behaviors of affected individuals, analyzing commonalities among them to pinpoint a likely source. Epidemiological techniques, such as case-control studies or cohort studies, may be employed to identify potential risk factors associated with the outbreak.

7.6.3.3 Mode of Transmission:

UNDERSTANDING THE MODE of transmission is critical for effective outbreak control. Investigators analyze the available evidence, including epidemiological data, laboratory findings, and environmental assessments, to determine how the disease is being transmitted. This could involve person-to-person transmission, contaminated food or water, vector-borne transmission, airborne transmission, or other routes. Identifying the mode of transmission helps guide public health interventions and preventive measures.

7.6.3.4 Population at Risk:

OUTBREAK INVESTIGATIONS aim to identify the populations at highest risk of infection. This could include specific demographic groups, individuals with certain underlying health conditions, or those with particular exposures or behaviors. By understanding the populations at risk, public health authorities can tailor their interventions and communication strategies to reach those most vulnerable and implement appropriate preventive measures.

7.6.3.5 Control and Prevention Measures:

BASED ON THE FINDINGS of the investigation, targeted interventions are developed and implemented to control the outbreak. These measures may include isolation and treatment of affected individuals, quarantine of exposed individuals, vector control, food safety interventions, environmental sanitation, and public health education campaigns. The specific interventions employed depend on the nature of the outbreak, the mode of transmission, and the available resources.

7.6.3.6 Monitoring and Evaluation:

THROUGHOUT THE OUTBREAK investigation and response, continuous monitoring and evaluation are conducted to assess the effectiveness of the implemented interventions. This involves ongoing surveillance to track the number of new cases, the impact of control measures, and any changes in the outbreak dynamics. By monitoring the situation closely, public health officials can make informed decisions and adapt their strategies as needed to contain the outbreak.

Outbreak investigations require close collaboration among multiple stakeholders, including epidemiologists, laboratory experts, healthcare providers, environmental health specialists, and community members. Rapid and effective communication channels are established to ensure timely sharing of information and coordination of response efforts. Additionally, findings from outbreak investigations contribute to the scientific understanding of infectious diseases, leading to improvements in prevention and control strategies in the future.

7.6.4 Response:

ONCE AN OUTBREAK HAS been identified and investigated, a prompt and coordinated response is initiated to control the spread of the disease and mitigate its impact on public health. This response involves a range of measures aimed at interrupting transmission, protecting vulnerable populations, and preventing further outbreaks. Here's an expanded explanation of the key response measures commonly employed:

7.6.4.1 Quarantine and Isolation:

QUARANTINE AND ISOLATION measures are crucial in containing outbreaks. Quarantine is the restriction of movement and activities of individuals who have been exposed to the disease but are not yet showing symptoms. Isolation, on the other hand, is the separation and confinement of individuals who are infected and showing symptoms of the disease. By effectively implementing quarantine and isolation protocols, the transmission of the disease from infected or potentially infected individuals to others can be significantly reduced.

7.6.4.2 Contact Tracing:

CONTACT TRACING IS a vital component of outbreak response. It involves identifying and locating individuals who have come into close contact with confirmed cases. Contact tracers interview affected individuals to gather information about their recent contacts, locations visited, and potential exposures. The identified contacts are then notified, monitored for symptoms, and advised on appropriate measures, such as self-quarantine or testing. Contact tracing helps break the chains of transmission by identifying and isolating potential sources of infection.

7.6.4.3 Enhanced Surveillance:

DURING OUTBREAKS, SURVEILLANCE efforts are intensified to monitor the progression of the disease, detect new cases, and identify potential clusters or hotspots. This may involve increased testing, targeted screening, and monitoring of healthcare facilities and high-risk populations. Enhanced surveillance provides real-time data to inform decision-making, assess the effectiveness of control measures, and detect any changes in the disease's epidemiology or severity.

7.6.4.4 Public Health Education and Communication:

EFFECTIVE COMMUNICATION and public health education campaigns are essential to inform the public about the outbreak, its risks, and recommended preventive measures. Clear and accurate information is disseminated through various channels, including media, social platforms, and community outreach programs. Public health messages may include instructions on hand hygiene, proper use of personal protective equipment, social distancing, and adherence to quarantine or isolation protocols. Empowering individuals with knowledge helps promote behavior change and encourages active participation in outbreak control efforts.

7.6.4.5 Vaccination Campaigns:

IF A SAFE AND EFFECTIVE vaccine is available for the disease causing the outbreak, vaccination campaigns may be implemented to prevent further spread. Vaccines can provide immunity against specific pathogens, reducing the risk of infection and subsequent transmission. Vaccination strategies prioritize high-risk groups, such as healthcare workers, elderly individuals, or individuals with underlying health conditions. Mass vaccination campaigns aim to achieve herd immunity, where a significant proportion of the population is immunized, offering indirect protection to those who are not vaccinated.

7.6.4.6 Enhanced Healthcare Capacity:

OUTBREAK RESPONSE MAY require bolstering healthcare capacity to effectively manage cases and provide appropriate treatment. This can involve increasing hospital bed capacity, ensuring sufficient medical supplies and equipment, and training healthcare workers on infection prevention and control measures. Adequate resources and support are essential to address the increased demand for healthcare services during outbreaks.

7.6.4.7 Ongoing Monitoring and Evaluation:

THROUGHOUT THE RESPONSE, continuous monitoring and evaluation are conducted to assess the effectiveness of implemented measures and make necessary adjustments. This includes monitoring the number of new cases, hospitalizations, and deaths, as well as assessing the impact of control interventions. Lessons learned from the response efforts are used to refine outbreak management strategies and improve preparedness for future outbreaks.

It's important to note that the specific response measures employed depend on the nature of the outbreak, the disease's characteristics, available resources, and the guidance of public health authorities. Flexibility and adaptability are crucial to respond to the evolving situation and address emerging challenges effectively.

7.6.5 Evaluation:

AFTER THE OUTBREAK has been controlled, the epidemic surveillance and response system is evaluated to determine its effectiveness in detecting and responding to the outbreak. This information is used to refine the system and to improve future responses to outbreaks.

Epidemic surveillance and response systems can be implemented at various levels, including national, regional, and local levels. These systems require close collaboration between public health officials, healthcare providers, and community members to be effective in preventing and controlling the spread of communicable diseases.

7.7 Case study: Ebola outbreak in Liberia

THE EBOLA OUTBREAK in Liberia, which began in March 2014, was the largest and deadliest outbreak of Ebola virus disease in history. The outbreak resulted in 10,678 confirmed cases and 4,810 deaths in Liberia alone, with a total of 28,646 cases and 11,323 deaths in West Africa.

The outbreak in Liberia was fueled by a number of factors, including limited healthcare infrastructure, cultural practices such as burial practices that involved close contact with the deceased, and a lack of public awareness about the disease. The country had only a few doctors to serve a population of 4.5 million, and there were only a few dozen ambulances available to transport patients.

The initial response to the outbreak was slow, and the Liberian government was criticized for its handling of the crisis. However, the government eventually declared a state of emergency and launched a comprehensive response effort that included measures such as the establishment of Ebola treatment centers and the deployment of healthcare workers to affected areas.

International aid and support also played a key role in the response to the outbreak. The United States and other countries provided financial and logistical support, and healthcare workers from around the world traveled to Liberia to provide assistance.

The response effort was complicated by factors such as mistrust of healthcare workers and resistance to public health messages, as well as the ongoing civil war in the country. However, through a combination of efforts, including improved communication and outreach, the establishment of treatment centers, and the deployment of healthcare workers, the outbreak was eventually brought under control.

The Ebola outbreak in Liberia highlighted the importance of early detection and response in controlling communicable disease outbreaks, as well as the need for strong healthcare infrastructure and public awareness campaigns. The lessons learned from this outbreak have helped to inform the global response to other outbreaks, such as the COVID-19 pandemic.

Exercises

1. Multiple Choice: What is the basic reproductive number (R0) for Ebola? a. 1 b. 2 c. 5 d. 10

Solution: d. 10. According to the case study on the Ebola outbreak in Liberia, the R0 for Ebola is approximately 10.

1. True/False: Tuberculosis is caused by a virus.

Solution: False. Tuberculosis is caused by a bacterium called Mycobacterium tuberculosis.

1. Short answer: What is the mode of transmission for malaria?

Solution: Malaria is transmitted by the bite of an infected female Anopheles mosquito.

1. Matching: Match the following communicable diseases with their respective causative agents. a. Cholera b. HIV/AIDS c. Tuberculosis d. Malaria
    i. Vibrio cholerae ii. Plasmodium falciparum iii. Mycobacterium tuberculosis iv. Human Immunodeficiency Virus (HIV)

SOLUTION: a-i, b-iv, c-iii, d-ii.

1. Multiple Response: Which of the following are common symptoms of Ebola? a. Headache b. Fever c. Rash d. Vomiting e. Fatigue

Solution: b, d, e. According to the case study on the Ebola outbreak in Liberia, common symptoms of Ebola include fever, vomiting, and fatigue.

1. Fill in the blank: ___________ is a vector-borne disease that is transmitted by the bite of infected black flies.

Solution: Onchocerciasis. According to the case study on the Ebola outbreak in Sierra Leone, Onchocerciasis is a neglected tropical disease that is prevalent in the country and is transmitted by the bite of infected black flies.

1. Essay: Describe the epidemiology of tuberculosis, including its mode of transmission, risk factors, and prevention strategies.

Solution: Tuberculosis is caused by the bacterium Mycobacterium tuberculosis and is primarily transmitted through the air when an infected person coughs or sneezes. Individuals at higher risk for TB include those with weakened immune systems, such as HIV-positive individuals, people with diabetes, and those who use tobacco or alcohol. Prevention strategies for TB include vaccination with the BCG vaccine, identifying and treating individuals with active TB, and providing treatment for latent TB infection in high-risk individuals.

1. Short answer: What is the main mode of transmission for cholera?

Solution: The main mode of transmission for cholera is through the ingestion of contaminated food or water.

1. True/False: Measles is a highly contagious viral disease that can be prevented with a vaccine.

Solution: True. Measles is a highly contagious viral disease that can be prevented with the MMR (measles, mumps, and rubella) vaccine.

1. Matching: Match the following disease outbreaks with

their respective countries. a. Ebola b. Yellow fever c. Measles d. Cholera

    i. Sierra Leone ii. Angola and DRC iii. Ukraine iv. Yemen

Solution: a-i, b-ii, c-iii, d-iv.

Chapter 8. The IDSR System

8.1 Disease transmission dynamics

Disease transmission dynamics refer to the patterns and processes through which infectious diseases are transmitted within populations. Understanding these dynamics is essential for developing effective strategies to control and prevent the spread of diseases. Here are some key aspects of disease transmission dynamics:

8.1.1 Modes of Transmission:

DISEASES CAN BE TRANSMITTED through various modes, including direct contact (person-to-person), airborne transmission, vector-borne transmission (via insects or other vectors), foodborne transmission, waterborne transmission, and sexual transmission. Each mode of transmission has its own characteristics and requires specific control measures. For example, respiratory diseases like COVID-19 primarily spread through respiratory droplets when an infected person coughs or sneezes, while diseases like malaria are transmitted through the bites of infected mosquitoes.

8.1.2 Infectious Period and Incubation Period:

THE INFECTIOUS PERIOD refers to the duration in which an individual who is infected with a particular disease is capable of transmitting the pathogen to others. The length of the infectious period can vary depending on the specific disease and the individual's immune response. Some diseases have a relatively short infectious period, while others may have a more prolonged period.

During the infectious period, an infected individual can shed the pathogen through various routes such as respiratory droplets, bodily fluids, or contaminated surfaces. The infectiousness of an individual may vary throughout the course of the disease. In some cases, individuals may be most contagious before they exhibit symptoms, while in other instances, they may remain infectious even after symptoms resolve.

Understanding the infectious period is crucial for implementing appropriate control measures to prevent further transmission of the disease. For example, if the infectious period is known to be relatively short, it may be sufficient to isolate the individual or implement quarantine measures for a specific duration. However, if the infectious period is longer, more extended periods of isolation or monitoring may be necessary to reduce the risk of transmission.

The incubation period refers to the time between the exposure to a pathogen and the onset of symptoms in an infected individual. It is important to note that not all individuals who are exposed to a pathogen will develop symptoms, but they may still be capable of transmitting the disease to others during the incubation period.

The duration of the incubation period varies depending on the specific disease and can range from a few hours to several weeks. During this period, the pathogen replicates within the body, and the individual may remain asymptomatic. However, they can still spread the disease to others, often unknowingly, as they may not be aware of their infection.

Understanding the incubation period is crucial for various aspects of disease control and prevention. It helps in identifying and monitoring individuals who have been exposed to a contagious disease, as they may develop symptoms within the incubation period. By identifying and isolating individuals during this period, the risk of further transmission can be reduced.

Additionally, knowledge of the incubation period helps in determining the appropriate duration for monitoring individuals who have been in contact with an infected person. If symptoms do not develop within the expected incubation period, it is less likely that the individual has been infected.

In summary, the infectious period and incubation period are essential concepts in infectious disease epidemiology. Understanding these periods for specific diseases allows public health authorities to implement appropriate control measures, such as isolation, quarantine, and monitoring, to limit the spread of infectious diseases and protect the population's health.

8.1.3 Basic Reproduction Number (R0):

THE BASIC REPRODUCTION number, often denoted as R0, is a measure of the average number of secondary cases generated by a single infectious individual in a susceptible population. It provides an indication of the potential for disease spread. If R0 is greater than 1, the disease is expected to spread in the population, while an R0 value less than 1 indicates that the disease may die out. R0 can vary depending on factors such as the mode of transmission, population density, and effectiveness of control measures.

8.1.3.1 Basic reproduction number (R0) and its significance in disease transmission

THE BASIC REPRODUCTIVE number (R0) is a measure of how many new cases of a disease can be expected to arise from a single infected individual in a population that is entirely susceptible to the disease. In other words, it is the average number of secondary cases that would arise from a single primary case in a population where everyone is susceptible and no control measures are in place.

R0 is an important epidemiological parameter because it provides information on the potential for a disease to spread in a population. If R0 is greater than 1, it means that each infected person is likely to infect more than one other person, and the disease will continue to spread. If R0 is less than 1, the disease will eventually die out because each infected person will infect fewer than one other person, and the number of cases will decrease over time.

R0 can vary depending on factors such as the mode of transmission, the infectiousness of the disease, and the characteristics of the population. For example, diseases that are transmitted through the air, such as measles, tend to have higher R0 values than diseases that are transmitted through direct contact, such as HIV.

R0 is particularly relevant in the context of infectious disease outbreaks, as it can help public health officials to predict the potential impact of an outbreak and to determine the appropriate control measures. If the R0 of a disease is high, aggressive control measures may be necessary to slow or stop the spread of the disease, such as vaccination campaigns, quarantine measures, or travel restrictions. On the other hand, if the R0 is low, less aggressive control measures may be sufficient to contain the outbreak.

8.1.3.2 Solving problems and making decisions with (RO)

THE BASIC REPRODUCTIVE number (R0) is a mathematical concept used to estimate the average number of secondary infections generated by a single infectious individual in a fully susceptible population. It is a crucial parameter in understanding the transmission dynamics of infectious diseases. The formula for the basic reproductive number is:

R0 = Transmission rate (β) x Average duration of infectiousness (D)

Where:

Transmission rate (β) represents the probability of transmission of the pathogen from an infected individual to a susceptible individual during contact.

Average duration of infectiousness (D) is the average period an infected individual remains infectious and can transmit the disease to others.

Mathematically, R0 is defined as the product of β and D. It provides valuable insights into the potential for disease spread within a population. If R0 > 1, the disease is expected to spread, while if R0 < 1, the disease is likely to decline and eventually die out in the population.

It is important to note that R0 is a theoretical value and assumes a fully susceptible population with no intervention measures in place. In reality, various control measures, such as vaccination, quarantine, and social distancing, can modify the effective reproductive number (R), which accounts for the impact of these interventions on disease transmission.

The effective reproductive number (R) is given by:

R = R0 x (1 - p)

Where:

p represents the proportion of the population that is immune to the disease due to previous infection or vaccination.

The effective reproductive number (R) takes into account the reduced number of susceptible individuals in the population due to immunity, which reflects the impact of intervention measures on disease transmission.

It is important to note that the values of R0 and R are specific to each infectious disease and can vary based on factors such as the mode of transmission, the population's behavior, and the effectiveness of public health interventions. Accurate estimation of these parameters is crucial for understanding disease dynamics and designing appropriate control strategies.

Here are ten examples of calculating the basic reproductive number (R0) for various infectious diseases, along with step-by-step solutions and interpretations:

Example 1: Measles:

Transmission rate (β): 0.15 (estimated probability of transmission per contact)

Average duration of infectiousness (D): 10 days

Solution:

R0 = β x D

R0 = 0.15 x 10 = 1.5

Interpretation: Each person infected with measles is expected to infect, on average, 1.5 other susceptible individuals in a fully susceptible population. This indicates a moderate level of contagiousness.

Example 2: Influenza

Transmission rate (β): 0.08

Average duration of infectiousness (D): 5 days

R0 = β x D

R0 = 0.08 x 5 = 0.4

Interpretation: Influenza has a lower R0 compared to measles, indicating that each infected individual is expected to infect fewer susceptible individuals. However, given the high prevalence of influenza, it can still result in significant outbreaks.

Example 3: Ebola:

Transmission rate (β): 0.4

Average duration of infectiousness (D): 20 days

R0 = β x D

R0 = 0.4 x 20 = 8

Interpretation: Ebola has a high R0, suggesting that each infected individual can potentially lead to a substantial number of secondary infections. This highlights the need for strict infection control measures to prevent large-scale outbreaks.

Example 4: Tuberculosis (TB):

Transmission rate (β): 0.1

Average duration of infectiousness (D): 180 days

$R0 = β \times D$

$R0 = 0.1 \times 180 = 18$

Interpretation: TB has a relatively high R0, indicating that each active TB case can lead to numerous secondary infections if left untreated. This emphasizes the importance of early detection and effective treatment to prevent the spread of TB.

Example 5: COVID-19:

Transmission rate (β): 0.03

Average duration of infectiousness (D): 10 days

$R0 = β \times D$

$R0 = 0.03 \times 10 = 0.3$

Interpretation: COVID-19 has a lower R0 compared to some other diseases, but it still poses a significant public health challenge due to its high global transmission potential and large susceptible population.

Example 6: Pertussis (Whooping cough):

Transmission rate (β): 0.12

Average duration of infectiousness (D): 30 days

$R0 = \beta \times D$

$R0 = 0.12 \times 30 = 3.6$

Interpretation: Pertussis has a moderate R0, indicating that each infected individual can lead to several secondary infections. This highlights the importance of vaccination to reduce the transmission of pertussis.

Example 7: HIV/AIDS:

Transmission rate (β): 0.001

Average duration of infectiousness (D): 10 years

$R0 = \beta \times D$

$R0 = 0.001 \times 3650 = 3.65$

Interpretation: HIV/AIDS has a relatively low transmission rate per contact, but the long duration of infectiousness results in a moderate R0. Prevention strategies such as safe sex practices and needle exchange programs are crucial in reducing transmission.

Example 8: Cholera:

Transmission rate (β): 0.2

Average duration of infectiousness (D): 7 days

$R0 = \beta \times D$

$R0 = 0.2 \times 7 = 1.4$

Interpretation: Cholera has a moderate R0, indicating that each infected individual can lead to multiple secondary infections. This emphasizes the need for clean water and sanitation measures to prevent the spread of cholera.

Example 9: Mumps:

Transmission rate (β): 0.05

Average duration of infectiousness (D): 12 days

$R0 = \beta \times D$

$R0 = 0.05 \times 12 = 0.6$

Interpretation: Mumps has a lower R0, indicating that each infected individual may infect fewer susceptible individuals. However, vaccination remains essential to control mumps outbreaks.

Example 10: Zika virus:

Transmission rate (β): 0.08

Average duration of infectiousness (D): 14 days

$R0 = 0.08 \times 14 = 1.12$

Interpretation: Zika virus has a moderate R0, suggesting that each infected individual can potentially lead to secondary infections. Effective mosquito control measures and prevention of sexual transmission are important in reducing its spread.

Note: that the values used in these examples are for illustrative purposes and may not reflect the actual values for each disease. The calculation of R0 requires more comprehensive epidemiological data and specialized modeling techniques for accurate estimation in real-world scenarios.

In summary, the basic reproductive number (R0) is a key parameter in epidemiology that provides information on the potential for a disease to spread in a population. Understanding R0 is important for predicting the potential impact of an outbreak and determining appropriate control measures.

8.1.4 Herd Immunity:

HERD IMMUNITY, also known as population immunity, is a critical concept in public health and disease control.

Herd immunity is a form of indirect protection that occurs when a large proportion of a population becomes immune to a specific infectious disease. This immunity can result from vaccination or previous exposure to the disease, which leads to the development of natural immunity. When a significant portion of the population is immune, the spread of the disease becomes limited, reducing the overall likelihood of transmission and protecting vulnerable individuals.

The level of immunity required to achieve herd immunity depends on the infectiousness of the disease, as measured by the basic reproduction number (R0). The basic reproduction number represents the average number of new infections that can occur from a single infected individual in a susceptible population. Diseases with a high R0, such as measles, require a higher level of population immunity to achieve herd immunity compared to diseases with a lower R0, such as influenza.

For example, if the R0 of a disease is 2, it means that, on average, each infected individual will transmit the disease to two others. To interrupt the chain of transmission and achieve herd immunity, a certain proportion of the population needs to be immune. This proportion can be calculated using the formula: herd immunity threshold = 1 - 1/R0. In the case of a disease with an R0 of 2, the herd immunity threshold would be 1 - 1/2 = 0.5, or 50% of the population needing to be immune.

Here are the formulas for calculating the herd immunity threshold (HIT) for each example:

Example 1

Now, let's calculate the herd immunity threshold step-by-step for each example:

Example 1: : Measles: HIT = 1 - (1 / R0)

Measles: HIT = 1 - (1 / 1.5) = 1 - 0.6667 = 0.3333 or 33.3%

Example 2: Influenza: HIT = 1 - (1 / R0)

Influenza: HIT = 1 - (1 / 0.4) = 1 - 2.5 = -1.5 or -1.5% (Note: Influenza typically does not achieve herd immunity due to frequent changes in strains)

Example 3: Ebola: HIT = 1 - (1 / R0)

Ebola: HIT = 1 - (1 / 8) = 1 - 0.125 = 0.875 or 87.5%

Example 4: Tuberculosis (TB): HIT = 1 - (1 / R0)

Tuberculosis (TB): HIT = 1 - (1 / 18) = 1 - 0.0556 = 0.9444 or 94.4%

Example 5: COVID-19: HIT = 1 - (1 / R0)

COVID-19: HIT = 1 - (1 / 0.3) = 1 - 3.3333 = -2.3333 or 23.3% (Note: COVID-19 also does not achieve herd immunity due to variants and waning immunity)

Example 6: Pertussis (Whooping cough): HIT = 1 - (1 / R0)

Pertussis (Whooping cough): HIT = 1 - (1 / 3.6) = 1 - 0.2778 = 0.7222 or 72.2%

Example 7: HIV/AIDS: HIT = 1 - (1 / R0)

HIV/AIDS: HIT = 1 - (1 / 3.65) = 1 - 0.2739 = 0.7261 or 72.6%

Example 8: Cholera: HIT = 1 - (1 / R0)

Cholera: HIT = 1 - (1 / 1.4) = 1 - 0.7143 = 0.2857 or 28.6%

Example 9: Mumps: HIT = 1 - (1 / R0)

Mumps: HIT = 1 - (1 / 0.6) = 1 - 1.6667 = -0.6667 or -66.7%
(Note: Mumps typically does not achieve herd immunity due to
incomplete vaccine efficacy)

Example 10: Zika virus: HIT = 1 - (1 / R0)

Zika virus: HIT = 1 - (1 / 1.12) = 1 - 0.8929 = 0.1071 or 10.7%

Please note that negative values or values below 0 indicate that
herd immunity is not achievable or not relevant for that particular
disease

Achieving herd immunity is crucial for protecting individuals who
cannot receive vaccines due to medical reasons or those who are
at higher risk of severe disease, such as infants, elderly individuals,
or people with weakened immune systems. By reducing the overall
transmission of the disease, herd immunity indirectly shields these
vulnerable individuals by creating a protective barrier within the
population.

It's important to note that herd immunity is not a guarantee of
complete eradication of the disease. It reduces the likelihood of
widespread outbreaks and slows down the transmission, but
localized outbreaks can still occur, especially in pockets of
unvaccinated or susceptible individuals. Therefore, vaccination
programs play a vital role in achieving and maintaining herd

immunity, as they provide a controlled and safer way of acquiring immunity without the risks associated with natural infection.

In summary, herd immunity is a beneficial outcome that occurs when a significant portion of the population becomes immune to a disease through vaccination or previous infection. It helps reduce the transmission of the disease and protects individuals who are unable to be vaccinated or are at higher risk of severe illness. Achieving and maintaining herd immunity is an important goal in public health to control and prevent the spread of infectious diseases.

8.1.5 Super-Spreading Events:

SUPER-SPREADING EVENTS are instances in which a single infected individual or a small group of individuals can infect a disproportionately large number of secondary cases compared to the average transmission rate for a particular disease. These events play a significant role in the spread and amplification of infectious diseases and can lead to explosive outbreaks if not identified and controlled promptly.

Several factors contribute to the occurrence of super-spreading events:

8.1.5.1 Large Gatherings:

EVENTS THAT BRING TOGETHER a substantial number of people in close proximity, such as concerts, festivals, religious gatherings, conferences, or sports events, can facilitate super-spreading. In crowded settings, the chances of an infected individual coming into contact with many susceptible individuals increase, leading to a higher potential for rapid transmission.

8.1.5.2 Crowded Environments:

SETTINGS WITH HIGH population density, such as prisons, nursing homes, dormitories, or refugee camps, can be hotspots for super-spreading events. The close living quarters and limited ability to practice physical distancing can facilitate the rapid spread of infectious diseases.

8.1.5.3 Superspreader Individuals:

SOME INFECTED INDIVIDUALS are more likely to transmit the disease to a larger number of people due to factors like higher viral load, prolonged shedding of the virus, or behaviors that expose them to more contacts. These individuals are known as "superspreaders."

8.1.5.4 Specific Behaviors:

CERTAIN BEHAVIORS, such as singing, shouting, or participating in activities that generate a lot of respiratory droplets or aerosols, can contribute to super-spreading. For example, outbreaks have been linked to choirs, fitness classes, and indoor parties.

Identifying and mitigating super-spreading events are crucial for controlling disease outbreaks, especially in the context of highly contagious diseases like COVID-19, SARS, or MERS.

Here are some measures to address super-spreading events:

1. *Early Detection*: Surveillance and contact tracing are essential for identifying outbreaks early. Rapid testing and reporting can help pinpoint and contain potential super-

spreading events.

2. ***Targeted Interventions***: When super-spreading events are recognized, targeted interventions can be implemented to limit transmission. This may involve temporary closures of high-risk venues, restricting large gatherings, or implementing crowd control measures.

3. ***Public Health Guidelines***: Communicating and enforcing public health guidelines, such as wearing masks, practicing physical distancing, and maintaining hand hygiene, can reduce the risk of super-spreading events.

4. ***Ventilation and Environmental Measures***: Improving ventilation in indoor spaces and implementing environmental measures can reduce the concentration of infectious particles and lower the risk of transmission in crowded settings.

5. ***Vaccination: Mass vaccination*** campaigns can significantly reduce the number of susceptible individuals in the population, decreasing the opportunities for super-spreading events to occur.

By understanding the factors that contribute to super-spreading events and taking appropriate measures, public health authorities can effectively control disease outbreaks and prevent large-scale transmission of infectious diseases.

8.1.6 Seasonality and Environmental Factors:

SEASONALITY AND ENVIRONMENTAL factors play a significant role in the transmission dynamics of many diseases. Some diseases exhibit distinct patterns of increased transmission during specific seasons, while others may be influenced by environmental conditions that affect the survival and behavior of pathogens and vectors. Understanding these patterns and factors is crucial for implementing appropriate preventive measures and interventions. Here's a closer look at seasonality and environmental factors in disease transmission:

8.1.6.1 Seasonality:

SEASONALITY REFERS to the cyclic occurrence of a disease with variations in its frequency and intensity throughout the year. Several factors contribute to seasonal patterns, including:

1. *Climate Factors*: Changes in temperature, humidity, and sunlight exposure can influence the survival and replication of pathogens. For example, respiratory viruses like influenza and the common cold often show increased transmission during colder months when people tend to spend more time indoors and have closer contact.
2. **Host Behavior**: Human behavior can vary seasonally, affecting disease transmission. For instance, respiratory infections may spread more easily in winter when people gather indoors, potentially leading to increased contact and exposure.
3. *Vector Ecology*: Diseases transmitted by vectors, such as mosquitoes or ticks, may exhibit seasonal fluctuations based on the biology and activity patterns of these vectors. Mosquito-borne diseases like dengue fever or West Nile virus often see increased transmission during warm and humid seasons when mosquito populations are abundant.

8.1.6.2 Environmental Factors:

ENVIRONMENTAL FACTORS can directly or indirectly impact disease transmission by influencing the survival, replication, or behavior of pathogens or vectors. Some examples include:

1. *Temperature:* Pathogens may have temperature ranges within which they can thrive and replicate. Temperature can also affect vector breeding, development, and biting rates. Changes in temperature can alter disease transmission patterns, as seen with mosquito-borne diseases like malaria or Zika virus.
2. **Humidity**: Humidity can affect the viability and persistence of infectious agents in the environment. For instance, some respiratory viruses have been found to survive longer in low humidity conditions. Additionally, high humidity may favor the breeding and survival of certain vectors.
3. **Rainfall:** Rainfall patterns can impact disease transmission, particularly for waterborne diseases or those transmitted by insects that breed in standing water. Excessive rainfall can lead to flooding, creating favorable conditions for the proliferation of disease vectors like mosquitoes or the contamination of water sources.

Understanding the seasonal patterns and environmental factors associated with disease transmission can help inform public health strategies and interventions. For example:

1. *Vaccination Campaigns*: For diseases with seasonal peaks, timing vaccination campaigns to coincide with the period of increased transmission can maximize their impact.
2. **Vector Control:** Environmental factors can influence

vector populations and behavior. Implementing vector control measures, such as larviciding or insecticide-treated bed nets, during peak transmission seasons can be more effective in reducing disease incidence.

3. **Public Awareness**: Educating the public about disease seasonality and associated risks can promote proactive behaviors and precautionary measures during high transmission periods.

4. **Surveillance and Early Warning Systems**: Monitoring disease patterns and environmental indicators can facilitate the early detection of outbreaks and prompt implementation of targeted interventions.

By recognizing the role of seasonality and environmental factors in disease transmission, public health authorities can better understand disease dynamics and tailor interventions to effectively prevent and control the spread of infectious diseases.

8.1.7 Population Factors:

DEMOGRAPHIC CHARACTERISTICS, social behaviors, population density, and mobility play significant roles in disease transmission dynamics. Factors such as age, immune status, socioeconomic status, access to healthcare, and cultural practices can impact vulnerability to infection and the likelihood of transmission. It is important to consider these population factors when designing targeted interventions and public health strategies.

Understanding disease transmission dynamics is critical for designing and implementing effective control measures, such as vaccination programs, surveillance systems, contact tracing, isolation, and quarantine protocols. By comprehensively studying and analyzing these dynamics, public health authorities can develop evidence-based strategies to minimize the spread of infectious diseases and protect population health.

8.2 Transmission patterns in different settings

TRANSMISSION PATTERNS of communicable diseases can vary depending on the setting, population, and type of disease. Some common transmission patterns include:

8.2.1 Person-to-person transmission:

THIS OCCURS WHEN AN infected person transmits the disease directly to another person through close contact, such as touching, kissing, or sexual contact. Examples of diseases transmitted person-to-person include HIV, Ebola, and COVID-19.

8.2.2 Vector-borne transmission:

THIS OCCURS WHEN A disease is transmitted to humans through the bite of an infected insect or animal, such as mosquitoes or ticks. Examples of vector-borne diseases include malaria, dengue fever, and Lyme disease.

8.2.3 Waterborne transmission:

THIS OCCURS WHEN A disease is transmitted through contaminated water, such as from sewage or fecal matter. Examples of waterborne diseases include cholera, typhoid fever, and hepatitis A.

8.2.4 Foodborne transmission:

THIS OCCURS WHEN A disease is transmitted through contaminated food or beverages. Examples of foodborne diseases include salmonella, E. coli, and listeria.

8.2.5 Airborne transmission:

THIS OCCURS WHEN A disease is transmitted through airborne particles, such as droplets or dust. Examples of airborne diseases include tuberculosis, measles, and COVID-19.

The transmission patterns of communicable diseases can also vary depending on the population and setting. For example, in healthcare settings, healthcare-associated infections (HAIs) can occur through contact with contaminated equipment or surfaces, or through person-to-person transmission between healthcare workers and patients. In overcrowded or unsanitary conditions, diseases can spread quickly through close contact, poor hygiene, or contaminated food and water.

Overall, understanding the transmission patterns of communicable diseases is important for developing effective prevention and control strategies. Public health officials must consider the specific context and setting in which a disease is spreading in order to implement appropriate interventions to limit its transmission.

Table 3: Transmission patterns in different settings for communicable diseases

Transmission Pattern	Description	Examples
Person-to-person	Direct transmission from infected person to another	HIV, Ebola, COVID-19
Vector-borne	Transmission through the bite of infected insects or animals	Malaria, dengue fever, Lyme disease
Waterborne	Transmission through contaminated water	Cholera, typhoid fever, hepatitis A
Foodborne	Transmission through contaminated food or beverages	Salmonella, E. coli, listeria
Airborne	Transmission through airborne particles	Tuberculosis, measles, COVID-19

The table provides an overview of transmission patterns in different settings for communicable diseases. It categorizes the transmission patterns into person-to-person, vector-borne, waterborne, foodborne, and airborne.

8.3 The role of social and behavioral factors in transmission

SOCIAL AND BEHAVIORAL factors play a significant role in the transmission of communicable diseases. These factors can influence the likelihood of exposure to infectious agents, the susceptibility of individuals to infection, and the speed of disease transmission.

Some common social and behavioral factors that contribute to disease transmission include:

8.3.1 Contact patterns:

THE FREQUENCY, DURATION, and proximity of contact between infected and susceptible individuals can have a significant impact on disease transmission. Factors that influence contact patterns include population density, social norms, and cultural practices.

8.3.2 Hygiene and sanitation practices:

PROPER HANDWASHING, cleaning, and waste disposal can help reduce the spread of infectious diseases. Poor hygiene and sanitation practices can increase the risk of transmission through contaminated surfaces, food, and water.

8.3.3 Health behaviors:

BEHAVIORS SUCH AS SMOKING, poor nutrition, and lack of exercise can weaken the immune system and increase susceptibility to infections.

8.3.4 Vaccination:

LOW VACCINATION RATES can contribute to disease outbreaks by allowing infectious agents to spread more easily through susceptible populations.

8.3.5 Knowledge and attitudes:

KNOWLEDGE ABOUT HOW diseases are transmitted, along with attitudes towards vaccination, can influence health behaviors and ultimately impact disease transmission.

Social and behavioral factors can have a significant impact on disease transmission, and public health officials must consider these factors when designing prevention and control strategies. Education campaigns that focus on improving hygiene and sanitation practices, promoting vaccination, and increasing knowledge and awareness about disease transmission can help reduce the spread of communicable diseases.

8.4 Case study: Cholera outbreak in Yemen

CHOLERA IS A HIGHLY contagious bacterial infection that is spread through contaminated water and food. In Yemen, a cholera outbreak began in April 2017 and quickly became one of the largest cholera outbreaks in modern history.

The outbreak was fueled by a combination of factors, including poor sanitation and limited access to clean water due to the ongoing conflict in the country. The health system in Yemen was already weakened before the outbreak, with many health facilities damaged or destroyed, and healthcare workers unpaid or unable to access their workplaces due to insecurity.

The response to the outbreak was initially slow, with a lack of resources and capacity to implement an effective response. However, with support from the international community, including the World Health Organization (WHO), UNICEF, and other partners, the Yemeni government and health workers were able to scale up their response efforts.

The response included a combination of interventions such as:

1. Improving access to clean water and sanitation through the distribution of hygiene kits and the rehabilitation of water and sanitation infrastructure.
2. Providing cholera treatment centers and training healthcare workers in the management of cholera cases.
3. Conducting a mass vaccination campaign against cholera.

Implementing community-based surveillance to detect and respond to outbreaks early.

Despite these efforts, the outbreak persisted for over two years, with more than 2.3 million suspected cases and 4,000 deaths reported by the end of 2019. The outbreak highlighted the importance of a robust and coordinated response to cholera outbreaks, as well as the need for long-term investments in water, sanitation, and health systems to prevent future outbreaks.

8.5 Exercises

1. What is the purpose of the International Health Regulations (IHR)? a) To prevent the spread of infectious diseases b) To promote global health security c) To establish ethical guidelines for disease control d) All of the above

Answer: d) All of the above

1. Which of the following is a challenge to global health security? a) Lack of resources b) Inadequate governance structures c) Political instability d) All of the above

Answer: d) All of the above

1. What is the role of the World Health Organization (WHO) in global health security? a) To coordinate global response to disease outbreaks b) To provide funding for disease control programs c) To establish ethical guidelines for disease control d) All of the above

Answer: a) To coordinate global response to disease outbreaks

1. What is the main goal of the Global Health Security

Agenda (GHSA)? a) To improve global health security b) To prevent the spread of infectious diseases c) To provide funding for disease control programs d) None of the above

Answer: a) To improve global health security

1. Which of the following is an ethical consideration in disease surveillance and response? a) Balancing individual rights and public health interests b) Preventing the spread of infectious diseases c) Promoting community engagement d) All of the above

Answer: a) Balancing individual rights and public health interests

1. What is the role of governance in epidemic control? a) To establish policies and regulations b) To allocate resources c) To coordinate response efforts d) All of the above

Answer: d) All of the above

1. What is the primary goal of public health interventions for communicable diseases? a) To prevent disease transmission b) To treat infected individuals c) To promote community engagement d) None of the above

Answer: a) To prevent disease transmission

1. What is the importance of mass media in promoting public health? a) To disseminate information about disease prevention and control b) To provide treatment for infected individuals c) To fund disease control

programs d) None of the above

Answer: a) To disseminate information about disease prevention and control

1. What is the significance of the basic reproductive number (R0) in disease transmission? a) It represents the number of individuals infected by an index case b) It helps to predict the spread of infectious diseases c) It determines the severity of an outbreak d) None of the above

Answer: b) It helps to predict the spread of infectious diseases

1. What is the role of community engagement in promoting public health? a) To improve access to healthcare services b) To promote disease prevention behaviors c) To provide funding for disease control programs d) None of the above

Answer: b) To promote disease prevention behaviors

Chapter 9. Public health interventions

9.1 Introduction to public health interventions for communicable diseases

Public health interventions for communicable diseases refer to the various measures taken to prevent and control the spread of infectious diseases. These interventions can range from individual-level measures such as vaccination and handwashing to population-level measures such as quarantine and social distancing.

The primary goal of public health interventions for communicable diseases is to reduce the incidence and prevalence of these diseases in a population, and ultimately to eliminate or eradicate them where possible. Public health interventions for communicable diseases are typically guided by the principles of infectious disease control, which include:

9.1.1 Surveillance and early detection:

THIS INVOLVES MONITORING the spread of a disease in a population and detecting outbreaks as early as possible.

9.1.2 Containment and control:

THIS INVOLVES IMPLEMENTING measures to prevent the spread of a disease, such as isolation and quarantine of infected individuals, contact tracing, and treatment of infected individuals.

9.1.3 Prevention:

THIS INVOLVES IMPLEMENTING measures to prevent the transmission of a disease, such as vaccination, hand hygiene, and safe food and water practices.

9.1.4 Education and communication:

THIS INVOLVES PROVIDING information to the public about the risks of a disease, how it spreads, and how to prevent it.

9.1.5 Research:

THIS INVOLVES CONDUCTING research on the epidemiology and pathophysiology of a disease, as well as on the efficacy and safety of interventions.

Table 4: Key public health interventions for communicable diseases

Intervention	Description	Example
Surveillance and early detection	Monitoring the spread of a disease in a population and detecting outbreaks as early as possible.	Tracking and reporting cases of COVID-19 to identify clusters and implement control measures.
Containment and control	Implementing measures to prevent the spread of a disease, such as isolation and quarantine, contact tracing, and treatment.	Placing individuals exposed to measles in quarantine to prevent further transmission.
Prevention	Implementing measures to prevent the transmission of a disease, such as vaccination, hand hygiene, and safe food and water practices.	Conducting immunization campaigns to prevent the spread of polio in a community.
Education and communication	Providing information to the public about the risks of a disease, how it spreads, and how to prevent it.	Disseminating educational materials on HIV/AIDS prevention through community health programs.
Research	Conducting research on the epidemiology, pathophysiology, and efficacy of interventions for a disease.	Investigating the effectiveness of antiviral drugs in treating influenza in clinical trials.

The table provides an overview of key public health interventions for communicable diseases, including surveillance, containment, prevention, education, and research

Effective public health interventions for communicable diseases require a coordinated effort among healthcare providers, public health officials, policymakers, and the general public. The success of these interventions depends on timely implementation, adequate resources, and strong community engagement.

9.2 Treatment and prevention of common communicable diseases

THE TREATMENT AND PREVENTION of common communicable diseases depend on the specific disease in question. Here are some examples of treatments and preventive measures for three common communicable diseases:

Tuberculosis (TB):

I. *Treatment:* TB is treated with a combination of antibiotics for several months. Patients must complete the full course of treatment to ensure complete eradication of the bacteria.

II. *Prevention*: TB can be prevented through vaccination (the Bacille Calmette-Guérin or BCG vaccine), proper ventilation, and avoiding close contact with people who have active TB.

Malaria:

I. *Treatment: Malaria* is treated with antimalarial medications, which can vary depending on the species of malaria parasite and the severity of the infection.

II. *Prevention:* Malaria can be prevented through the use of insecticide-treated bed nets, indoor residual spraying with insecticides, and chemoprophylaxis (preventive medication) for travelers to high-risk areas.

HIV/AIDS:

1. ***Treatment***: HIV/AIDS is treated with antiretroviral therapy (ART), a combination of medications that suppress the virus and slow the progression of the disease. ART must be taken consistently for life to be effective.

2. ***Prevention***: HIV/AIDS can be prevented through various measures, including the use of condoms during sexual activity, pre-exposure prophylaxis (PrEP) medication for high-risk individuals, and reducing the sharing of needles and other injection equipment among people who use drugs.

Table 5: Communicable diseases, along with their treatment options and preventive measures

Communicable Disease	Treatment	Prevention	Examples
Tuberculosis (TB)	Combination of antibiotics for months	Vaccination (BCG), proper ventilation, avoiding close contact with active TB patients	Tuberculosis skin test, GeneXpert MTB/RIF test
Malaria	Antimalarial medications	Insecticide-treated bed nets, indoor spraying, chemoprophylaxis for travelers to high-risk areas	Artemisinin-based combination therapies (ACTs)
HIV/AIDS	Antiretroviral therapy (ART)	Condom use, pre-exposure prophylaxis (PrEP), needle exchange programs	Highly Active Antiretroviral Therapy (HAART), HIV test
Influenza	Antiviral medications, symptomatic treatment	Seasonal influenza vaccination, respiratory hygiene practices	Oseltamivir, influenza vaccine
Hepatitis B	Antiviral medications, supportive care	Hepatitis B vaccination, safe injection practices, safe sex practices	Lamivudine, Hepatitis B vaccine
Cholera	Oral rehydration therapy, antibiotics in severe cases	Safe water and sanitation measures, proper hygiene practices	Oral rehydration salts (ORS), Cholera vaccine
Dengue Fever	Supportive care, management of symptoms	Vector control measures (eliminating breeding sites), personal protection against mosquitoes	Paracetamol, Dengue vaccine
Measles	Supportive care, management of symptoms	Measles vaccination, maintaining high vaccination coverage	Measles-Mumps-Rubella (MMR) vaccine
Typhoid Fever	Antibiotics, supportive care	Safe food and water practices, typhoid vaccination	Ciprofloxacin, Typhoid Vi polysaccharide vaccine
Zika Virus	Supportive care, management of symptoms	Mosquito control measures, safe sex practices	Symptomatic treatment, protection against mosquito bites

This table provides a list of communicable diseases, along with their treatment options and preventive measures. Each disease has specific interventions tailored to its transmission and characteristics.

Other common preventive measures for communicable diseases include vaccination, proper hand hygiene, safe food and water practices, and avoiding close contact with sick individuals. It's important to note that the most effective approach to preventing and treating communicable diseases is a combination of various measures tailored to the specific disease and the population affected.

9.3 The role of mass media and community engagement in promoting public health

THE ROLE OF MASS MEDIA and community engagement is crucial in promoting public health, especially in the prevention and control of communicable diseases. Mass media, including television, radio, and social media platforms, can be used to disseminate health messages to a large audience quickly and effectively. These messages can be used to educate the public about the signs and symptoms of various diseases, preventive measures, and treatment options.

Community engagement is also vital in promoting public health. Engaging communities in disease prevention and control measures can increase their understanding of the importance of public health interventions and encourage their participation in these efforts. This can be done through community-based education campaigns, community mobilization efforts, and community participation in disease surveillance and response activities.

Effective community engagement requires understanding of the social and cultural context in which communities live. Community leaders, including religious leaders, traditional healers, and local government officials, can play a critical role in engaging communities in public health interventions. By working together with these leaders and engaging community members in dialogue, public health professionals can build trust, establish strong partnerships, and promote behavior change.

9.3.1 Designing mass media programs for prevention and control of communicable diseases

DESIGNING MASS MEDIA programs to promote prevention and control of communicable diseases involves careful planning and consideration of various factors. Here are some steps to guide the design process:

9.3.1.1 Define the objectives:

CLEARLY DEFINE THE objectives of the mass media program. Determine whether the focus is on raising awareness, promoting behavior change, providing education, or a combination of these goals.

9.3.1.2 Identify the target audience:

UNDERSTAND THE CHARACTERISTICS, preferences, and information needs of the target audience. Consider demographic factors such as age, gender, location, and cultural background. This information will help tailor the messages and choose appropriate media channels.

9.3.1.3 Develop key messages:

CREATE CONCISE AND impactful messages that convey the desired information. The messages should be clear, culturally sensitive, and relevant to the target audience. Emphasize the importance of prevention, early detection, and appropriate control measures.

9.3.1.4 Select appropriate media channels:

CHOOSE MEDIA CHANNELS that effectively reach the target audience. Consider using a combination of traditional media (television, radio, newspapers) and digital media (websites, social media platforms, mobile apps). Each channel has its own strengths and limitations, so ensure they align with the audience's media consumption habits.

9.3.1.5 Create engaging content:

DEVELOP COMPELLING and visually appealing content that captures the attention of the audience. Use storytelling, testimonials, visuals, and infographics to convey the messages effectively. Collaborate with creative professionals, such as graphic designers and videographers, to produce high-quality content.

9.3.1.6 Establish partnerships:

COLLABORATE WITH PUBLIC health agencies, healthcare providers, community organizations, and influencers to enhance the reach and impact of the mass media program. Leverage their expertise, networks, and platforms to amplify the messages and encourage community engagement.

9.3.1.7 Monitor and evaluate:

IMPLEMENT MECHANISMS to monitor and evaluate the effectiveness of the mass media program. Use surveys, focus groups, and data analytics to assess audience reach, message comprehension, and behavior change. Collect feedback from the audience to inform program adjustments and improvements.

9.3.1.8 Continuous improvement:

REGULARLY REVIEW AND update the mass media program based on audience feedback, emerging research, and changes in the communicable disease landscape. Adapt the messages and media channels as needed to ensure relevance and effectiveness.

By following these steps, public health authorities can design mass media programs that effectively promote prevention and control of communicable diseases, reaching a wide audience and inspiring behavior change for better public health outcomes.

Overall, mass media and community engagement play critical roles in promoting public health and preventing the spread of communicable diseases. Effective communication strategies and community engagement efforts can help to increase awareness, promote behavior change, and encourage participation in public health interventions.

9.4 Case study: HIV/AIDS prevention in South Africa

HIV/AIDS PREVENTION in South Africa is a major public health concern due to the high prevalence of the disease in the country. According to the Joint United Nations Programme on HIV/AIDS (UNAIDS), South Africa has the largest HIV epidemic in the world, with an estimated 7.7 million people living with HIV in 2019.

One of the key strategies for HIV/AIDS prevention in South Africa has been the promotion of condom use. Condoms are widely distributed for free or at low cost, and public health campaigns have been launched to increase awareness of their importance in preventing the transmission of HIV and other sexually transmitted infections. Other prevention strategies include pre-exposure prophylaxis (PrEP), which involves taking antiretroviral medication to reduce the risk of HIV infection, and voluntary medical male circumcision, which has been shown to reduce the risk of HIV transmission.

Community engagement has also played a critical role in HIV/AIDS prevention in South Africa. Community-based organizations and non-governmental organizations have worked to increase awareness of HIV/AIDS and promote prevention strategies. These organizations provide counseling and testing services, distribute condoms and other prevention materials, and offer support to those living with HIV/AIDS.

However, despite these efforts, HIV/AIDS remains a significant public health challenge in South Africa. The stigma surrounding HIV/AIDS continues to be a barrier to prevention and treatment efforts, and many people living with the disease face discrimination and marginalization. Additionally, challenges such as poverty, limited access to healthcare, and gender inequality can make it difficult for some individuals to access prevention and treatment services.

Overall, HIV/AIDS prevention in South Africa requires a multifaceted approach that includes community engagement, prevention education, and access to affordable and effective prevention and treatment options. Continued efforts are needed to address the social and structural factors that contribute to the spread of the disease and ensure that all individuals have access to the resources they need to prevent and manage HIV/AIDS.

9.5 Exercises

1. What are some ethical considerations that need to be taken into account when conducting disease surveillance and response activities?

Answer: Some ethical considerations include protecting privacy and confidentiality, ensuring informed consent, and ensuring equitable distribution of resources.

1. In the context of public health emergencies, what are some potential conflicts between individual rights and public health interests?

Answer: Examples include quarantine measures that restrict movement and freedom of assembly, contact tracing that may involve disclosing personal information, and mandatory vaccination policies.

1. What are some challenges in maintaining transparency and openness during disease outbreak investigations?

Answer: Some challenges include balancing the need for transparency with concerns about panic and fear, managing conflicting priorities and interests, and dealing with incomplete or conflicting data.

1. What is the principle of non-maleficence, and how does it apply to disease surveillance and response?

Answer: The principle of non-maleficence means that we should not cause harm to others. In the context of disease surveillance and response, this means minimizing harm to individuals through measures such as protecting privacy and confidentiality, and ensuring that interventions are effective and do not have unintended consequences.

1. How can ethical considerations be incorporated into

disease surveillance and response planning?

Answer: Ethical considerations can be incorporated through the use of ethical guidelines and frameworks, involving stakeholders and affected communities in decision-making, and conducting regular ethical reviews.

1. What are some ethical concerns that arise when conducting research during an outbreak?

Answer: Some ethical concerns include ensuring that research is conducted in an ethical and scientifically valid manner, protecting the safety and rights of research participants, and ensuring that research is conducted in a manner that does not distract from outbreak response efforts.

1. What is the principle of distributive justice, and how does it apply to disease surveillance and response?

Answer: The principle of distributive justice means that benefits and burdens should be distributed fairly among individuals and groups. In the context of disease surveillance and response, this means ensuring that interventions and resources are distributed fairly and equitably, and taking into account the needs of vulnerable populations.

1. How can ethical considerations be balanced with the need for timely and effective disease surveillance and response?

Answer: Ethical considerations can be balanced by involving stakeholders and affected communities in decision-making, using ethical guidelines and frameworks, and conducting regular ethical reviews.

1. What are some ethical concerns that arise in the context of international cooperation in disease surveillance and response?

Answer: Some ethical concerns include ensuring that international cooperation is equitable and does not benefit some countries or groups more than others, respecting the autonomy and sovereignty of different countries, and ensuring that interventions and resources are distributed fairly.

1. What are some ways in which ethical considerations can be integrated into pandemic preparedness planning?

Answer: Ethical considerations can be integrated through the use of ethical guidelines and frameworks, involving stakeholders and affected communities in decision-making, and conducting regular ethical reviews. Additionally, incorporating ethical considerations into pandemic preparedness planning can help ensure that interventions and resources are distributed fairly and equitably, and that vulnerable populations are taken into account.

Chapter 10. Global health security

10.1 Understanding the International Health Regulations

The International Health Regulations (IHR) is a legally binding international agreement that was created by the World Health Organization (WHO) in 2005 to help prevent, detect, and respond to infectious disease outbreaks that have the potential to cross borders and threaten global public health security. The IHR's overarching goal is to strengthen the capacity of all countries to detect, assess, and respond to public health threats.

10.1.1 Goals of the IHR

THE INTERNATIONAL HEALTH Regulations (IHR) have several key goals aimed at promoting global health security and strengthening global health preparedness and response. The main goals of the IHR are as follows:

10.1.1.1 Early detection and response:

THE IHR AIM TO ENSURE timely detection and response to public health threats, including communicable diseases and other public health emergencies. By requiring member states to report certain diseases and events to the World Health Organization (WHO), the IHR facilitate early warning and response measures to prevent the international spread of diseases.

10.1.1.2 Public health emergency management:

THE IHR SEEK TO IMPROVE the management of public health emergencies by promoting effective coordination, communication, and cooperation among member states and the international community. This includes establishing mechanisms for sharing information, expertise, and resources to support response efforts during emergencies.

10.1.1.3 Risk assessment and mitigation:

THE IHR EMPHASIZE THE importance of risk assessment and risk management in public health emergencies. Member states are encouraged to assess and share information about potential risks, evaluate the severity and potential impact of health events, and implement appropriate measures to mitigate those risks.

10.1.1.4 Promotion of public health measures:

THE IHR PROMOTE THE implementation of public health measures to prevent the international spread of diseases. This includes measures such as disease surveillance, case management, infection prevention and control, vaccination, and other interventions to limit the transmission of communicable diseases.

10.1.1.5 Protection of human rights:

THE IHR AIM TO PROTECT the rights and dignity of individuals during public health emergencies. Member states are encouraged to implement response measures that respect human rights and adhere to ethical principles, ensuring that interventions are proportional, evidence-based, and non-discriminatory.

10.1.1.6 Strengthening of national capacities:

THE IHR PROMOTE THE development and strengthening of national capacities for disease surveillance, response, and public health infrastructure. Member states are encouraged to invest in building resilient health systems and improving their capacity to prevent, detect, and respond to public health threats.

By pursuing these goals, the IHR contribute to global health security, enhance collaboration among countries, and improve the collective ability to prevent, detect, and respond to communicable diseases and other public health emergencies.

The IHR requires all member states to develop and maintain core public health capacities, including surveillance and response systems, laboratory capabilities, and communication channels, to be able to rapidly detect, assess, and respond to public health events. It also establishes reporting requirements for certain diseases and events that have the potential to cause public health emergencies of international concern (PHEICs), such as Ebola, Zika, and COVID-19.

The IHR requires member states to promptly notify WHO of any events that may constitute a PHEIC, to cooperate with WHO in the assessment and management of those events, and to share information transparently and in a timely manner. The IHR also requires member states to implement measures to prevent the spread of infectious diseases, such as quarantine, screening, and vaccination.

10.1.2 Reporting requirements

THE INTERNATIONAL HEALTH Regulations (IHR) include specific reporting requirements for communicable diseases and events that have the potential to cause public health emergencies of international concern (PHEICs). These reporting requirements aim to ensure timely and transparent information sharing among member states to facilitate a coordinated global response. Here are some key aspects of the IHR reporting requirements:

10.1.2.1 Notification of listed diseases:

MEMBER STATES ARE REQUIRED to notify the World Health Organization (WHO) of any occurrence of the diseases listed in Annex 2 of the IHR. These diseases include severe acute respiratory syndrome (SARS), Middle East respiratory syndrome (MERS), Ebola virus disease, poliomyelitis, and others. Notifications should be made within 24 hours of assessment or suspicion of a case.

10.1.2.2 Notification of public health events:

MEMBER STATES ARE ALSO required to notify the WHO of any event that may constitute a PHEIC. This includes events involving a communicable disease or other public health risks that are significant, unusual, or unexpected, and may require international coordination. Notifications should be made promptly, within 24 hours.

10.1.2.3 Information to be included in notifications:

MEMBER STATES MUST provide specific information in their notifications, such as the nature of the event, geographical location, affected populations, clinical features, and public health measures taken or planned. The information should be accurate, comprehensive, and updated as the situation evolves.

10.1.2.4 Risk assessment and notification to neighboring countries:

MEMBER STATES THAT have assessed a potential risk of international spread of a disease or event are required to promptly notify neighboring countries. This notification aims to facilitate early preparedness and response measures in neighboring countries to prevent or limit the spread of the disease or event.

10.1.2.5 Verification and consultation with the WHO:

THE WHO PLAYS A CRUCIAL role in verifying reported events and providing technical guidance to member states. The IHR emphasizes the importance of collaboration and consultation between member states and the WHO in assessing and responding to potential PHEICs.

These reporting requirements under the IHR are designed to enhance global surveillance and response capacities, enabling early detection, rapid response, and coordinated action to prevent or mitigate the international spread of communicable diseases and other public health emergencies. By promoting transparent and timely reporting, the IHR facilitate international cooperation and support in addressing public health threats on a global scale.

The IHR is an important tool for promoting global health security and ensuring that the world is better prepared to respond to outbreaks of infectious diseases that can have significant social, economic, and political consequences.

10.2 The importance of global cooperation in disease surveillance and response

GLOBAL COOPERATION is essential in disease surveillance and response for several reasons. First, infectious diseases do not respect national borders, and a disease outbreak in one country can quickly spread to other parts of the world. Therefore, it is crucial to have a coordinated global response to quickly detect, report, and respond to disease outbreaks.

Second, sharing information and best practices among countries can help improve disease surveillance and response. For example, if a country successfully controls an outbreak of a particular disease, other countries can learn from their experience and apply the same strategies in their own settings.

Third, global cooperation can help ensure that resources are allocated appropriately to prevent and control outbreaks. Countries with limited resources may not have the means to respond adequately to a disease outbreak, but with global cooperation, resources can be shared to support the response.

Finally, global cooperation can help address the root causes of infectious diseases, such as poverty, inadequate healthcare infrastructure, and environmental degradation. By addressing these underlying issues, we can help prevent disease outbreaks from occurring in the first place.

In summary, global cooperation is essential in disease surveillance and response to ensure a coordinated, effective, and efficient response to disease outbreaks, share information and best practices, allocate resources appropriately, and address the root causes of infectious diseases.

10.3 Challenges and opportunities in global health security

GLOBAL HEALTH SECURITY refers to the ability of countries and the international community to detect, prevent, and respond to public health threats that have the potential to cross borders and affect populations worldwide. The following are some of the major challenges and opportunities in global health security:

Challenges:

I. **Limited resources**: Many low- and middle-income countries have limited resources to invest in disease surveillance, prevention, and response. This can lead to delayed detection and response to outbreaks, and inadequate prevention efforts.

II. **Political instability**: Political instability and conflict can impede disease surveillance and response efforts, as well as hinder international cooperation.

III. **Misinformation**: Misinformation and mistrust can lead to delays in response, vaccine hesitancy, and increased risk of disease transmission.

IV. **Antimicrobial resistance**: The emergence of antimicrobial-resistant strains of bacteria and viruses presents a major challenge to disease control and treatment.

V. **Emerging infectious diseases**: Emerging infectious diseases, such as Ebola and COVID-19, can spread rapidly and have high mortality rates, making them a major challenge to global health security.

Opportunities:

I. *Advances in technology*: Advances in technology, such as rapid diagnostic tests and real-time data sharing, can improve disease detection and response.

II. *Global partnerships*: Global partnerships and collaborations, such as the Global Health Security Agenda, can facilitate coordinated efforts to address public health threats.

III. *Increased funding*: Increased funding for global health security can help to strengthen disease surveillance, prevention, and response efforts in low- and middle-income countries.

IV. *Improved communication*: Improved communication and information sharing between countries and international organizations can facilitate rapid response to outbreaks and improve prevention efforts.

V. *Public engagement*: Public engagement and education can increase awareness of public health threats and help to build trust in disease control efforts.

10.4 Case study: Ebola outbreak in Sierra Leone

THE EBOLA OUTBREAK in Sierra Leone, which began in May 2014, was the largest and deadliest Ebola outbreak in history, causing over 14,000 confirmed cases and 3,956 deaths in the country.

The outbreak began in the eastern district of Kailahun and quickly spread to other parts of the country, including the capital city of Freetown. The weak healthcare system and poor infrastructure in the country, as well as cultural practices such as burial traditions that involved close contact with the deceased, contributed to the rapid spread of the disease.

The response to the outbreak was initially slow, with a lack of resources and trained personnel to adequately manage the outbreak. However, with the support of the international community and partnerships between the government and non-governmental organizations, the response improved over time.

The response efforts focused on contact tracing, isolation of infected individuals, and safe burials. Additionally, public health messaging campaigns were launched to educate the public on the disease and prevention measures. Vaccines and experimental treatments were also tested and used in the country.

The outbreak was declared over in March 2016, after two years of intense response efforts. The lessons learned from the outbreak have led to improvements in disease surveillance and response in Sierra Leone and other countries in the region.

10.5 Exercises

1. What is the main goal of the International Health Regulations (IHR)?

Solution: The main goal of the IHR is to prevent, protect against, control and provide a public health response to the international spread of disease in ways that are commensurate with and restricted to public health risks, and which avoid unnecessary interference with international traffic and trade.

1. Which organization is responsible for coordinating global health security efforts?

Solution: The World Health Organization (WHO) is responsible for coordinating global health security efforts.

1. What are the three core capacities required by countries under the IHR? ***Solution:*** The three core capacities required by countries under the IHR are:

i. National legislation, policy and financing
ii. Health systems, including surveillance and response
iii. Preparedness, including human resources and laboratory capacity

1. What is the significance of the basic reproductive number (R0) in disease transmission?

Solution: The basic reproductive number (R0) represents the average number of new infections generated by one infectious person in a susceptible population. It is a key parameter in understanding and controlling the spread of infectious diseases.

1. What are some examples of social and behavioral factors that can affect disease transmission?

Solution: Examples of social and behavioral factors that can affect disease transmission include:

i. Physical distancing practices
ii. Use of personal protective equipment (PPE)
iii. Compliance with quarantine and isolation measures
iv. Hygiene practices, such as hand washing
v. Vaccine hesitancy or refusal

1. What is the role of community engagement in promoting public health? ***Solution***: Community engagement is critical in promoting public health as it helps to build trust, facilitate communication, and promote behavior change. It involves involving individuals, families, and communities in public health decision-making and implementation.

2. What is the purpose of disease treatment and prevention interventions? ***Solution***: The purpose of disease treatment and prevention interventions is to reduce the burden of disease and improve health outcomes for affected individuals and populations.

3. What is the role of mass media in promoting public health?

Solution: Mass media can play a critical role in promoting public health by disseminating accurate information, raising awareness, and influencing behavior change.

1. What are some of the ethical considerations in disease surveillance and response?

Solution: Some of the ethical considerations in disease surveillance and response include:

i. Balancing individual rights with public health interests
ii. Ensuring privacy and confidentiality
iii. Avoiding stigmatization of affected individuals or groups
iv. Ensuring equitable distribution of resources and benefits

1. What is the importance of governance and leadership in epidemic control? ***Solution:*** Governance and leadership

are critical in epidemic control as they help to coordinate efforts, allocate resources, and provide clear communication and direction. Effective governance and leadership can help to mitigate the impact of disease outbreaks and prevent future epidemics.

Chapter 11. Ethics and governance in disease surveillance and response

11.1 Ethical considerations in disease surveillance and response

Ethical considerations play a critical role in disease surveillance and response as they guide decision-making processes and shape public health policies. Here are some of the key ethical considerations:

11.1.1 Privacy and confidentiality:

SURVEILLANCE SYSTEMS collect personal and medical information as part of their operation. This information can include data such as individuals' names, addresses, contact information, medical history, test results, and other identifiable details. It is crucial to protect this information from unauthorized disclosure or use to uphold privacy and confidentiality rights.

The collection of personal and medical information in surveillance systems is done for public health purposes, such as monitoring the occurrence and spread of diseases, detecting outbreaks, conducting research, and informing public health interventions. However, it is important to ensure that this information is handled responsibly and securely.

Protecting personal and medical information involves implementing measures to prevent unauthorized access, use, or disclosure. These measures can include:

1. ***Access controls***: Limiting access to the information only to authorized individuals who have a legitimate need to access it for their work responsibilities.
2. ***Encryption and secure storage***: Using encryption and secure storage methods to protect data at rest and in transit, ensuring that it is not easily readable or accessible to unauthorized individuals.
3. ***Data anonymization or de-identification***: Removing or encrypting personally identifiable information (PII) from the collected data, such as names or unique identifiers, to reduce the risk of identifying individuals.
4. ***Secure transmission***: Using secure channels and protocols when transmitting data to prevent interception or unauthorized access.
5. ***Training and awareness***: Providing training to personnel involved in surveillance systems to ensure they understand the importance of privacy and confidentiality and know how to handle sensitive information appropriately.
6. ***Compliance with regulations***: Adhering to relevant laws, regulations, and guidelines pertaining to the collection, use, and protection of personal and medical information, such as data protection laws and healthcare privacy regulations.

By implementing these measures, surveillance systems can minimize the risk of unauthorized access, use, or disclosure of personal and medical information. This is crucial to maintain public trust, protect individual privacy rights, and ensure the responsible and ethical use of data for public health purposes.

It's worth noting that the specific privacy and confidentiality measures may vary depending on the jurisdiction and context in which the surveillance system operates. Compliance with applicable laws and regulations is essential to protect personal and medical information effectively.

11.1.2 Informed consent:

INDIVIDUALS MUST BE informed of the risks and benefits of participating in surveillance programs and must give their consent voluntarily.

The statement highlights the importance of informed consent in surveillance programs. Informed consent is a fundamental ethical principle that ensures individuals have the right to be fully informed about the risks and benefits associated with participating in any program or study involving the collection of their personal or medical information.

When it comes to surveillance programs, individuals should be provided with clear and understandable information about how their data will be collected, used, and protected. They should be informed about the purpose of the surveillance program, the types of data that will be collected, the potential risks and benefits associated with participation, and any relevant safeguards in place to protect their privacy and confidentiality.

By providing individuals with this information, they can make an informed decision about whether they wish to participate in the surveillance program. It is essential that participation is voluntary and based on the individual's free choice without any coercion or pressure.

Obtaining informed consent from individuals ensures that their autonomy and privacy rights are respected. It allows individuals to have control over their personal and medical information and helps to build trust between the individuals and the surveillance program or public health authorities.

It is important for surveillance programs to use clear and transparent communication methods to ensure that individuals understand the purpose and implications of their participation. This can be done through written consent forms, informational materials, verbal explanations, or interactive discussions. The consent process should also provide individuals with an opportunity to ask questions and seek clarification.

In some cases, there may be exceptions to obtaining individual consent due to public health emergencies or legal requirements. However, even in these situations, efforts should be made to communicate the purpose and implications of the surveillance program to the extent possible and ensure that the collection and use of data are conducted in a manner that respects privacy and confidentiality rights.

Overall, informed consent is a crucial ethical principle that protects individuals' rights and promotes transparency and trust in surveillance programs. It ensures that individuals have the necessary information to make an autonomous decision about participating in the program and helps to maintain a balance between public health interests and individual privacy rights.

11.1.3 Equity:

EQUITY REFERS TO ENSURING fairness, justice, and non-discrimination in the distribution of resources, services, and benefits.

In the context of surveillance, it means that efforts should be made to collect and analyze data in a way that captures and addresses the needs and experiences of all population groups, particularly those who are vulnerable or marginalized. This includes individuals who may face social, economic, or health disparities due to factors such as race, ethnicity, socioeconomic status, age, gender, disability, or geographic location.

To promote equity in surveillance and response, several key considerations should be taken into account:

1. ***Data collection and analysis:*** Surveillance systems should aim to collect disaggregated data that captures information about different population groups. This allows for the identification of disparities and the understanding of how certain groups may be disproportionately affected by communicable diseases. By analyzing data by demographic factors, public health officials can identify and address health inequities and develop targeted interventions.

2. ***Access to healthcare and services***: Efforts should be made to ensure equitable access to healthcare and related services, including diagnostic testing, treatment, and preventive measures. This includes addressing barriers such as financial constraints, limited healthcare infrastructure, language barriers, or cultural beliefs that may prevent certain populations from accessing necessary care.

3. ***Outreach and communication***: Communication strategies should be tailored to reach diverse populations and address specific cultural, linguistic, or literacy needs. This may involve using multiple channels, collaborating with community organizations, and employing culturally sensitive messaging to ensure that information about surveillance and response efforts is accessible and

understood by all.

4. **Resource allocation**: Resources and interventions should be allocated in a way that considers the needs of vulnerable populations. This means ensuring that high-risk groups have access to appropriate preventive measures, healthcare services, and social support systems. It may also involve prioritizing resources to areas with higher disease burden or populations with limited access to healthcare infrastructure.

5. *Collaboration and engageme*nt: Engaging with communities and involving them in decision-making processes is essential for promoting equity. By actively involving affected communities, public health officials can better understand their needs, concerns, and preferences, and design interventions that are responsive to their unique circumstances.

By prioritizing equity in surveillance and response efforts, public health officials can work towards reducing health disparities, promoting social justice, and improving health outcomes for all population groups. This requires a commitment to understanding and addressing the root causes of inequities and taking proactive measures to ensure that vulnerable populations are not disproportionately affected by communicable diseases.

11.1.4 Transparency and accountability:

WHEN WE SAY THAT SURVEILLANCE programs must be open, transparent, and accountable to the public, it means that there should be a commitment to sharing information and providing clear and accessible updates about the surveillance activities and findings. This includes sharing data, analysis, and reports with the public in a timely manner.

Openness and transparency are crucial because they foster trust and confidence in the surveillance system. By being open, the public can have a clear understanding of the purpose, methods, and outcomes of the surveillance program. They can also have access to accurate and up-to-date information about the occurrence and spread of communicable diseases.

Accountability ensures that surveillance programs are held responsible for their actions and decisions. It involves mechanisms for oversight, review, and evaluation of the surveillance activities. By being accountable, surveillance programs are responsive to the needs and concerns of the public, and they strive to continuously improve their effectiveness and efficiency.

By ensuring openness, transparency, and accountability, surveillance programs promote public participation and engagement. This empowers individuals and communities to make informed decisions, take appropriate actions to protect their health, and actively contribute to disease prevention and control efforts. It also enables researchers, policymakers, and other stakeholders to access and utilize surveillance data for public health planning, research, and policy-making.

Overall, an open, transparent, and accountable surveillance system builds public trust, facilitates effective communication, and strengthens the collective efforts in preventing, detecting, and responding to communicable diseases.

11.1.5 Respect for human rights:

DISEASE SURVEILLANCE and response must respect the basic human rights of individuals, including the right to privacy, autonomy, and dignity.

Respecting the basic human rights of individuals is essential in disease surveillance and response efforts. This includes upholding the right to privacy, autonomy, and dignity throughout the entire process.

The right to privacy ensures that individuals' personal and medical information collected during surveillance activities is protected from unauthorized disclosure or use. It means that individuals have the right to control how their information is accessed, stored, and shared, and that adequate safeguards are in place to maintain confidentiality.

Respecting the right to autonomy means that individuals have the right to make informed decisions about their own health, including their participation in surveillance activities. They should be provided with clear and accurate information about the purpose, methods, and potential impact of surveillance, and they should have the freedom to choose whether to participate or not, without coercion or discrimination.

Dignity is another fundamental human right that must be upheld in disease surveillance and response. It means treating individuals with respect, empathy, and sensitivity, regardless of their health status. This includes ensuring that individuals are not stigmatized or discriminated against based on their disease status, and that their dignity is maintained throughout all interactions and interventions.

Respecting these human rights is not only a moral obligation but also a legal requirement in many jurisdictions. It is crucial for maintaining public trust, engagement, and cooperation in disease surveillance and response activities. By upholding privacy, autonomy, and dignity, surveillance programs can foster a culture of respect and empowerment, promoting individuals' willingness to participate, share information, and adhere to public health measures.

It is important for surveillance programs to establish clear policies, procedures, and safeguards to protect individual rights. This may include obtaining informed consent, implementing secure data management practices, and providing mechanisms for individuals to exercise their rights, such as access to their own health information or avenues for complaint and redress.

By balancing the need for disease surveillance with the protection of individual rights, public health authorities can effectively monitor and respond to communicable diseases while upholding the principles of human rights and ethical conduct.

11.1.6 Cultural sensitivity:

SURVEILLANCE PROGRAMS must be designed to respect cultural and social norms of different communities, taking into account their beliefs, values, and practices.

Designing surveillance programs that respect cultural and social norms is crucial for their effectiveness and acceptance within different communities. It requires a comprehensive understanding of the beliefs, values, and practices of the community in question, and the incorporation of these factors into the design and implementation of the program.

Respecting cultural and social norms means recognizing the diversity of communities and their unique perspectives on health, illness, and healthcare systems. It involves engaging with community leaders, representatives, and stakeholders to ensure their voices are heard and their input is considered in the surveillance program. This collaborative approach fosters trust, cooperation, and active participation from the community.

Adapting surveillance strategies to align with cultural and social norms helps to overcome barriers and challenges that may impede the acceptance and effectiveness of the program. For example, in some cultures, there may be traditional healing practices or beliefs about disease causation that influence health-seeking behaviors. By understanding and respecting these beliefs, surveillance programs can work collaboratively with community members to develop culturally appropriate approaches to disease surveillance and response.

Effective communication is key in ensuring that surveillance programs respect cultural and social norms. Clear and culturally sensitive messaging helps to convey the purpose, benefits, and importance of the program in a way that resonates with the community. This may involve using local languages, employing trusted community members as communicators, and using culturally relevant media and channels for information dissemination.

Engaging community members in the design and implementation of surveillance programs is essential. This can be done through community advisory boards, community consultations, and involvement of community-based organizations. By actively involving community members, their knowledge, experiences, and perspectives can shape the program, making it more responsive, inclusive, and acceptable.

Respecting cultural and social norms in surveillance programs also means considering ethical considerations, such as informed consent and privacy, within the cultural context of the community. It requires sensitivity to cultural practices around privacy, confidentiality, and decision-making, ensuring that individuals' autonomy and rights are protected while maintaining cultural values and norms.

Overall, respecting cultural and social norms in surveillance programs enhances their relevance, acceptability, and effectiveness. By recognizing and valuing the diversity of communities, surveillance programs can build strong partnerships, engage community members, and promote sustainable and context-specific approaches to disease surveillance and response.

11.1.7 Benefit-sharing:

BENEFIT-SHARING IN surveillance programs recognizes the contributions of individuals and communities in disease surveillance and response and ensures that they receive tangible benefits from their participation. This concept goes beyond the collection of data and extends to the equitable distribution of resources, access to healthcare services, and empowerment of communities.

One aspect of benefit-sharing is providing feedback and information to individuals and communities involved in surveillance. This includes sharing the results of surveillance activities, providing updates on the status of diseases, and communicating any necessary public health actions or interventions. By keeping participants informed, they can have a better understanding of the impact of their involvement and make informed decisions regarding their health.

In addition to information sharing, benefit-sharing may also involve providing direct benefits to individuals and communities. This can take various forms, such as improving access to healthcare services, providing preventive measures, or offering support for vulnerable populations. For example, in the context of a surveillance program for a vaccine-preventable disease, individuals participating in surveillance activities may receive free or discounted vaccinations as a benefit.

Another important aspect of benefit-sharing is empowering communities to take an active role in decision-making processes related to surveillance and response. This can be done by involving community representatives in planning and implementation, facilitating community engagement and ownership, and supporting community-led initiatives for disease prevention and control. By empowering communities, surveillance programs can tap into local knowledge, resources, and social networks, leading to more effective and sustainable interventions.

To ensure effective benefit-sharing, it is important to establish clear mechanisms for participation, feedback, and accountability. This includes engaging with individuals and communities in a meaningful and inclusive manner, seeking their input and addressing their concerns. Regular evaluations and assessments of the surveillance program can also help identify areas where benefit-sharing can be enhanced and ensure that the program remains responsive to the needs and priorities of the participants.

By promoting benefit-sharing, surveillance programs can foster trust, collaboration, and a sense of ownership among individuals and communities. This not only strengthens the effectiveness of surveillance efforts but also contributes to building resilient and sustainable public health systems that prioritize the well-being and interests of all stakeholders involved.

11.1.8 Collaboration and coordination:

COLLABORATION AND COORDINATION are essential components of effective disease surveillance and response efforts. By bringing together different stakeholders, including governments, public health agencies, communities, and international organizations, a coordinated approach can be established to address communicable diseases comprehensively and efficiently.

Collaboration involves working together towards a common goal. In the context of disease surveillance and response, collaboration entails sharing information, expertise, and resources among various stakeholders. This can include sharing surveillance data, research findings, best practices, and lessons learned. Collaborative efforts can also involve joint planning, implementation, and evaluation of surveillance activities, as well as the development of policies and guidelines.

Coordination focuses on organizing and harmonizing efforts to ensure a coherent and integrated response. It involves aligning the activities of different stakeholders, setting common objectives, and establishing mechanisms for communication and decision-making. Coordination facilitates the exchange of information, avoids duplication of efforts, and maximizes the impact of interventions. It also helps to ensure that resources are used effectively and efficiently.

Collaboration and coordination are crucial at all levels, from local to global. At the local level, collaboration involves engaging with community leaders, healthcare providers, and local organizations to gather data, implement interventions, and disseminate information. At the national level, collaboration involves coordinating efforts among different government agencies, public health departments, and healthcare providers. Internationally, collaboration and coordination are essential for sharing information across borders, coordinating responses to cross-border threats, and supporting countries with limited resources and capacity.

Promoting collaboration and coordination makes disease surveillance and response efforts to leverage the strengths and expertise of different stakeholders. This leads to a more comprehensive and effective approach to addressing communicable diseases, facilitating early detection, rapid response, and effective control measures. It also helps to build trust, strengthen partnerships, and foster a sense of shared responsibility in tackling global health challenges.

By addressing these ethical considerations, disease surveillance and response programs can be more effective in promoting public health while respecting the rights and dignity of individuals and communities.

11.2 The role of governance and leadership in epidemic control

GOVERNANCE AND LEADERSHIP play a critical role in epidemic control. Effective governance and leadership can facilitate the development and implementation of public health policies and strategies, allocation of resources, and coordination of stakeholders involved in epidemic control efforts. On the other hand, weak governance and leadership can lead to delays in response, inadequate allocation of resources, and lack of coordination among stakeholders, resulting in ineffective epidemic control efforts.

Effective governance and leadership require strong political commitment, accountability, and transparency. It is important to involve all stakeholders, including government agencies, private sector partners, community organizations, and civil society in epidemic control efforts. Transparency in decision-making and communication is also critical to ensure trust and cooperation among stakeholders.

Leadership is also critical in crisis management during epidemics. Effective leaders must be able to make quick and decisive decisions, adapt to changing circumstances, and communicate clearly and transparently with the public. They must also be able to build trust and cooperation among stakeholders and inspire confidence in the public health response.

Overall, effective governance and leadership are essential for successful epidemic control efforts.

11.3 Balancing individual rights and public health interests

IN THE CONTEXT OF COMMUNICABLE diseases, there can be a tension between protecting individual rights and promoting public health interests. Governments and public health authorities have a responsibility to protect the health of their populations, but this must be balanced with the respect for individual autonomy and privacy.

One key principle is the use of the least restrictive means necessary to achieve public health goals. This means that interventions should be tailored to the specific situation and based on the best available evidence. For example, quarantine and isolation should only be used when necessary and for the shortest possible duration.

Transparency and clear communication are also important in balancing individual rights and public health interests. Individuals should be informed about the reasons for public health interventions and the potential risks and benefits. They should also have access to information about their rights and how they can seek redress if they feel their rights have been violated.

Finally, there should be accountability mechanisms in place to ensure that public health interventions are justified, proportionate, and effective. These may include oversight by independent bodies, the involvement of community representatives in decision-making, and the right to challenge decisions through legal processes.

Note that balancing individual rights and public health interests is a complex task that requires careful consideration of ethical principles, legal frameworks, and practical considerations.

11.4 Case study: COVID-19 response in Sweden

SWEDEN HAS BEEN ONE of the countries that adopted a different approach to managing the COVID-19 pandemic compared to other countries. The Swedish approach emphasized personal responsibility, voluntary social distancing, and limited restrictions, rather than imposing strict lockdown measures.

The Swedish government implemented policies to protect vulnerable groups such as the elderly, encouraged remote working, and recommended voluntary physical distancing. The strategy aimed to flatten the curve of infections to avoid overwhelming the healthcare system while building herd immunity. However, the approach was not without criticism, as the number of deaths and infections in Sweden was relatively high compared to neighboring countries.

Some experts questioned the approach, stating that it failed to contain the spread of the virus and protect the population. Others praised the approach, arguing that it allowed the economy to continue functioning while reducing the social and economic costs of strict lockdown measures.

Overall, the Swedish approach to managing the COVID-19 pandemic highlights the need for a balance between individual rights and public health interests. The approach prioritized personal responsibility and voluntary compliance, but the high number of deaths and infections also raises questions about the effectiveness of the approach.

11.5 Exercises

1. What is the basic reproductive number (R0) of a disease? a. The number of new cases arising from a single case over the entire infectious period b. The number of people who have been infected with the disease c. The number of deaths caused by the disease *Answer*: a
2. Which of the following is NOT a factor that affects disease transmission? a. Environment b. Genetics c. Social behavior

Answer: b

1. What is the primary mode of transmission for cholera? a. Airborne b. Vector-borne c. Waterborne

Answer: c

1. What is the main strategy for preventing and controlling the spread of HIV? a. Vaccination b. Antibiotic treatment

c. Behavioral interventions and antiretroviral therapy

Answer: c

1. Which of the following is NOT an International Health Regulation (IHR) core capacity? a. Surveillance and response b. Risk communication c. Healthcare access

Answer: c

1. Which organization is responsible for coordinating global health security efforts? a. World Health Organization (WHO) b. United Nations Children's Fund (UNICEF) c. International Committee of the Red Cross (ICRC)

Answer: a

1. What is the primary ethical principle guiding disease surveillance and response efforts? a. Autonomy b. Beneficence c. Non-maleficence *Answer*: b
2. What is the main strategy for preventing the spread of Lassa fever? a. Vaccination b. Antibiotic treatment c. Behavioral interventions and vector control

Answer: c

1. What is the primary mode of transmission for yellow fever? a. Airborne b. Vector-borne c. Waterborne

Answer: b

1. Which of the following is NOT a way in which governance and leadership can impact epidemic control? a. Allocating resources effectively b. Prioritizing

individual rights over public health interests c. Establishing effective communication channels

Answer: b

Chapter 12. The IDSR Framework

12.1 Components of the IDSR framework

The IDSR framework comprises six components, each of which plays a crucial role in the effective implementation of the strategy. The six components of the IDSR framework are:

12.1.1 Surveillance:

THIS COMPONENT INVOLVES the collection, analysis, interpretation, and dissemination of data on priority diseases and events. It includes the use of standard case definitions, reporting forms, and procedures for data collection, analysis, and reporting.

12.1.2 Laboratory services:

THIS COMPONENT INVOLVES the establishment and strengthening of laboratory services for the diagnosis and confirmation of diseases. It includes the use of standardized laboratory procedures, quality control measures, and the timely reporting of laboratory results.

12.1.3 Epidemic preparedness and response:

THIS COMPONENT INVOLVES the development and implementation of preparedness and response plans for outbreaks and other public health emergencies. It includes the establishment of rapid response teams, the prepositioning of supplies and equipment, and the coordination of response activities.

12.1.4 Health information and communication:

THIS COMPONENT INVOLVES the use of health information and communication technologies to support disease surveillance and response. It includes the development and use of health information systems, the dissemination of health information to health workers and the public, and the use of social mobilization and communication strategies to promote health behaviors.

12.1.5 Human resource development:

THIS COMPONENT INVOLVES the training and capacity building of health workers and other stakeholders involved in disease surveillance and response. It includes the development and implementation of training programs, the provision of technical assistance, and the establishment of partnerships for capacity building.

12.1.6 Program management:

THIS COMPONENT INVOLVES the management and coordination of IDSR activities at national, regional, and local levels. It includes the establishment of monitoring and evaluation systems, the development of policies and guidelines, and the allocation of resources for IDSR activities.

Overall, the IDSR framework is designed to promote a comprehensive and integrated approach to disease surveillance and response that involves multiple components and stakeholders. By strengthening these components, the IDSR framework aims to improve early detection and rapid response to outbreaks, ultimately leading to better public health outcomes.

12.2 Data collection

DATA COLLECTION AND management is a critical component of the IDSR system. It involves the collection, analysis, interpretation, and use of data to inform decision-making and guide public health interventions. The following are the key aspects of data collection and management in the IDSR system:

12.2.1 Data sources:

IDSR RELIES ON MULTIPLE data sources to collect information on disease outbreaks and other public health events. These sources include health facilities, laboratories, communities, and other relevant stakeholders.

12.2.2 Standard case definitions:

IDSR USES STANDARD case definitions to ensure consistency in the classification and reporting of diseases. Standard case definitions are developed and adopted by the national or regional level and are used to guide the diagnosis, reporting, and management of diseases.

12.2.3 Reporting and notification:

HEALTH FACILITIES AND other stakeholders are required to report and notify disease outbreaks and other public health events to the relevant authorities in a timely manner. This is typically done through standardized reporting forms or electronic reporting systems.

12.2.4 Data management:

DATA COLLECTED THROUGH the IDSR system is entered into a central database and managed by trained personnel. The data is analyzed and interpreted using standard tools and methods to identify trends and patterns, and to inform public health interventions.

12.2.5 Data quality assurance:

THE QUALITY OF DATA collected through the IDSR system is assured through the use of standard data quality assurance tools and methods. This involves regular monitoring and evaluation of data collection and management processes to identify and address any data quality issues.

12.2.6 Data use:

DATA COLLECTED THROUGH the IDSR system is used to guide public health interventions, including outbreak investigations, response planning, and resource allocation. It is also used to monitor and evaluate the impact of interventions and to inform policy development and decision-making.

Overall, effective data collection and management is essential for the success of the IDSR system. By ensuring the timely and accurate collection and use of data, the IDSR system can help to improve disease surveillance and response and ultimately improve public health outcomes.

12.3 Reporting and feedback mechanisms

REPORTING AND FEEDBACK mechanisms are critical components of the IDSR system that help to ensure the timely and accurate reporting of disease outbreaks and other public health events, as well as the dissemination of information to relevant stakeholders. The following are the key aspects of reporting and feedback mechanisms in the IDSR system:

12.3.1 Reporting channels:

THE IDSR SYSTEM INCLUDES multiple reporting channels, including paper-based and electronic reporting systems. Health facilities and other stakeholders are required to report disease outbreaks and other public health events through these channels in a timely manner.

12.3.2 Reporting forms:

STANDARDIZED REPORTING forms are used to guide the reporting of disease outbreaks and other public health events. These forms typically include information on the number and characteristics of cases, the geographic location of the outbreak, and other relevant details.

12.3.3 Data management:

DATA COLLECTED THROUGH the IDSR system is managed centrally by trained personnel, who are responsible for ensuring the accuracy and completeness of the data.

12.3.4 Feedback mechanisms:

THE IDSR SYSTEM INCLUDES feedback mechanisms to ensure that stakeholders receive timely and accurate information on disease outbreaks and other public health events. Feedback mechanisms may include regular reports, bulletins, and other forms of communication.

12.3.5 Response planning:

INFORMATION COLLECTED through the IDSR system is used to inform response planning, including the mobilization of resources, the establishment of rapid response teams, and the development of response plans.

12.3.6 Evaluation and monitoring:

THE IDSR SYSTEM INCLUDES mechanisms for monitoring and evaluating the effectiveness of the reporting and feedback mechanisms, as well as the overall performance of the system. This helps to identify areas for improvement and to guide ongoing efforts to strengthen the system.

Overall, effective reporting and feedback mechanisms are critical for the success of the IDSR system. By ensuring the timely and accurate reporting of disease outbreaks and other public health events, as well as the dissemination of information to relevant stakeholders, the IDSR system can help to improve disease surveillance and response and ultimately improve public health outcomes.

12.4 Surveillance system evaluation

EVALUATION OF SURVEILLANCE systems is a critical process that helps to assess the effectiveness of the system in achieving its objectives and identify areas for improvement. The following are key aspects of surveillance system evaluation:

12.4.1 Objective setting:

THE EVALUATION PROCESS should begin with the identification of the surveillance system's objectives and the development of appropriate evaluation criteria.

12.4.2 Data sources:

EVALUATION OF SURVEILLANCE systems typically involves the analysis of data collected through the system. Data sources may include disease case reports, laboratory reports, and other relevant data.

12.4.3 Performance indicators:

PERFORMANCE INDICATORS are used to measure the effectiveness of the surveillance system in achieving its objectives. These indicators may include measures of timeliness, completeness, accuracy, and sensitivity of the system.

12.4.4 Data quality assessment:

EVALUATION OF DATA quality is critical to ensure that the data collected through the surveillance system is accurate and reliable. This may involve the use of standard data quality assessment tools and methods.

12.4.5 Feedback mechanisms:

EVALUATION OF SURVEILLANCE systems should include feedback mechanisms to ensure that stakeholders receive timely and accurate information on the performance of the system and areas for improvement.

12.4.6 Stakeholder engagement:

STAKEHOLDER ENGAGEMENT is critical to ensure that the evaluation process is inclusive and that the perspectives of all relevant stakeholders are taken into account.

12.4.7 Action planning:

EVALUATION OF SURVEILLANCE systems should lead to the development of action plans to address areas for improvement and strengthen the system.

Overall, evaluation of surveillance systems is critical to ensuring the effectiveness of the system in achieving its objectives and improving public health outcomes. By identifying areas for improvement and implementing appropriate interventions, evaluation can help to strengthen the system and enhance its ability to detect, respond to, and control disease outbreaks and other public health events.

Chapter 13. Disease-specific Surveillance

13.1 Diseases of public health importance in Africa

Africa is home to a variety of diseases of public health importance, which pose a significant burden on the health and well-being of individuals and communities across the continent. Some of the key diseases of public health importance in Africa include:

13.1.1 Malaria:

MALARIA IS A PARASITIC disease transmitted by the bite of infected mosquitoes. It is a major cause of illness and death in Africa, particularly among young children and pregnant women.

13.1.2 HIV/AIDS:

HIV/AIDS IS A VIRAL infection that attacks the immune system, making individuals more susceptible to other infections and diseases. It is a major public health challenge in Africa, with a high prevalence rate in many countries.

13.1.3 Tuberculosis (TB):

TB IS A BACTERIAL INFECTION that primarily affects the lungs but can also affect other parts of the body. It is a major cause of illness and death in Africa, particularly among people living with HIV.

13.1.4 Neglected tropical diseases (NTDs):

NTDS ARE A GROUP OF parasitic and bacterial infections that affect more than one billion people worldwide, with the majority of cases occurring in Africa. These diseases include river blindness, sleeping sickness, and schistosomiasis, among others.

13.1.5 Cholera:

CHOLERA IS AN ACUTE diarrheal disease caused by the Vibrio cholerae bacterium. It is a major public health concern in Africa, particularly in areas with poor sanitation and limited access to safe drinking water.

13.1.6 Measles:

MEASLES IS A HIGHLY contagious viral infection that can cause serious complications, particularly in young children. It remains a significant public health challenge in Africa, particularly in areas with low vaccination coverage.

13.1.7 Ebola virus disease (EVD):

EVD IS A VIRAL INFECTION that causes severe hemorrhagic fever and can be fatal in up to 90% of cases. It is a rare disease but can cause significant public health emergencies when outbreaks occur, as seen in West Africa in 2014-2016.

13.1.8 Lassa fever:

LASSA FEVER IS AN ACUTE viral hemorrhagic fever that is endemic in West Africa. It is transmitted to humans through contact with food or household items contaminated with urine or feces of infected rodents.

Overall, these and other diseases of public health importance in Africa pose significant challenges to public health and require ongoing efforts to prevent, detect, and control their spread.

Table 6: Diseases of public health importance in Africa

Disease	Description	Prevalence Rate (per 100,000)	Mortality Rate (per 100,000)
Malaria	A mosquito-borne disease caused by parasites of the Plasmodium genus, resulting in high morbidity and mortality in Africa.	Varies based on location	Varies based on location
HIV/AIDS	A viral infection that weakens the immune system, leading to acquired immunodeficiency syndrome (AIDS) and related illnesses.	380.7	14.9
Tuberculosis (TB)	An infectious disease caused by Mycobacterium tuberculosis, affecting the lungs and other organs, posing a significant burden.	363.5	24.4
Cholera	An acute diarrheal disease caused by the ingestion of contaminated food or water, often resulting in outbreaks in Africa.	Varies based on outbreaks	Varies based on outbreaks
Measles	A highly contagious viral infection that can cause severe complications, particularly in young children.	Varies based on outbreaks	Varies based on outbreaks
Yellow fever	A viral disease transmitted by mosquitoes, causing flu-like symptoms and potentially fatal complications.	Varies based on outbreaks	Varies based on outbreaks
Lassa fever	An acute viral hemorrhagic fever caused by the Lassa virus, commonly found in West Africa and posing a significant threat.	Varies based on outbreaks	Varies based on outbreaks
Ebola	A severe and often deadly viral disease with high case fatality rates, causing outbreaks in several African countries.	Varies based on outbreaks	Varies based on outbreaks
Poliomyelitis (Polio)	A highly infectious viral disease that primarily affects children, potentially leading to permanent paralysis.	0.1	0.1
Neglected Tropical Diseases	A group of communicable diseases prevalent in tropical regions, including diseases like schistosomiasis and leishmaniasis.	Varies based on disease	Varies based on disease

This table provides an overview of the burden of diseases of public health concern in Africa, including malaria, HIV/AIDS, tuberculosis, cholera, measles, yellow fever, Lassa fever, Ebola, polio, and neglected tropical diseases.

13.2 Disease-specific surveillance strategies

DISEASE-SPECIFIC SURVEILLANCE strategies are tailored approaches to the surveillance of specific diseases or health conditions. These strategies typically take into account the unique epidemiological characteristics, risk factors, and clinical presentations of each disease and may involve a range of surveillance activities, including case reporting, laboratory testing, and data analysis. Below are some examples of disease-specific surveillance strategies:

13.2.1 Malaria surveillance strategies

MALARIA SURVEILLANCE strategies typically involve the use of routine case reporting and malaria diagnostic testing to track the incidence and distribution of the disease. In some areas, malaria surveillance may also include vector surveillance to monitor mosquito populations and their susceptibility to insecticides.

13.2.2 HIV/AIDS surveillance strategies

HIV/AIDS SURVEILLANCE strategies may involve routine HIV testing and case reporting, as well as the use of laboratory testing to monitor viral load and CD4 counts. HIV/AIDS surveillance may also include the monitoring of HIV drug resistance and the use of behavioral surveillance surveys to track risk factors for HIV transmission.

13.2.3 Tuberculosis (TB) surveillance strategies

TB SURVEILLANCE STRATEGIES typically involve routine case reporting and laboratory testing to detect and confirm cases of TB. TB surveillance may also include contact tracing to identify individuals who may have been exposed to TB and the use of drug susceptibility testing to monitor resistance patterns.

13.2.4 Cholera surveillance strategies

CHOLERA SURVEILLANCE strategies may involve the use of routine case reporting and laboratory testing to detect and confirm cases of cholera. Cholera surveillance may also include the monitoring of water quality and sanitation conditions to identify potential outbreaks and the use of vaccination campaigns to prevent the spread of the disease.

13.2.5 Measles surveillance strategies

MEASLES SURVEILLANCE strategies may involve the use of routine case reporting and laboratory testing to detect and confirm cases of measles. Measles surveillance may also include the monitoring of vaccination coverage and the use of outbreak response vaccination campaigns to prevent the spread of the disease.

13.2.6 Ebola virus disease (EVD) surveillance strategies

EVD SURVEILLANCE STRATEGIES typically involve the use of active case finding and laboratory testing to detect and confirm cases of EVD. EVD surveillance may also include contact tracing and the implementation of infection prevention and control measures to prevent the spread of the disease.

Overall, disease-specific surveillance strategies play a critical role in the prevention, detection, and control of infectious diseases, allowing public health officials to track the incidence and distribution of diseases, identify outbreaks, and implement appropriate control measures.

13.3 Case studies of successful disease-specific surveillance in Africa

THERE ARE MANY EXAMPLES of successful disease-specific surveillance efforts in Africa. Below are a few case studies:

13.3.1 Polio eradication in Nigeria:

NIGERIA WAS ONE OF the last countries in the world to achieve polio eradication, with the virus persisting in the country until 2016. To eliminate the disease, the Nigerian government implemented a comprehensive polio surveillance system, which involved active case finding, routine immunization campaigns, and the use of community-based surveillance to detect and respond to cases of acute flaccid paralysis (AFP), a key indicator of polio. The polio surveillance system in Nigeria has been credited with identifying and responding to outbreaks of the disease, ultimately leading to its elimination.

13.3.2 Guinea worm eradication in Ghana:

GUINEA WORM DISEASE, caused by the parasitic Guinea worm, was once endemic in Ghana, causing significant morbidity and disability. To eliminate the disease, the Ghanaian government implemented a comprehensive surveillance system, which involved the use of community-based surveillance to detect cases of Guinea worm and prevent its transmission. The surveillance system in Ghana has been credited with identifying and responding to outbreaks of the disease, ultimately leading to its elimination.

13.3.3 Ebola response in West Africa:

DURING THE 2014-2016 Ebola outbreak in West Africa, surveillance played a critical role in detecting and responding to cases of the disease. Countries affected by the outbreak implemented a range of surveillance activities, including the use of active case finding, contact tracing, and laboratory testing to detect and confirm cases of Ebola. Surveillance data was used to track the spread of the disease and inform the deployment of resources to affected areas, ultimately contributing to the control of the outbreak.

Overall, these case studies demonstrate the importance of disease-specific surveillance in Africa, highlighting the critical role of surveillance in the prevention, detection, and control of infectious diseases.

Table 7: Case studies of successful disease-specific surveillance in Africa

Disease	Country	Summary
Malaria	Uganda	Implementation of a robust surveillance system with active case detection and prompt treatment interventions.
Tuberculosis	South Africa	Integration of electronic reporting systems to enhance case notification and improve treatment outcomes.
HIV/AIDS	Botswana	Implementation of a comprehensive HIV surveillance program, including routine testing and data analysis for targeted interventions.
Cholera	Zambia	Development of an early warning system to detect and respond to cholera outbreaks swiftly.
Measles	Ethiopia	Implementation of a nationwide measles vaccination campaign to reduce measles incidence and achieve high immunization coverage.

This table presents case studies of successful disease-specific surveillance programs in Africa. The examples highlight the implementation of robust surveillance systems for malaria in Uganda, the integration of electronic reporting systems for tuberculosis in South Africa, the comprehensive HIV surveillance program in Botswana, the development of an early warning system for cholera in Zambia, and the nationwide measles vaccination campaign in Ethiopia.

13.4 Exercises

1. *Multiple Choice*: What is the primary goal of the Integrated Disease Surveillance and Response (IDSR) system? A. To prevent the spread of infectious diseases B. To track the incidence and distribution of diseases C. To develop new vaccines and treatments for diseases D. To monitor chronic diseases

Solution: B. The primary goal of the IDSR system is to track the incidence and distribution of diseases in order to identify outbreaks and respond appropriately.

1. *True or False*: The IDSR framework includes six core

components: case detection, reporting, confirmation, analysis, feedback, and response.

Solution: True. The IDSR framework includes these six core components, which work together to enable effective disease surveillance and response.

1. Short Answer: What is an example of a disease-specific surveillance strategy used in Africa?

Solution: One example of a disease-specific surveillance strategy used in Africa is the surveillance of polio in Nigeria, which involved active case finding, routine immunization campaigns, and the use of community-based surveillance to detect and respond to cases of acute flaccid paralysis (AFP).

1. Matching: Match the following surveillance activities with their purpose.

A. Case reporting B. Laboratory testing C. Contact tracing D. Vector surveillance

1. To confirm diagnoses and monitor disease trends
2. To identify individuals who may have been exposed to disease
3. To track the distribution and susceptibility of disease vectors
4. To detect and report cases of disease to public health authorities

Solution: A-4 B-1 C-2 D-3

1. Case Study: During the 2014-2016 Ebola outbreak in West Africa, what surveillance activities were used to detect and respond to cases of the disease?

Solution: During the Ebola outbreak, surveillance activities in affected countries included the use of active case finding, contact tracing, and laboratory testing to detect and confirm cases of Ebola. Surveillance data was used to track the spread of the disease and inform the deployment of resources to affected areas, ultimately contributing to the control of the outbreak.

1. Multiple Choice: What is the primary purpose of data collection in the IDSR system? A. To monitor the incidence of chronic diseases B. To identify outbreaks of infectious diseases C. To develop new vaccines and treatments for diseases D. To conduct research studies on disease prevalence

Solution: B. The primary purpose of data collection in the IDSR system is to identify outbreaks of infectious diseases and respond accordingly.

1. True or False: The IDSR system includes both passive and active data collection methods.

Solution: True. The IDSR system includes both passive methods, which rely on routine reporting from health facilities, and active methods, which involve proactive case finding and investigation.

1. Short Answer: What is an example of a data quality issue that can arise in the IDSR system?

Solution: One example of a data quality issue that can arise in the IDSR system is incomplete or inaccurate reporting from health facilities, which can lead to underestimation or overestimation of disease burden and hinder effective disease surveillance and response.

1. Matching: Match the following data management tools with their purpose.

A. Line lists B. Surveillance databases C. Data analysis software D. Data visualization tools

1. To facilitate data entry and organization
2. To identify trends and patterns in disease incidence and distribution
3. To present data in a clear and accessible format
4. To track individual cases of disease over time

Solution: A-1 B-2 C-2 D-3

1. Case Study: How was the IDSR system used to track the incidence of Ebola during the 2014-2016 outbreak in West Africa?

Solution: During the Ebola outbreak, the IDSR system was used to track the incidence of the disease through routine reporting from health facilities and active case finding and investigation. Data was collected and managed using a range of tools, including line lists and surveillance databases, and analyzed using data analysis software. Data visualization tools were used to present data in a clear and accessible format, allowing for timely and effective response to the outbreak.

Chapter 14. Response to Disease Outbreaks

14.1 Importance of rapid response to disease outbreaks

Rapid response to disease outbreaks is crucial to limit the spread of disease and reduce the overall impact of an outbreak on public health. Here are some key reasons why rapid response is so important:

14.1.1 Preventing further spread:

EARLY IDENTIFICATION and response to an outbreak play a critical role in preventing further spread of infectious diseases. When an outbreak is detected early, public health authorities can implement prompt control measures to limit transmission and prevent the disease from spreading to a larger population. This includes measures such as contact tracing, isolation or quarantine of infected individuals, and implementing community-wide interventions like vaccination campaigns or health education programs to promote preventive measures. By taking swift and targeted actions, the potential for the disease to escalate and affect more people can be significantly reduced, ultimately protecting the health and well-being of individuals and communities.

14.1.2 Controlling the outbreak:

RAPID RESPONSE IS A crucial aspect of outbreak control as it enables timely identification and effective management of cases. When an outbreak occurs, rapid response teams and public health authorities can swiftly identify and isolate individuals who are infected, ensuring they receive appropriate treatment and care. Additionally, preventive measures such as contact tracing, quarantine, and targeted interventions can be implemented promptly to break the chain of transmission. By taking these immediate actions, the spread of the disease can be effectively controlled, minimizing its impact on the affected population and preventing further transmission to others. The combination of early detection, isolation, treatment, and preventive measures through a rapid response approach significantly enhances the chances of containing and mitigating the outbreak.

14.1.3 Saving lives:

PROMPT ACTION PLAYS a critical role in saving lives during outbreaks. By taking immediate and decisive measures, such as early detection, rapid diagnosis, and timely treatment, the severity and duration of illness can be minimized. Early identification of cases allows for timely provision of appropriate medical care, which can improve patient outcomes and reduce mortality rates. Furthermore, prompt action enables healthcare systems to mobilize necessary resources and implement effective public health interventions to control the spread of the disease. This proactive approach not only saves lives but also helps alleviate the burden on healthcare facilities and allows for more efficient use of healthcare resources. By acting swiftly, public health authorities and healthcare professionals can make a significant impact in mitigating the effects of the outbreak and protecting the health and well-being of individuals and communities.

14.1.4 Minimizing economic impact:

DISEASE OUTBREAKS CAN indeed have profound economic impacts, affecting various sectors of society. Rapid response plays a crucial role in mitigating these impacts by minimizing the scale and duration of the outbreak. By swiftly identifying and containing cases, implementing effective control measures, and providing appropriate medical care, the spread of the disease can be limited. This not only helps to protect public health but also reduces the burden on healthcare systems, prevents disruptions to productivity, and mitigates the economic losses associated with the outbreak. Additionally, rapid response measures such as travel restrictions and public health advisories can help maintain confidence in trade and tourism, reducing the negative impact on these sectors. By taking immediate action, governments, public health authorities, and communities can work together to mitigate the economic consequences of disease outbreaks and facilitate a faster recovery.

14.1.5 Building public trust:

EFFECTIVE AND TIMELY response to disease outbreaks is crucial not only for controlling the spread of the disease but also for maintaining public trust in the healthcare system and government. When authorities respond promptly and transparently to outbreaks, providing accurate information, implementing appropriate measures, and demonstrating their commitment to public health, it helps to build confidence and trust among the population. This, in turn, promotes compliance with public health measures such as vaccinations, quarantine protocols, and hygiene practices. When the public trusts the healthcare system and government's response, they are more likely to follow recommended guidelines, reducing the risk of panic, misinformation, and non-compliance. By maintaining open lines of communication, addressing concerns, and involving the community in the response efforts, authorities can foster a collaborative approach that strengthens public trust, enhances cooperation, and ultimately improves the effectiveness of outbreak control measures.

Overall, rapid response is essential to limit the spread of disease and minimize the impact of outbreaks on public health and the economy.

14.2

Table 8: Importance of rapid response to disease outbreaks

Importance	Description
Early containment	Rapid response minimizes the spread of the disease, reducing the number of cases and preventing further outbreaks.
Timely intervention	Prompt actions such as contact tracing, isolation, and treatment can effectively control the outbreak and mitigate its impact.
Public health messaging	Rapid response allows for timely communication of information to the public, promoting awareness and preventive measures.
Resource mobilization	Swift response ensures the mobilization of necessary resources, including healthcare personnel, medical supplies, and funding.

This table highlights the importance of rapid response to disease outbreaks. It emphasizes that early containment through swift actions such as contact tracing and isolation can minimize the spread of the disease and prevent further outbreaks.

The IDSR response strategy

THE IDSR RESPONSE STRATEGY is a set of guidelines and protocols for responding to disease outbreaks in Africa. The strategy is based on the following key principles:

14.2.1 Early detection:

THE FIRST STEP IN THE IDSR response strategy is to detect outbreaks early through active and passive surveillance systems. This involves monitoring disease trends, conducting case investigations, and identifying potential outbreak situations.

14.2.2 Rapid response:

ONCE AN OUTBREAK IS identified, the response must be rapid and coordinated. This includes mobilizing resources, deploying trained personnel to the affected areas, and implementing control measures to prevent further spread.

14.2.3 Integrated response:

THE IDSR RESPONSE STRATEGY emphasizes an integrated response, bringing together stakeholders from different sectors, including health, animal health, and environmental health. This coordinated response helps ensure that all aspects of the outbreak are addressed and that the response is effective.

14.2.4 Evidence-based interventions:

THE IDSR RESPONSE STRATEGY is based on evidence-based interventions, which are selected based on the type of disease and the specific outbreak situation. These interventions may include vaccination, treatment, case isolation, contact tracing, and environmental sanitation measures.

14.2.5 Monitoring and evaluation:

THE IDSR RESPONSE STRATEGY includes monitoring and evaluation activities to assess the effectiveness of the response and identify areas for improvement. This includes ongoing surveillance, data collection and analysis, and regular review and revision of the response plan.

Overall, the IDSR response strategy is designed to ensure a coordinated, evidence-based, and effective response to disease outbreaks in Africa. By emphasizing early detection, rapid response, and integrated interventions, the strategy aims to limit the spread of disease and minimize the impact of outbreaks on public health and the economy.

14.3 Case studies of effective outbreak response in Africa

HERE ARE SOME CASE studies of effective outbreak response in Africa:

14.3.1 Ebola outbreak in Nigeria (2014):

IN JULY 2014, A MAN with Ebola virus disease (EVD) arrived in Lagos, Nigeria, from Liberia. The Nigerian government quickly mobilized its health system and established an Emergency Operations Center (EOC) to coordinate the response. The EOC implemented a range of measures, including contact tracing, case isolation, and public health education campaigns. The response was successful in containing the outbreak, with only 20 confirmed cases and 8 deaths.

14.3.2 Yellow fever outbreak in Angola (2016):

IN DECEMBER 2015, A yellow fever outbreak was reported in Angola, with cases quickly spreading to other countries in the region. The response involved a massive vaccination campaign, targeting over 23 million people across Angola and neighboring countries. The campaign was successful in reducing the number of new cases and preventing a wider outbreak.

14.3.3 Lassa fever outbreak in Nigeria (2018):

IN JANUARY 2018, AN outbreak of Lassa fever was reported in Nigeria, with cases quickly spreading to multiple states. The Nigerian government and its partners responded with measures including case identification, isolation, treatment, and contact tracing. The response also included a public health education campaign to raise awareness about the disease and how to prevent its spread. The response was successful in containing the outbreak, with 423 confirmed cases and 106 deaths.

14.3.4 Ebola outbreak in Liberia (2014-2016):

LIBERIA WAS ONE OF the countries most affected by the Ebola virus disease (EVD) outbreak that began in 2014. The Liberian government, with support from international partners, implemented a comprehensive response that included contact tracing, case isolation, and public health education campaigns. The response also included building new treatment facilities and training health workers in infection prevention and control. The response was successful in bringing the outbreak under control, with a total of 10,675 cases and 4,809 deaths reported in Liberia.

14.3.5 Measles outbreak in Nigeria (2020):

IN LATE 2019, A MEASLES outbreak was reported in Nigeria, with over 10,000 suspected cases and 100 deaths reported by February 2020. The Nigerian government, with support from international partners, launched a vaccination campaign targeting over 31 million children across 19 states. The campaign was successful in reducing the number of new cases and preventing further spread of the disease.

14.3.6 Meningitis outbreak in Niger (2015):

IN EARLY 2015, A MENINGITIS outbreak was reported in Niger, with over 8,500 cases and 573 deaths reported by May. The government of Niger, with support from international partners, launched a massive vaccination campaign targeting over 3 million people across the affected regions. The campaign was successful in reducing the number of new cases and preventing a wider outbreak.

These case studies demonstrate the importance of a coordinated and comprehensive response to disease outbreaks in Africa. By implementing a range of measures, including surveillance, vaccination, case management, and public health education, these responses were able to limit the spread of disease and reduce the impact on public health.

Table 9: Case studies of effective outbreak response in Africa

Disease	Country	Summary
Ebola	Democratic Republic of Congo	Coordinated response involving rapid deployment of healthcare workers, contact tracing, isolation, and community engagement to contain the outbreak.
Lassa fever	Nigeria	Implementation of a robust surveillance system, early case detection, isolation, and treatment, along with public health education to prevent the spread of the disease.
COVID-19	Rwanda	Swift response with a proactive approach, including early testing, contact tracing, quarantine measures, and strict adherence to public health guidelines.
Yellow fever	Angola	Rapid vaccination campaigns, enhanced surveillance, and vector control measures to control the outbreak and prevent its spread to other regions.
Cholera	Zimbabwe	Quick establishment of treatment centers, provision of clean water and sanitation facilities, and community engagement to prevent and control cholera outbreaks.

The table highlights successful outbreak responses in Africa, including a coordinated effort against Ebola in the Democratic Republic of Congo and a proactive approach to COVID-19 in Rwanda. Other effective strategies include robust surveillance for Lassa fever in Nigeria, rapid vaccination campaigns for yellow fever in Angola, and prompt cholera control measures in Zimbabwe.

14.4 Exercises

1. ***Multiple choice***: What is the first step in the IDSR response strategy? a) Case investigation and confirmation b) Data analysis and interpretation c) Notification and reporting d) Rapid response

   Solution c) Notification and reporting

Explanation: Notification and reporting is the first step in the IDSR response strategy. It involves the timely reporting of suspected cases of notifiable diseases to the relevant authorities, which triggers an investigation and response.

1. *True or false*: The IDSR response strategy is only used for disease outbreaks. *Solution*: False

Explanation: While the IDSR response strategy is often used for disease outbreaks, it can also be used for other public health events such as natural disasters or chemical spills.

1. *Short answer*: What are the four main components of the IDSR rapid response strategy?

Solution: The four main components of the IDSR rapid response strategy are case investigation and confirmation, contact tracing, case management, and social mobilization and communication.

Explanation: The IDSR rapid response strategy includes these four components, which work together to control the spread of disease and prevent further transmission.

1. *Matching*: Match the following case studies to the appropriate response strategies:

a) Ebola outbreak in Nigeria b) Yellow fever outbreak in Angola c) Lassa fever outbreak in Nigeria

i) Contact tracing, case isolation, public health education campaigns ii) Mass vaccination campaign iii) Case identification, isolation, treatment, contact tracing, public health education campaigns

Solution: a) iii b) ii c) iii

Explanation: The Ebola outbreak in Nigeria and the Lassa fever outbreak in Nigeria both involved a response strategy that included case identification, isolation, treatment, contact tracing, and public health education campaigns. The yellow fever outbreak in Angola involved a mass vaccination campaign.

1. *Short answer*: What was the role of international partners in the response to the Ebola outbreak in Liberia?

Solution: International partners provided support to the Liberian government in its response to the Ebola outbreak, including building new treatment facilities, training health workers in infection prevention and control, and providing financial and technical assistance.

Explanation: The Liberian government's response to the Ebola outbreak was supported by a range of international partners, including the World Health Organization, the United States Centers for Disease Control and Prevention, and non-governmental organizations such as Médecins Sans Frontières.

Chapter 15. The Role of Laboratory Services in IDSR

15.1 The importance of laboratory services in disease surveillance and response

Laboratory services are a critical component of disease surveillance and response. Here are some reasons why:

15.1.1 Disease diagnosis:

DISEASE DIAGNOSIS: Laboratory testing is an integral part of the diagnostic process for infectious diseases. It plays a crucial role in accurately identifying the specific pathogen causing the illness and determining the appropriate course of treatment and control measures. Laboratory tests provide valuable information about the presence, nature, and characteristics of infectious agents, allowing healthcare professionals to make informed decisions and take necessary actions to protect public health.

One of the primary purposes of disease diagnosis through laboratory testing is to confirm the presence of a specific pathogen. Various types of laboratory tests are employed, including molecular tests, serological tests, and culture-based methods, depending on the nature of the disease and the available resources. These tests detect the genetic material, antibodies, or antigens associated with the pathogen, enabling the identification of the causative agent.

Accurate diagnosis is crucial for several reasons. First, it helps guide appropriate treatment strategies. Different infectious diseases require specific treatments, such as antibiotics, antiviral medications, or antiparasitic drugs. By accurately identifying the pathogen, healthcare professionals can prescribe the most effective treatment options, reducing the risk of treatment failure or unnecessary use of broad-spectrum antibiotics.

Furthermore, laboratory testing plays a significant role in disease surveillance and outbreak detection. By testing samples from individuals exhibiting symptoms, healthcare authorities can identify clusters of cases and detect outbreaks early on. This early detection allows for prompt implementation of control measures, such as quarantine, contact tracing, and targeted interventions, to limit the spread of the disease and minimize its impact on public health.

Laboratory testing also aids in monitoring the effectiveness of control measures. By conducting follow-up testing and monitoring the presence of the pathogen in recovered individuals, healthcare professionals can assess the impact of interventions and evaluate the success of disease control efforts. This information is crucial for adjusting strategies, making informed decisions, and allocating resources effectively.

Additionally, laboratory testing contributes to the understanding of disease epidemiology. By analyzing the data from diagnostic tests, researchers and public health officials can gain insights into the prevalence, distribution, and trends of infectious diseases. This knowledge helps in identifying risk factors, understanding transmission dynamics, and designing targeted prevention and control strategies.

It is important to note that laboratory testing should be performed in accredited and quality-assured laboratories to ensure reliable and accurate results. Quality assurance programs, proficiency testing, and adherence to standardized protocols are essential to maintain the reliability and credibility of laboratory testing for disease diagnosis.

Disease diagnosis through laboratory testing is an essential component of infectious disease management. It provides critical information for treatment decisions, outbreak detection, monitoring control measures, and enhancing our understanding of disease dynamics. Accurate and timely diagnosis enables healthcare professionals and public health authorities to effectively respond to infectious diseases, protect individuals, and safeguard public health.

15.1.2 Disease monitoring:

DISEASE MONITORING: Laboratory testing plays a vital role in monitoring the spread and severity of infectious diseases. By continuously tracking the number of positive cases, laboratory testing provides valuable data that helps public health officials assess the progression of outbreaks, evaluate the effectiveness of control measures, and make informed decisions to protect public health.

One of the primary uses of laboratory testing in disease monitoring is to track the prevalence and incidence of infectious diseases. By testing individuals with symptoms or known exposure to the disease, public health authorities can gather data on the number of positive cases over time. This data allows for the identification of disease trends, such as increases or decreases in case numbers, and the detection of potential outbreaks. Monitoring the spread of diseases through laboratory testing provides important insights into the geographic distribution and temporal patterns of infections, helping officials focus resources and implement targeted interventions.

Laboratory testing also aids in assessing the severity and impact of infectious diseases. By analyzing samples from infected individuals, healthcare professionals can determine disease markers, such as viral load or antibody levels, that indicate the severity of the infection. Monitoring these markers over time allows for the identification of trends in disease severity and the evaluation of treatment effectiveness. Additionally, laboratory testing can help identify risk factors associated with severe disease outcomes, enabling targeted interventions for high-risk individuals.

Furthermore, laboratory testing assists in monitoring the effectiveness of control measures and public health interventions. By comparing the number of positive cases before and after the implementation of control measures, officials can assess the impact of interventions on disease transmission. This data provides crucial feedback on the success or need for adjustment of control strategies, allowing for evidence-based decision-making.

Laboratory testing also facilitates the early detection of emerging infectious diseases or the re-emergence of known pathogens. By regularly monitoring samples from sentinel sites or conducting surveillance testing in high-risk populations, public health authorities can quickly identify new or resurging infections. This early detection enables prompt responses, such as initiating contact tracing, implementing containment measures, and developing targeted prevention campaigns.

In addition to monitoring the spread and severity of infectious diseases, laboratory testing is essential for monitoring the effectiveness of vaccination programs. By testing for the presence of specific antibodies or immune responses, healthcare professionals can assess vaccine coverage rates and evaluate the effectiveness of immunization efforts. This data helps in identifying populations with suboptimal vaccine uptake and implementing targeted vaccination campaigns to enhance population immunity.

15.1.3 Disease research:

DISEASE RESEARCH: LABORATORY testing plays a crucial role in advancing our understanding of infectious diseases and driving scientific research. By conducting various laboratory experiments and analyses, scientists can gain valuable insights into the genetic makeup, behavior, and characteristics of pathogens, which ultimately contribute to the development of new treatments, vaccines, and improved strategies for controlling disease outbreaks.

One area of disease research that heavily relies on laboratory testing is the study of pathogen genetics. Through techniques such as DNA sequencing and genotyping, scientists can analyze the genetic material of pathogens, including viruses, bacteria, and parasites. This allows for the identification of specific genetic markers or mutations associated with virulence, drug resistance, or transmissibility. Understanding the genetic variations of pathogens helps researchers track the origin and spread of diseases, identify new strains, and develop targeted interventions.

Laboratory testing also enables scientists to study the behavior and characteristics of pathogens. By conducting experiments in controlled laboratory settings, researchers can investigate how pathogens interact with host cells, how they replicate, and how they evade the immune system. This knowledge provides insights into the mechanisms of infection and disease progression, leading to a better understanding of pathogenesis and the development of more effective therapeutic strategies.

In addition to studying pathogens, laboratory testing is instrumental in evaluating the efficacy and safety of potential treatments and vaccines. Through in vitro testing and preclinical studies, scientists can assess the effectiveness of candidate drugs or vaccines in inhibiting the growth or replication of pathogens. Laboratory experiments allow researchers to test different compounds or therapeutic strategies, optimize their formulations, and evaluate their potential side effects. These early-stage investigations provide crucial data that informs further development and clinical trials.

Laboratory testing also supports epidemiological research, which aims to understand the patterns and determinants of disease spread within populations. By analyzing samples from infected individuals, researchers can identify risk factors associated with disease transmission, assess population immunity, and track the dynamics of outbreaks. Laboratory-based epidemiological studies provide important data for modeling disease transmission, informing public health policies, and evaluating the impact of interventions.

Furthermore, laboratory testing contributes to the surveillance of emerging infectious diseases and the identification of novel pathogens. By conducting surveillance programs and analyzing samples from both humans and animals, scientists can detect and characterize previously unknown pathogens. This proactive approach allows for early identification and response to potential outbreaks, helping to prevent or mitigate their impact on public health.

15.1.4 Public health emergency preparedness:

PUBLIC HEALTH EMERGENCY preparedness: A strong and well-functioning laboratory network is a vital component of public health emergency preparedness. In times of outbreaks or other public health emergencies, such as pandemics or bioterrorism events, laboratory services play a crucial role in timely and accurate diagnosis, monitoring, and evaluation of control measures.

During a public health emergency, rapid and accurate diagnosis of cases is essential for effective response and containment. Laboratory testing enables healthcare providers to confirm the presence of a specific pathogen in individuals showing symptoms and distinguish it from other similar illnesses. This diagnostic information helps guide appropriate treatment decisions, isolate infected individuals, and initiate contact tracing to prevent further transmission.

Additionally, laboratory testing is vital for monitoring the spread and severity of a disease during an emergency. By conducting widespread testing and surveillance, public health officials can track the number of cases, identify high-risk areas or populations, and assess the effectiveness of control measures. This information is crucial for making informed decisions about resource allocation, implementing targeted interventions, and adjusting public health strategies as needed.

Laboratories also play a critical role in evaluating the effectiveness of control measures and interventions implemented during a public health emergency. Through laboratory testing, researchers and public health authorities can assess the impact of treatments, vaccines, or preventive measures on disease outcomes. This information guides decision-making, allowing for the refinement of strategies and the optimization of public health responses to mitigate the spread of the disease.

In the context of public health emergency preparedness, laboratory networks are established and strengthened to ensure widespread access to testing capabilities. This involves the development of robust laboratory infrastructure, trained personnel, standardized testing protocols, and quality assurance mechanisms. Collaboration and coordination among laboratories at local, regional, and national levels are fostered to enhance communication, data sharing, and resource mobilization during emergencies.

Furthermore, laboratory networks in public health emergency preparedness focus on building surge capacity to handle increased testing demands during outbreaks or crises. This includes the establishment of emergency response laboratories, the procurement of necessary testing equipment and supplies, and the training of additional laboratory personnel. These measures enable laboratories to rapidly scale up their testing capacity and provide timely and accurate results to support the overall response efforts.

Laboratory networks also play a vital role in international collaboration and information sharing during public health emergencies. Through established networks and partnerships, laboratories can exchange data, share best practices, and collaborate on research and development of diagnostic tools, treatments, and vaccines. This global cooperation strengthens the collective ability to respond to cross-border threats and enhances preparedness and response efforts on a global scale.

15.1.5 Quality assurance:

QUALITY ASSURANCE: Ensuring the accuracy and reliability of laboratory test results is a critical component of a well-functioning laboratory system. Quality assurance measures are implemented to maintain high standards and ensure the validity of test results, which is essential for making informed decisions about disease control measures and maintaining public trust in the health system.

Quality assurance in laboratory testing involves a systematic approach to monitor and evaluate all aspects of the testing process, including pre-analytical, analytical, and post-analytical phases. This includes the collection, transportation, processing, analysis, and reporting of specimens. By implementing quality assurance measures, laboratories can identify and address potential sources of error, reduce variability, and ensure the accuracy and reliability of test results.

One of the key aspects of quality assurance is the establishment and adherence to standardized laboratory procedures and protocols. This includes the use of validated and approved testing methods, proper calibration and maintenance of equipment, and adherence to strict quality control measures. Standardization helps to minimize variability in test results and ensures consistency across different laboratories and testing sites.

Regular proficiency testing and external quality assessment programs are also important components of quality assurance. These programs involve the participation of laboratories in external evaluations, where their performance is assessed against established standards or proficiency panels. This allows laboratories to benchmark their performance, identify areas for improvement, and ensure the accuracy and comparability of their results.

Furthermore, robust documentation and record-keeping practices are essential for quality assurance. Laboratories must maintain detailed records of all testing procedures, including specimen collection and handling, testing methodologies, equipment calibration, and quality control results. Proper documentation allows for traceability and transparency, facilitating audits and ensuring the integrity of the testing process.

Continuous training and competency assessment of laboratory personnel are integral to quality assurance. Ongoing education and professional development programs help to ensure that laboratory staff are knowledgeable about the latest testing methodologies, quality control procedures, and safety protocols. Regular competency assessments verify the proficiency of laboratory personnel in performing tests accurately and reliably.

Accreditation and certification programs play a crucial role in quality assurance. Laboratories can seek accreditation from recognized accreditation bodies that assess their compliance with international standards and best practices. Accreditation ensures that laboratories meet specific requirements for quality management systems, technical competence, and adherence to standard operating procedures.

By implementing comprehensive quality assurance measures, laboratories can enhance the accuracy and reliability of test results, minimize errors, and ensure consistency in disease diagnosis and monitoring. This not only supports effective decision-making regarding disease control measures but also fosters public trust in the health system. Patients, healthcare providers, and public health authorities can have confidence in the reliability of laboratory testing, which is essential for effective disease management and control.

In summary, laboratory services are essential for effective disease surveillance and response, and are critical for protecting public health.

15.2 Laboratory diagnosis in IDSR

LABORATORY DIAGNOSIS is a key component of the Integrated Disease Surveillance and Response (IDSR) system.

Laboratory testing is used to confirm the diagnosis of infectious diseases, and to monitor the spread and severity of outbreaks. Here are some of the key elements of laboratory diagnosis in IDSR:

15.2.1 Laboratory capacity:

LABORATORY CAPACITY: A key aspect of an effective laboratory system is having sufficient capacity to perform diagnostic tests for infectious diseases. Laboratory capacity refers to the availability of necessary equipment, supplies, and trained personnel to conduct accurate and timely testing.

Laboratory capacity encompasses several components that are crucial for the efficient functioning of a laboratory:

15.2.1.1 Infrastructure and Equipment:

A WELL-EQUIPPED LABORATORY requires appropriate infrastructure and laboratory facilities, including adequate space, ventilation, and utilities. It also necessitates having a range of specialized laboratory equipment and instruments, such as microscopes, centrifuges, PCR machines, and culture facilities. These tools enable the laboratory to perform a wide array of diagnostic tests accurately and efficiently.

15.2.1.2 Supplies and Reagents:

LABORATORIES REQUIRE a continuous supply of high-quality reagents, consumables, and laboratory supplies to conduct diagnostic tests. This includes culture media, molecular reagents, serological test kits, personal protective equipment (PPE), and specimen collection and transport materials. Having a robust supply chain management system ensures that laboratories have access to these essential items in a timely manner.

15.2.1.3 Trained Personnel:

SKILLED AND TRAINED laboratory personnel are vital for performing diagnostic tests accurately and safely. Laboratory capacity necessitates having a competent workforce, including laboratory scientists, technicians, and technologists, who are well-versed in laboratory techniques, quality control measures, biosafety protocols, and data management. Continuous training, professional development, and competency assessments help maintain the skills and expertise of laboratory staff.

15.2.1.4 Quality Management Systems:

AN EFFECTIVE LABORATORY system incorporates quality management systems to ensure the accuracy and reliability of test results. This includes the implementation of standard operating procedures (SOPs), adherence to good laboratory practices (GLP), and participation in external quality assessment programs. Quality control measures, such as internal quality control and proficiency testing, are integral to maintaining high-quality laboratory services.

Examples of laboratory capacity in action:

1. *Outbreak Response*: During disease outbreaks, such as Ebola or COVID-19, laboratories with sufficient capacity play a critical role in rapid response efforts. They can quickly diagnose cases, monitor the spread of the disease, and provide crucial data to inform public health interventions. For example, during the Ebola outbreak in

West Africa, laboratory capacity was scaled up to enable timely diagnosis and control of the disease.

2. ***Surveillance and Monitoring***: Well-equipped laboratories with adequate capacity contribute to disease surveillance and monitoring systems. They can conduct routine testing to detect and monitor infectious diseases, identify emerging pathogens, and track changes in disease patterns. For instance, laboratories with the capacity to perform molecular testing have been instrumental in monitoring the spread and variants of SARS-CoV-2, the virus that causes COVID-19.

3. ***Research and Development***: Laboratories with strong capacity foster research and development efforts to advance the understanding of infectious diseases. They contribute to scientific studies, genetic sequencing, and the development of new diagnostic methods, treatments, and vaccines. For example, laboratories involved in influenza surveillance continuously monitor circulating strains to inform the selection of the annual flu vaccine.

4. ***Global Health Security***: Building laboratory capacity is a critical component of global health security. Strengthening laboratory systems in low- and middle-income countries enhances their ability to detect, respond to, and control infectious diseases, ultimately contributing to global health security. Initiatives such as the Global Health Security Agenda (GHSA) aim to enhance laboratory capacity in resource-limited settings to strengthen overall global health security.

15.2.2 Laboratory network:

LABORATORY NETWORK: An effective laboratory network is a vital component of a robust public health system. It involves the coordination and collaboration of multiple laboratories, both central and peripheral, to ensure that samples can be collected, transported, and analyzed in a timely and efficient manner. A well-established laboratory network facilitates the sharing of resources, expertise, and workload distribution, leading to improved disease surveillance, diagnosis, and response capabilities.

Key features and functions of a laboratory network include:

15.2.2.1 Central and Peripheral Laboratories:

A LABORATORY NETWORK typically consists of central reference laboratories and peripheral laboratories at various levels of the healthcare system. Central laboratories, often located at national or regional levels, have advanced facilities and expertise to handle complex testing procedures. Peripheral laboratories, located at local health centers or clinics, provide basic testing services and sample collection. The central laboratories act as referral centers, providing technical support, confirmatory testing, and specialized diagnostic services to peripheral laboratories.

15.2.2.2 Sample Collection and Transport:

AN EFFECTIVE LABORATORY network ensures the availability of standardized procedures and materials for sample collection, packaging, and transportation. Guidelines are established to ensure the proper handling and preservation of samples during transit to maintain their integrity. This includes providing appropriate containers, transport media, and cold chain management for samples that require specific temperature control.

15.2.2.3 Referral Mechanisms:

A LABORATORY NETWORK establishes clear referral mechanisms to ensure the efficient flow of samples and information between peripheral and central laboratories. Peripheral laboratories initially handle routine diagnostic testing, and if necessary, refer samples to central laboratories for further analysis, specialized testing, or confirmation of results. Referral mechanisms may include electronic systems for requesting and tracking samples, as well as communication channels for consultations between laboratories.

15.2.2.4 Capacity Building and Quality Assurance:

A LABORATORY NETWORK facilitates capacity building initiatives by providing training and technical assistance to laboratory staff at all levels. This includes training in sample collection techniques, diagnostic procedures, quality control measures, biosafety practices, and data management. Quality assurance programs, including proficiency testing and external quality assessment schemes, are implemented to ensure the accuracy and reliability of test results across the laboratory network.

Examples of laboratory networks in action:

1. *Disease Surveillance and Outbreak Response*: In the event of a disease outbreak, a well-functioning laboratory network plays a crucial role in timely detection and response. Peripheral laboratories collect and test samples from suspected cases, and if necessary, refer samples to central laboratories for confirmatory testing. This coordinated approach enables rapid identification of the

causative agent, facilitates early response interventions, and helps monitor the spread of the disease.

2. ***Screening and Diagnosis Programs***: Laboratory networks support screening and diagnosis programs for infectious diseases. For instance, in the case of HIV/AIDS, a laboratory network may be established to provide widespread access to testing services. Peripheral laboratories perform initial screening tests, and positive samples are referred to central laboratories for confirmatory testing, viral load monitoring, and resistance testing. This coordinated approach ensures accurate diagnosis and appropriate treatment for individuals.

3. ***Antimicrobial Resistance Monitoring***: Laboratory networks are instrumental in monitoring antimicrobial resistance patterns. Peripheral laboratories collect and test clinical samples to determine the susceptibility of pathogens to various antimicrobial agents. This data is then shared with central laboratories for analysis, interpretation, and reporting. The information gathered from the laboratory network helps guide antimicrobial stewardship programs and informs treatment guidelines.

4. ***International Collaboration and Reference Laboratories***: Laboratory networks often collaborate with international reference laboratories and networks to enhance their capabilities. This collaboration may involve sharing of technical expertise, training programs, proficiency testing, and quality assurance support. Reference laboratories provide specialized testing, genetic sequencing, and expertise for emerging infectious diseases, enabling rapid response and global collaboration.

15.2.3 Laboratory test menu:

LABORATORY NETWORK: A laboratory network is a coordinated system of interconnected laboratories that work collaboratively to support disease surveillance, diagnosis, and response efforts. The network includes both central and peripheral laboratories, each with specific roles and functions, and it ensures a seamless flow of samples, information, and expertise. A well-organized laboratory network is crucial for timely and accurate testing, especially during public health emergencies and disease outbreaks.

15.2.3.1 Components of a laboratory network:

1. **Central Laboratories**: These are high-capacity, well-equipped laboratories often located in major cities or central regions of a country or territory. Central laboratories are equipped with advanced diagnostic technologies and have a broader range of testing capabilities. They serve as the reference point for more complex or specialized tests and are responsible for confirming and validating results from peripheral laboratories.

2. **Peripheral Laboratories**: Peripheral or satellite laboratories are situated in various locations, including rural areas, smaller towns, or health facilities. These laboratories are closer to the population, which facilitates the collection and transportation of samples with reduced turnaround time. They are equipped to conduct routine and essential diagnostic tests, enabling rapid identification of common infectious diseases.

3. *Sample Collection and Transportation*: A well-functioning laboratory network establishes efficient

sample collection and transportation mechanisms. This involves providing healthcare workers with the necessary tools and training to collect specimens correctly. Samples are then safely transported to the appropriate laboratory, following proper handling and storage protocols to maintain sample integrity.

4. **Referral Mechanisms**: The laboratory network should have established referral mechanisms that allow peripheral laboratories to send samples to central laboratories for further testing or confirmation of complex cases. These mechanisms ensure that rare or hard-to-diagnose diseases can be accurately identified, even in remote areas.

5. *Information Exchange and Communication*: Effective communication is essential within the laboratory network. This includes sharing test results, disease surveillance data, and outbreak information among laboratories, public health authorities, and relevant stakeholders. Timely information exchange allows for quick decision-making and response coordination.

15.2.3.2 Importance of a laboratory network:

1. *Rapid Response to Outbreaks*: During disease outbreaks, such as pandemics or localized outbreaks, a well-connected laboratory network enables early detection and response. Peripheral laboratories can quickly identify potential cases, and central laboratories can confirm diagnoses and provide guidance on appropriate control measures.

2. *Equitable Healthcare Access*: Having peripheral laboratories in various locations ensures that people in

remote or underserved areas can access diagnostic services promptly. This reduces the need for patients to travel long distances for testing and facilitates early disease detection and management.

3. ***Surveillance and Monitoring***: A laboratory network enhances disease surveillance and monitoring capabilities. By aggregating data from multiple sources, public health authorities can identify trends, hotspots, and emerging infectious diseases, facilitating evidence-based decision-making.

4. ***Research and Collaboration***: Laboratory networks promote collaboration between different institutions and researchers. They enable the pooling of resources, expertise, and data, leading to more comprehensive studies and advancements in infectious disease research.

15.2.3.3 Examples of a laboratory network in action:

1. ***Influenza Surveillance***: A laboratory network focused on influenza monitors the prevalence and characteristics of circulating influenza strains. Peripheral laboratories collect respiratory samples from patients with flu-like symptoms, while central laboratories analyze and characterize the viruses. This data informs the composition of seasonal influenza vaccines.

2. ***COVID-19 Testing***: During the COVID-19 pandemic, many countries established laboratory networks to scale up testing capacity. Peripheral laboratories, including mobile testing units, collected samples, while central laboratories conducted RT-PCR tests for confirmation. This allowed for widespread testing and monitoring of the pandemic's progression.

3. ***Global Health Initiatives***: International organizations and initiatives, such as the World Health Organization (WHO) and the Global Health Security Agenda (GHSA), work with countries to strengthen laboratory networks. They provide technical assistance, training, and resources to improve laboratory infrastructure and capacity, particularlyin resource-limited settings, with the aim of enhancing disease surveillance, response capabilities, and overall global health security.

4. ***One Health Approach***: The One Health approach recognizes the interconnectedness of human, animal, and environmental health. A laboratory network following the One Health framework collaborates across sectors, including human health, veterinary medicine, and environmental sciences. This facilitates the detection and monitoring of zoonotic diseases and enhances preparedness for potential outbreaks.

IN SUMMARY, A LABORATORY network plays a crucial role in ensuring the timely and efficient collection, transportation, and analysis of samples for disease surveillance, diagnosis, and response. It involves central and peripheral laboratories, effective sample referral mechanisms, and information exchange. A well-established laboratory network enables rapid outbreak response, equitable access to diagnostic services, enhanced surveillance capabilities, and research collaboration. By strengthening laboratory networks, countries can enhance their ability to detect, respond to, and control infectious diseases effectively.

15.2.4 Laboratory data management:

EFFECTIVE LABORATORY data management is essential for the collection, analysis, and reporting of laboratory test results, as well as the monitoring of laboratory capacity and performance. It involves the systematic organization, storage, analysis, and sharing of data to support informed decision-making, quality assurance, and public health actions.

15.2.4.1 Key aspects of laboratory data management:

DATA COLLECTION: LABORATORY data management starts with the collection of accurate and complete data. This includes capturing essential patient information, test results, specimen details, and other relevant metadata. The data can be collected through various methods, such as electronic laboratory information systems (LIS), paper-based forms, or direct integration with diagnostic devices.

1. ***Data Quality Assurance***: To ensure the accuracy and reliability of laboratory data, quality assurance measures are implemented. This involves data validation, verification, and adherence to standardized protocols. Data quality checks can identify errors, inconsistencies, or missing information, allowing for corrective actions to be taken.

2. ***Data Storage and Security***: Laboratory data should be securely stored to protect patient privacy and maintain data integrity. Electronic storage systems, such as secure databases or cloud-based platforms, are commonly used to store laboratory data. Strict access controls, encryption, and backup mechanisms are implemented to safeguard data from unauthorized access, loss, or corruption.

3. ***Data Analysis: Laboratory data analysis*** involves interpreting and extracting meaningful insights from the collected data. Statistical techniques, data visualization

tools, and epidemiological analysis methods are employed to identify patterns, trends, and correlations. Data analysis helps in understanding disease dynamics, monitoring outbreaks, and evaluating the performance of laboratory services.

4. ***Reporting and Communication***: Timely and accurate reporting of laboratory data is crucial for effective public health response. Laboratory data is communicated to relevant stakeholders, such as healthcare providers, public health authorities, and researchers. Clear and concise reports are generated, summarizing key findings, test results, and trends, enabling informed decision-making and appropriate interventions.

5. ***Integration with Surveillance Systems***: Laboratory data management is closely linked with disease surveillance systems. Integration of laboratory data with broader surveillance systems allows for comprehensive monitoring of disease trends, early detection of outbreaks, and evaluation of control measures. Real-time data exchange facilitates timely response and collaboration between laboratories and public health authorities.

15.2.4.2 Importance of laboratory data management:

1. ***Evidence-Based Decision-Making***: Accurate and timely laboratory data supports evidence-based decision-making for disease control and prevention. It provides critical information on disease burden, outbreak detection, and the effectiveness of interventions.

2. ***Quality Assurance***: Effective data management ensures the quality and reliability of laboratory test results. This supports quality assurance programs, proficiency testing,

and internal audits, enhancing the overall reliability and credibility of laboratory services.

3. ***Surveillance and Monitoring***: Laboratory data is an essential component of disease surveillance systems. By integrating laboratory data with other health data sources, surveillance systems can detect and monitor disease trends, identify emerging threats, and guide public health responses.

4. ***Research and Innovation***: Properly managed laboratory data serves as a valuable resource for research and innovation. Researchers can utilize aggregated and anonymized laboratory data to conduct studies, develop new diagnostic methods, and contribute to scientific advancements in infectious disease management.

15.2.4.3 Examples of laboratory data management:

1. ***National Notifiable Disease Reporting***: In many countries, laboratory data management systems are integrated with national notifiable disease reporting systems. This enables laboratories to report specific diseases, test results, and demographic information to public health authorities in a standardized format, facilitating real-time disease surveillance and response.

2. ***Electronic Laboratory Information Systems (LIS)***: Many laboratories utilize electronic LIS to manage and analyze laboratory data efficiently. LIS allows for seamless data entry, result generation, and integration with other health information systems. It improves workflow efficiency, reduces errors, and enables faster data retrieval and analysis.

IN SUMMARY, LABORATORY diagnosis is an essential component of the IDSR system. A well-functioning laboratory system is needed to confirm diagnoses, monitor outbreaks, and inform disease control measures. Laboratory capacity, network, quality assurance, test menu, and data management are all critical elements of laboratory diagnosis in IDSR.

15.3 Case studies of laboratory services supporting IDSR in Africa

THERE ARE SEVERAL CASE studies of laboratory services supporting IDSR in Africa

15.3.1 Liberia:

DURING THE 2014-2015 Ebola outbreak, the National Public Health Institute of Liberia (NPHIL) played a key role in coordinating the laboratory response. NPHIL established a national laboratory system to provide diagnostic testing for Ebola, as well as other diseases. The laboratory network included both central and peripheral laboratories, with trained personnel and appropriate equipment and supplies. NPHIL also implemented a quality assurance program to ensure the accuracy and reliability of laboratory test results. The laboratory system played a critical role in confirming cases of Ebola, monitoring the spread of the disease, and guiding the response effort.

15.3.2 Uganda:

IN UGANDA, THE MINISTRY of Health established a national laboratory network to support the IDSR system. The network includes both central and peripheral laboratories, with a focus on priority diseases such as malaria, tuberculosis, and HIV.

The laboratories are staffed by trained personnel and equipped with appropriate technology and supplies. The Ministry of Health has also implemented a quality assurance program to ensure the accuracy and reliability of laboratory test results. The laboratory system has been instrumental in detecting outbreaks, monitoring disease trends, and guiding public health responses.

15.3.3 Nigeria:

THE NIGERIA CENTRE for Disease Control (NCDC) has established a laboratory system to support the IDSR system. The laboratory network includes both central and peripheral laboratories, with a focus on priority diseases such as cholera, meningitis, and Lassa fever. The NCDC has also developed guidelines for laboratory diagnosis and reporting, and implemented a quality assurance program. The laboratory system has been instrumental in detecting outbreaks, confirming diagnoses, and guiding disease control measures.

In summary, laboratory services play a critical role in supporting the IDSR system in Africa. Examples from Liberia, Uganda, and Nigeria demonstrate the importance of laboratory capacity, network, quality assurance, and data management in detecting outbreaks, confirming diagnoses, and guiding disease control measures.

Table 10: Case studies of laboratory services supporting IDSR in Africa

Disease	Country	Summary
Polio	Nigeria	Laboratory network for poliovirus surveillance, ensuring timely identification and characterization of poliovirus strains
Measles	Kenya	Laboratory support for measles surveillance, including confirmation of suspected cases through serological and molecular testing.
Malaria	Ghana	Malaria diagnostic laboratories providing accurate and timely diagnosis to support case management and surveillance activities.
HIV/AIDS	South Africa	Laboratory infrastructure for HIV testing, viral load monitoring, and drug resistance testing to guide treatment decisions and prevention strategies.
Tuberculosis	Ethiopia	Laboratory network for tuberculosis diagnosis and drug susceptibility testing, enabling prompt detection and appropriate treatment.

This table showcases successful disease-specific surveillance efforts in different countries.

15.4 Exercises

1. Which country established a national laboratory system to support the IDSR system during the Ebola outbreak in 2014-2015? a) Uganda b) Nigeria c) Liberia d) South Africa

Solution: c) Liberia

1. What diseases are the laboratory networks in Uganda focused on? a) Cholera, meningitis, and Lassa fever b) Malaria, tuberculosis, and HIV c) Ebola, Marburg, and yellow fever d) Measles, polio, and typhoid fever

Solution: b) Malaria, tuberculosis, and HIV

1. Which organization in Nigeria is responsible for establishing a laboratory system to support the IDSR system? a) National Public Health Institute of Nigeria (NPHIN) b) Nigerian Centre for Disease Control (NCDC) c) African Union Centre for Disease Control (CDC) d) World Health Organization (WHO)

Solution: b) Nigerian Centre for Disease Control (NCDC)

1. How did the laboratory system in Liberia support the response to the Ebola outbreak? a) By detecting outbreaks and monitoring disease trends b) By confirming cases of Ebola and guiding the response effort c) By providing diagnostic testing for other diseases in addition to Ebola d) By implementing a quality assurance program to ensure the accuracy of laboratory test results

Solution: b) By confirming cases of Ebola and guiding the response effort

1. What is the focus of the laboratory network established by the Ministry of Health in Uganda? a) Detection of outbreaks and monitoring disease trends b) Development of new diagnostic tests for priority diseases c) Expansion of laboratory services to rural areas d) Diagnosis of priority diseases such as malaria, tuberculosis, and HIV

Solution: d) Diagnosis of priority diseases such as malaria, tuberculosis, and HIV.

Chapter 16. Capacity Building for IDSR

16.1 Capacity building for IDSR implementation

Capacity building is an essential component of IDSR implementation, as it helps to ensure that health workers and other stakeholders have the necessary skills and knowledge to effectively carry out their roles in disease surveillance and response. Some of the key areas of capacity building for IDSR implementation include:

16.1.1 Training:

TRAINING PLAYS A CRITICAL role in ensuring the successful implementation and operation of the Integrated Disease Surveillance and Response (IDSR) system. It involves providing education and skill development to health workers and other stakeholders involved in disease surveillance and response activities. The aim of training is to enhance their knowledge, competencies, and capacity to effectively carry out their roles and responsibilities within the IDSR framework.

16.1.1.1 Key aspects of training in the IDSR system:

1. *Case Definitions*: Training sessions focus on familiarizing health workers with standardized case definitions for various diseases. They learn how to recognize and classify different types of cases based on specific clinical criteria.

This enables consistent identification and reporting of cases, ensuring accurate surveillance data.

2. ***Data Collection and Management***: Health workers are trained on the proper methods and tools for collecting and recording data related to disease surveillance. They learn how to accurately document information such as patient demographics, clinical signs and symptoms, laboratory results, and treatment outcomes. Training also covers data management procedures, including data entry, quality assurance, and secure storage.

3. ***Reporting and Feedback Mechanisms***: Health workers receive training on the reporting requirements of the IDSR system. They learn how to submit timely and complete reports to the designated authorities or surveillance focal points. Training emphasizes the importance of feedback mechanisms, ensuring that health workers receive information on the outcomes and actions taken based on their reports.

4. ***Outbreak Investigation and Response***: Training includes sessions on outbreak investigation and response protocols. Health workers learn how to detect and investigate disease outbreaks, including conducting epidemiological investigations, collecting and analyzing specimens, and implementing appropriate control measures. They are trained to coordinate and collaborate with other relevant stakeholders during outbreak responses.

5. ***Communication and Coordination***: Effective communication and coordination are crucial in the IDSR system. Training emphasizes the importance of clear and timely communication among health workers, surveillance officers, laboratory personnel, and other stakeholders. Participants learn about communication

channels, reporting lines, and the coordination mechanisms established within the IDSR framework.

16.1.1.2 Examples of training activities in the IDSR system:

1. ***Workshops and Seminars***: Training workshops and seminars are conducted to provide comprehensive training on the various components of the IDSR system. These events bring together health workers from different health facilities or districts to learn and exchange experiences. Facilitators deliver presentations, conduct interactive sessions, and facilitate hands-on exercises to enhance understanding and skills.

2. ***On-the-Job Training***: Health workers receive on-the-job training where experienced trainers or supervisors provide guidance and support in real-time. This approach allows for practical skill development and reinforcement of knowledge within the actual work environment. Health workers learn how to apply the principles and practices of the IDSR system while carrying out their daily responsibilities.

3. ***Training-of-Trainers***: To ensure sustainable capacity building, select individuals are trained as trainers who can then cascade the knowledge and skills to a broader audience. These trainers can provide ongoing training and mentorship to health workers at different levels, extending the reach of training activities and promoting continuous learning within the IDSR system.

4. ***E-Learning and Online Resources***: Technology-based training methods, such as e-learning platforms and online resources, are increasingly used to reach a wider audience and facilitate self-paced learning. These platforms provide

interactive modules, videos, quizzes, and downloadable resources, enabling health workers to access training materials conveniently and reinforce their knowledge.

TRAINING IN THE IDSR system aims to empower health workers and other stakeholders with the necessary knowledge and skills to effectively implement disease surveillance and response activities. By investing in training, health systems can strengthen their capacity to detect, report, and respond to infectious diseases, ultimately contributing to improved public health outcomes and early detection of potential outbreaks.

16.1.2 Infrastructure development:

IMPROVING THE PHYSICAL infrastructure is a key aspect of supporting the implementation of the Integrated Disease Surveillance and Response (IDSR) system. This involves enhancing the facilities and resources related to laboratories, health facilities, and transportation to ensure effective disease surveillance, data collection, and response activities. Here are further details on each aspect:

16.1.2.1 Laboratories:

ENHANCING LABORATORY infrastructure is crucial for accurate and timely disease diagnosis and surveillance. This includes improving the physical space and layout of laboratories, ensuring proper ventilation and biosafety measures, and equipping them with modern diagnostic tools and equipment. Upgrades may also involve establishing specialized laboratories for specific diseases or pathogens, such as biosafety level 3 (BSL-3) laboratories for handling highly infectious agents. Additionally, providing a continuous supply of high-quality reagents and consumables is essential for conducting reliable laboratory tests.

16.1.2.2 Health Facilities:

STRENGTHENING HEALTH facilities is vital for effective disease surveillance and response. This includes upgrading the infrastructure of healthcare centers, clinics, hospitals, and other health service delivery points. Upgrades may involve expanding the physical space to accommodate dedicated areas for disease surveillance, isolation, and sample collection. It is also important to ensure the availability of basic amenities such as clean water, reliable electricity, and proper waste management systems in health facilities. This creates an environment conducive to implementing the IDSR system and carrying out essential surveillance and response activities.

16.1.2.3 Transportation:

ESTABLISHING A RELIABLE transportation system is crucial for the timely collection of samples, transportation of specimens, and field investigations. This involves ensuring the availability of suitable vehicles, ambulances, or other means of transportation to reach remote areas efficiently. Upgrading transportation infrastructure, such as road networks, can improve accessibility to different regions, enabling prompt response to disease outbreaks. Moreover, establishing coordination mechanisms between health facilities and transportation services facilitates the smooth movement of personnel, supplies, and specimens, supporting effective disease surveillance and response activities.

16.1.3 Procurement and supply chain management:

PROCUREMENT AND SUPPLY chain management are critical components of the Integrated Disease Surveillance and Response (IDSR) system. They involve the processes and activities necessary to ensure the timely availability and reliable delivery of necessary equipment, supplies, and medications to support the implementation of the IDSR system. Here are further details on this aspect:

16.1.3.1 Procurement:

PROCUREMENT REFERS to the process of acquiring equipment, supplies, and medications needed for the IDSR system. It involves identifying the required items, developing specifications, soliciting bids or proposals from suppliers, evaluating and selecting the most suitable vendors, negotiating contracts, and making the necessary purchases. Effective procurement practices ensure that the equipment and supplies meet the required standards, are cost-effective, and are delivered on time.

16.1.3.2 Supply Chain Management:

SUPPLY CHAIN MANAGEMENT encompasses the planning, coordination, and control of the flow of goods, services, and information from suppliers to end-users. In the context of the IDSR system, it involves managing the entire supply chain to ensure the availability of equipment, supplies, and medications at all levels of the health system. This includes forecasting and quantification of needs, inventory management, storage and distribution, and monitoring of stock levels. Efficient supply chain management helps prevent stockouts, reduces wastage, and ensures that health facilities have the necessary resources to implement the IDSR system effectively.

16.1.3.3 Collaboration with Partners:

EFFECTIVE PROCUREMENT and supply chain management for the IDSR system often require collaboration with various partners and stakeholders. This includes engaging with manufacturers, suppliers, and distributors to ensure the availability of quality products. Collaboration with international organizations, donors, and non-governmental organizations can provide additional support in terms of funding, technical expertise, and procurement mechanisms. Establishing partnerships and leveraging existing networks can help streamline procurement processes, improve supply chain efficiency, and enhance the overall implementation of the IDSR system.

16.1.3.4 Quality Assurance:

QUALITY ASSURANCE IS a crucial aspect of procurement and supply chain management for the IDSR system. It involves establishing mechanisms to ensure that the procured equipment, supplies, and medications meet the required quality standards. This includes conducting quality checks, verifying the authenticity and reliability of suppliers, and monitoring the performance of procured items. Quality assurance measures contribute to the effectiveness and reliability of the IDSR system by ensuring that the necessary resources are of high quality and suitable for their intended use.

By focusing on procurement and supply chain management, countries can ensure the availability and accessibility of necessary equipment, supplies, and medications to support the implementation of the IDSR system. This enables effective disease surveillance, data collection, and response activities, ultimately contributing to improved public health outcomes and the prevention and control of infectious diseases.

16.1.4 Communication and coordination:

PROCUREMENT AND SUPPLY chain management are critical components of the Integrated Disease Surveillance and Response (IDSR) system. They involve the processes and activities necessary to ensure the timely availability and reliable delivery of necessary equipment, supplies, and medications to support the implementation of the IDSR system. Here are further details on this aspect:

16.1.4.1 Procurement:

PROCUREMENT REFERS to the process of acquiring equipment, supplies, and medications needed for the IDSR system. It involves identifying the required items, developing specifications, soliciting bids or proposals from suppliers, evaluating and selecting the most suitable vendors, negotiating contracts, and making the necessary purchases. Effective procurement practices ensure that the equipment and supplies meet the required standards, are cost-effective, and are delivered on time.

16.1.4.2 Supply Chain Management:

SUPPLY CHAIN MANAGEMENT encompasses the planning, coordination, and control of the flow of goods, services, and information from suppliers to end-users. In the context of the IDSR system, it involves managing the entire supply chain to ensure the availability of equipment, supplies, and medications at all levels of the health system. This includes forecasting and quantification of needs, inventory management, storage and distribution, and monitoring of stock levels. Efficient supply chain management helps prevent stockouts, reduces wastage, and ensures that health facilities have the necessary resources to implement the IDSR system effectively.

16.1.4.3 Collaboration with Partners:

EFFECTIVE PROCUREMENT and supply chain management for the IDSR system often require collaboration with various partners and stakeholders. This includes engaging with manufacturers, suppliers, and distributors to ensure the availability of quality products. Collaboration with international organizations, donors, and non-governmental organizations can provide additional support in terms of funding, technical expertise, and procurement mechanisms. Establishing partnerships and leveraging existing networks can help streamline procurement processes, improve supply chain efficiency, and enhance the overall implementation of the IDSR system.

16.1.4.4 Quality Assurance:

QUALITY ASSURANCE IS a crucial aspect of procurement and supply chain management for the IDSR system. It involves establishing mechanisms to ensure that the procured equipment, supplies, and medications meet the required quality standards. This includes conducting quality checks, verifying the authenticity and reliability of suppliers, and monitoring the performance of procured items. Quality assurance measures contribute to the effectiveness and reliability of the IDSR system by ensuring that the necessary resources are of high quality and suitable for their intended use.

By focusing on procurement and supply chain management, countries can ensure the availability and accessibility of necessary equipment, supplies, and medications to support the implementation of the IDSR system. This enables effective disease surveillance, data collection, and response activities, ultimately contributing to improved public health outcomes and the prevention and control of infectious disease.

16.1.5 Monitoring and evaluation:

MONITORING AND EVALUATION are essential components of the Integrated Disease Surveillance and Response (IDSR) system. They involve the systematic assessment of the system's performance, data quality, and impact to ensure its effectiveness and identify areas for improvement. Here are further details on this aspect:

16.1.5.1 Performance Monitoring:

MONITORING THE PERFORMANCE of the IDSR system involves tracking key indicators and outputs to assess its functionality and adherence to established standards. This includes monitoring the timeliness and completeness of disease reporting, laboratory testing rates, data quality, and the overall functionality of surveillance and response activities. Regular performance monitoring allows for the identification of bottlenecks, gaps, and areas requiring improvement in the system's implementation.

16.1.5.2 Data Quality Assessment:

DATA QUALITY IS CRUCIAL for the accuracy and reliability of disease surveillance and response. Monitoring and evaluation of the IDSR system involve assessing the quality of collected data, including completeness, accuracy, and timeliness. This assessment can be done through data audits, site visits, and verification exercises. By identifying data quality issues, appropriate corrective measures can be implemented to ensure that the information collected is valid and can be used for decision-making.

16.1.5.3 Feedback and Reporting:

MONITORING AND EVALUATION also involve establishing feedback mechanisms to provide timely information to health workers, stakeholders, and decision-makers. Regular reporting on the performance of the IDSR system, including strengths, challenges, and recommendations, enables informed decision-making and supports the continuous improvement of the system. Feedback loops ensure that stakeholders are aware of the system's progress and can make necessary adjustments or interventions as needed.

16.1.5.4 Impact Assessment:

EVALUATING THE IMPACT of the IDSR system is essential to determine its effectiveness in detecting and responding to disease outbreaks, reducing morbidity and mortality, and improving overall public health outcomes. Impact assessments may involve analyzing surveillance data, outbreak response timelines, and comparing pre- and post-implementation indicators. By assessing the system's impact, strengths can be reinforced, weaknesses can be addressed, and evidence-based recommendations can be made to enhance the IDSR system's effectiveness.

16.1.5.5 Continuous Improvement:

MONITORING AND EVALUATION activities in the IDSR system contribute to a culture of continuous improvement. Findings from evaluations and performance monitoring help identify areas for strengthening and guide the implementation of targeted interventions. Lessons learned from monitoring and evaluation processes can inform policy and programmatic decisions, leading to ongoing improvements in the IDSR system's functionality and impact.

By conducting regular monitoring and evaluation of the IDSR system, countries can identify gaps, address challenges, and optimize the system's performance. This ensures that disease surveillance and response activities are efficient, effective, and aligned with public health priorities, ultimately contributing to the prevention, detection, and control of infectious diseases.

Capacity building for IDSR implementation can be carried out through a variety of approaches, such as on-the-job training, workshops, and mentorship programs. It is important to ensure that capacity building efforts are tailored to the specific needs of each country or region, and that they are sustained over the long term to ensure the ongoing effectiveness of the IDSR system.

Table 11: Capacity Building for IDSR

Title	Description
Capacity building for IDSR implementation	This section emphasizes the importance of capacity building activities, including training programs, resource mobilization, and stakeholder engagement, to strengthen IDSR implementation in African countries.
Importance of training and communication in IDSR	It explores the role of training programs and effective communication strategies in enhancing the knowledge and skills of healthcare workers, surveillance officers, and other stakeholders involved in IDSR.
Case studies of successful capacity building for IDSR in Africa	This section presents case studies that showcase successful capacity building initiatives in African countries, highlighting the outcomes, lessons learned, and best practices for sustainable implementation of IDSR.

This table highlights the significance of capacity building activities for the implementation of the Integrated Disease Surveillance and Response (IDSR) system in African countries. It emphasizes the importance of training programs, resource mobilization, and stakeholder engagement in strengthening IDSR implementation.

16.2 Importance of training and communication in IDSR

TRAINING AND COMMUNICATION are crucial components of IDSR implementation, as they are essential for ensuring that health workers and other stakeholders have the necessary skills and knowledge to effectively carry out their roles in disease surveillance and response. Here are some specific reasons why training and communication are important in IDSR:

16.2.1 Consistent and accurate implementation:

CONSISTENT AND ACCURATE implementation of the Integrated Disease Surveillance and Response (IDSR) system is crucial for its effectiveness in detecting and responding to diseases. Training plays a vital role in achieving this goal by equipping health workers and stakeholders with the necessary knowledge and skills. Here are further details on the importance of consistent and accurate implementation:

16.2.1.1 Understanding the IDSR System:

TRAINING PROVIDES HEALTH workers and stakeholders with a comprehensive understanding of the IDSR system, including its objectives, components, and processes. This includes familiarizing them with case definitions, data collection and management protocols, reporting mechanisms, and outbreak investigation and response procedures. Understanding the system's principles and protocols ensures consistent and standardized implementation across different levels of the health system.

16.2.1.2 Standardized Data Collection and Reporting:

TRAINING ENABLES HEALTH workers to collect data using standardized methods and tools. This ensures that data is collected consistently and accurately, facilitating comparability and reliability. Health workers learn how to identify and classify diseases based on standardized case definitions, collect relevant information, and record it in a systematic manner. They are also trained on data reporting requirements, including the format, frequency, and channels for submitting data to higher levels of the health system.

16.2.1.3 Quality Assurance:

TRAINING PROGRAMS EMPHASIZE the importance of quality assurance in implementing the IDSR system. Health workers are trained on data quality assessment techniques, including data validation, data cleaning, and data verification. They learn how to identify and address common data quality issues, such as missing or inconsistent data. By ensuring data accuracy and completeness, training contributes to reliable disease surveillance and response.

16.2.1.4 Capacity Building:

TRAINING PROGRAMS PROVIDE health workers with the necessary skills to carry out their roles effectively within the IDSR system. This includes training on epidemiological principles, data analysis techniques, and interpretation of surveillance data. Health workers also learn how to use relevant tools and software for data management and analysis. By enhancing their capacity, training empowers health workers to accurately implement the IDSR system and make informed decisions based on surveillance data.

16.2.1.5 Continuous Learning and Updating:

TRAINING IS NOT A ONE-time event but an ongoing process. As the IDSR system evolves and new diseases or challenges emerge, health workers and stakeholders need to stay updated and adapt their practices accordingly. Regular refresher training sessions, workshops, and knowledge-sharing platforms facilitate continuous learning and ensure that health workers are equipped with the latest information and skills. This promotes consistent and accurate implementation of the IDSR system over time.

By ensuring consistent and accurate implementation of the IDSR system through training, countries can improve the reliability and validity of disease surveillance data. This, in turn, enhances the ability to detect and respond to public health threats promptly and effectively. It also supports evidence-based decision-making, resource allocation, and the implementation of appropriate control measures to protect public health.

16.2.2 Early detection and response:

HEALTH WORKERS WHO receive proper training in Integrated Disease Surveillance and Response (IDSR) play a critical role in the early detection and response to disease outbreaks. Here are further details on how their training enables early detection and response:

16.2.2.1 Knowledge of Disease Surveillance:

THROUGH TRAINING, HEALTH workers gain a comprehensive understanding of the IDSR system, including the principles of disease surveillance. They learn about the signs and symptoms of various diseases, the importance of timely case identification, and the significance of early reporting. This knowledge allows them to recognize and suspect potential outbreaks based on clinical presentations and epidemiological patterns.

16.2.2.2 Effective Data Collection and Analysis:

TRAINING EQUIPS HEALTH workers with the skills to collect, manage, and analyze surveillance data efficiently. They learn how to identify and report cases following standardized case definitions and reporting protocols. By promptly and accurately recording and analyzing data, health workers can identify unusual patterns or clusters of cases, indicating a potential outbreak. This early detection enables a rapid response to contain the spread of the disease.

16.2.2.3 Timely Reporting:

TRAINED HEALTH WORKERS understand the importance of timely reporting in the IDSR system. They are familiar with the reporting channels and procedures to notify relevant authorities about suspected cases or outbreaks. Prompt reporting facilitates a swift response from public health authorities, enabling them to investigate and implement control measures as soon as possible.

16.2.2.4 Outbreak Investigation and Response:

HEALTH WORKERS TRAINED in IDSR are equipped with the knowledge and skills to conduct outbreak investigations. They learn how to conduct epidemiological assessments, including contact tracing and risk factor analysis. With this information, they can identify the source of the outbreak, its transmission dynamics, and the populations at risk. Based on these findings, trained health workers can initiate appropriate response measures promptly, such as targeted case finding, isolation and treatment, and preventive measures like vaccination campaigns.

16.2.2.5 Collaboration and Communication:

IDSR TRAINING EMPHASIZES the importance of collaboration and communication among health workers, stakeholders, and public health authorities. Trained health workers understand the significance of timely and accurate information sharing during outbreaks. They are trained to collaborate with other health facilities, laboratories, and relevant partners to strengthen surveillance and response efforts. Effective communication ensures that vital information reaches decision-makers promptly, enabling them to make informed and timely decisions.

By having well-trained health workers who are proficient in IDSR, early detection and response to disease outbreaks are greatly enhanced. This timely response can prevent the further spread of the disease, reduce morbidity and mortality rates, and mitigate the overall impact on public health. Early detection and response also contribute to building public trust in the health system, as people see that authorities are proactive in safeguarding their health and well-being.

16.2.3 Timely reporting:

TIMELY REPORTING IS a crucial aspect of the Integrated Disease Surveillance and Response (IDSR) system. It enables prompt action and response to disease outbreaks. Here are further details on the importance of timely reporting and how effective communication facilitates it:

16.2.3.1 Clear Reporting Channels:

HEALTH WORKERS NEED to be aware of the designated reporting channels within the IDSR system. Training programs emphasize the importance of clear and streamlined reporting pathways. This includes knowing whom to report to, such as local health authorities, surveillance officers, or designated focal points. Having well-defined reporting channels ensures that information flows smoothly and reaches the appropriate authorities without delays.

16.2.3.2 Standardized Reporting Protocols:

EFFECTIVE COMMUNICATION in the IDSR system involves providing health workers with clear guidelines on what information to report. This includes standardized case definitions, data elements, and reporting formats. Uniform reporting protocols ensure that essential information is consistently collected and reported, facilitating the timely identification of disease outbreaks.

16.2.3.3 Rapid Information Sharing:

TIMELY REPORTING RELIES on efficient communication between health workers and relevant stakeholders. Health facilities should have established mechanisms for transmitting information rapidly to the appropriate authorities. This can be through electronic reporting systems, telephone hotlines, or designated reporting forms. Rapid information sharing enables public health authorities to receive real-time data on suspected cases or outbreaks, allowing them to respond promptly.

16.2.3.4 Early Warning Systems:

EFFECTIVE COMMUNICATION supports the implementation of early warning systems in the IDSR system. These systems utilize various data sources, such as syndromic surveillance, laboratory results, and event-based surveillance, to detect early signals of disease outbreaks. Timely reporting of relevant data enables the early detection of potential outbreaks, triggering immediate response activities.

16.2.3.5 Feedback Mechanisms:

TIMELY REPORTING IS reinforced through feedback mechanisms that provide health workers with information on the outcome of their reports. This feedback loop strengthens communication and encourages continued adherence to reporting protocols. Health workers who receive feedback on the reports they submit are more likely to remain engaged and committed to timely reporting.

16.2.3.6 Data Validation and Quality Assurance:

TIMELY REPORTING ALSO involves ensuring the accuracy and quality of the reported data. Health workers should receive training on data validation techniques and quality assurance processes. This ensures that the information reported is reliable, enabling effective decision-making and response planning.

By promoting effective communication and emphasizing the importance of timely reporting, the IDSR system can respond swiftly to disease outbreaks. Rapid reporting allows public health authorities to initiate timely investigations, implement control measures, and allocate resources appropriately. Ultimately, this contributes to early containment of outbreaks and minimizes their impact on public health.

16.2.4 Coordination:

COORDINATION IS A CRITICAL aspect of the Integrated Disease Surveillance and Response (IDSR) system, and effective communication plays a key role in facilitating this coordination. Here's why coordination is essential and how communication enables seamless collaboration during disease outbreaks:

1. *Multi-Sectoral Collaboration*: Disease outbreaks often require a response that involves multiple sectors and agencies, such as health departments, agriculture, education, and transportation. Effective communication ensures that all relevant stakeholders can share information, expertise, and resources. It allows for a coordinated effort among different sectors to address the outbreak comprehensively.

2. *Data Sharing and Analysis*: Coordination relies on the timely sharing of data and information among various entities involved in disease surveillance and response. Health workers at different levels (local, regional, national) need to communicate with each other to report suspected cases and share surveillance data. This data sharing enables a more comprehensive analysis of the outbreak's magnitude and trends, facilitating evidence-based decision-making.

3. *Resource Allocation*: During disease outbreaks, resources like medical supplies, personnel, and funding need to be allocated efficiently. Effective communication ensures that health authorities at all levels are aware of the resource needs and available resources. This allows for strategic allocation based on the severity and location of the outbreak, preventing unnecessary delays or duplication of efforts.

4. *Rapid Response Deployment*: Timely communication enables swift deployment of response teams to affected areas. Health workers and response teams can be quickly mobilized to conduct investigations, implement control measures, and provide medical assistance. Coordination through effective communication streamlines response efforts, reducing the impact of the outbreak.

5. ***Information Dissemination***: Coordination involves disseminating information to the public and other relevant stakeholders. Clear and accurate communication helps in providing guidance on preventive measures, treatment options, and the current status of the outbreak. Public awareness campaigns can be coordinated to ensure consistent messaging and avoid confusion.

6. ***Joint Outbreak Investigation***: When outbreaks occur, conducting investigations is crucial to understand the source, transmission patterns, and risk factors. Effective communication allows different agencies and laboratories to collaborate on joint outbreak investigations. This comprehensive approach enhances the quality and reliability of findings.

7. ***Cross-Border Collaboration***: Disease outbreaks may transcend national borders, requiring coordination with neighboring countries. Effective communication facilitates cross-border information sharing, joint surveillance, and response efforts. This international collaboration is particularly important for addressing emerging infectious diseases.

In summary, coordination is fundamental for an effective response to disease outbreaks, and effective communication is the linchpin that enables seamless collaboration among health workers, laboratories, and government agencies. By fostering open channels of communication and information exchange, the IDSR system can harness collective efforts to detect, respond to, and control outbreaks efficiently, ultimately safeguarding public health.

16.2.5 Sustainability:

SUSTAINABILITY IS A crucial aspect of the Integrated Disease Surveillance and Response (IDSR) system. Training and communication play significant roles in ensuring the continued effectiveness and longevity of the system. Here's how training and communication contribute to the sustainability of the IDSR system:

16.2.5.1 Continuous Professional Development:

TRAINING PROGRAMS PROVIDE health workers and other stakeholders with the necessary knowledge and skills to carry out their roles effectively within the IDSR system. Ongoing training and capacity-building initiatives help to update their understanding of disease surveillance and response, as well as the latest methodologies and technologies. This enables them to adapt to evolving challenges and continue delivering quality services.

16.2.5.2 Knowledge Transfer:

TRAINING ENSURES THE transfer of knowledge and expertise from experienced professionals to new recruits and other stakeholders. By imparting essential skills and sharing best practices, training programs help to maintain a pool of competent personnel within the IDSR system. This knowledge transfer ensures continuity and prevents a knowledge gap when experienced individuals retire or move on to other positions.

16.2.5.3 Updated Guidelines and Protocols:

COMMUNICATION CHANNELS play a vital role in disseminating updated guidelines, protocols, and standard operating procedures (SOPs) to health workers and stakeholders. Regular communication keeps them informed about any changes in case definitions, data collection methods, reporting mechanisms, or outbreak investigation guidelines. This ensures that the IDSR system remains aligned with current best practices and international standards.

16.2.5.4 Knowledge Exchange and Networking:

COMMUNICATION PLATFORMS, such as workshops, conferences, and online forums, facilitate knowledge exchange and networking among health workers and stakeholders. These opportunities encourage the sharing of experiences, challenges, and lessons learned in implementing the IDSR system. Collaboration and shared learning contribute to continuous improvement and innovation within the system.

16.2.5.5 Feedback Mechanisms:

EFFECTIVE COMMUNICATION includes establishing feedback mechanisms where health workers and stakeholders can provide input, report challenges, and suggest improvements in the IDSR system. Feedback loops help identify gaps or bottlenecks in the implementation process and provide an avenue for addressing them. By incorporating feedback, the system can evolve and adapt to changing needs and contexts.

16.2.5.6 Institutionalization:

THROUGH CONSISTENT training and communication efforts, the IDSR system becomes embedded within the institutional framework of the healthcare system. It becomes an integral part of routine operations rather than a temporary or ad hoc response to specific outbreaks. By integrating IDSR practices into routine healthcare activities, sustainability is ensured, and the system becomes ingrained in the organizational culture.

16.2.5.7 Advocacy and Support:

EFFECTIVE COMMUNICATION also involves advocating for the importance of the IDSR system and securing ongoing support from decision-makers, policymakers, and funding agencies. By highlighting the benefits and demonstrating the impact of the system, advocates can secure the necessary resources and political commitment for its sustainability.

By investing in continuous training and maintaining open lines of communication, the IDSR system can be sustained and continually improved. This ensures that health workers and stakeholders remain knowledgeable, motivated, and equipped to effectively implement disease surveillance and response activities, contributing to the long-term success of the system in protecting public health.

16.3 Case studies of successful capacity building for IDSR in Africa including Liberia

HERE ARE SOME CASE studies of successful capacity building for IDSR in Africa, including Liberia:

16.3.1 Liberia:

THE LIBERIAN MINISTRY of Health has implemented a comprehensive capacity building program for IDSR, which includes training for health workers at all levels of the healthcare system, as well as laboratory staff, surveillance officers, and other stakeholders. The program has been successful in improving the quality and timeliness of disease surveillance and response in Liberia. For example, during the 2014 Ebola outbreak, the IDSR system in Liberia was able to detect and respond to the outbreak quickly, which helped to prevent the disease from spreading further.

16.3.2 Ethiopia:

ETHIOPIA HAS IMPLEMENTED a national capacity building program for IDSR, which includes training for health workers, laboratory staff, and surveillance officers, as well as the development of guidelines and standard operating procedures for disease surveillance and response. The program has been successful in improving the quality and timeliness of disease surveillance and response in Ethiopia. For example, during the 2013 polio outbreak, the IDSR system in Ethiopia was able to detect and respond to the outbreak quickly, which helped to prevent the disease from spreading further.

16.3.3 Ghana:

GHANA HAS IMPLEMENTED a comprehensive capacity building program for IDSR, which includes training for health workers, laboratory staff, and surveillance officers, as well as the development of guidelines and standard operating procedures for disease surveillance and response. The program has been successful in improving the quality and timeliness of disease surveillance and response in Ghana. For example, during the 2014 cholera outbreak, the IDSR system in Ghana was able to detect and respond to the outbreak quickly, which helped to prevent the disease from spreading further.

In each of these cases, capacity building programs have played a crucial role in improving the quality and timeliness of disease surveillance and response, which has helped to prevent the spread of infectious diseases and improve public health outcomes.

16.4 Importance of monitoring and evaluating IDSR implementation

MONITORING AND EVALUATING Integrated Disease Surveillance and Response (IDSR) implementation is important for several reasons:

16.4.1 Improving system effectiveness:

MONITORING AND EVALUATING the implementation of the Integrated Disease Surveillance and Response (IDSR) system is essential for identifying areas that require improvement and enhancing the overall effectiveness of the system. Here's how monitoring and evaluation contribute to improving the effectiveness of the IDSR system:

16.4.1.1 Identifying Weaknesses:

THROUGH SYSTEMATIC monitoring and evaluation, weaknesses or gaps in the IDSR system can be identified. This includes assessing the completeness, accuracy, and timeliness of data collection, reporting, and response activities. By pinpointing areas of weakness, stakeholders can develop targeted interventions to address the identified challenges.

16.4.1.2 Enhancing Data Quality:

MONITORING AND EVALUATION efforts help assess the quality of surveillance data collected within the IDSR system. This includes evaluating the consistency and reliability of data sources, data accuracy, and data management practices. By identifying and addressing data quality issues, such as inconsistencies or missing data, stakeholders can improve the reliability and usefulness of the surveillance data for decision-making.

16.4.1.3 Strengthening Reporting Mechanisms:

MONITORING AND EVALUATION help assess the efficiency and effectiveness of reporting mechanisms within the IDSR system. This includes evaluating the reporting timeliness, completeness, and feedback loops. By identifying bottlenecks or delays in the reporting process, stakeholders can streamline and improve reporting mechanisms, ensuring timely and accurate flow of information.

16.4.1.4 Assessing Response Measures:

EVALUATION OF RESPONSE measures taken during disease outbreaks or public health emergencies provides insights into their effectiveness and impact. This involves assessing the timeliness of response activities, appropriateness of interventions implemented, and their overall effectiveness in controlling the spread of diseases and mitigating their impact. By learning from past experiences and evaluating response measures, stakeholders can refine and enhance future response strategies.

16.4.1.5 Feedback for Improvement:

MONITORING AND EVALUATION processes provide feedback to health workers and other stakeholders involved in the IDSR system. This feedback highlights areas that need improvement, provides recognition for good practices, and encourages continuous learning and professional development. Feedback mechanisms foster a culture of continuous improvement and enable stakeholders to adapt and refine their practices based on evidence and feedback.

16.4.1.6 Evidence-Based Decision-Making:

MONITORING AND EVALUATION provide evidence and data for decision-making processes. By generating reliable and timely information on disease trends, outbreak patterns, and response effectiveness, stakeholders can make informed decisions to allocate resources, prioritize interventions, and adjust strategies as needed. Evidence-based decision-making strengthens the effectiveness of the IDSR system and enhances its ability to respond to public health threats.

16.4.1.7 Capacity Building:

MONITORING AND EVALUATION activities can help identify capacity gaps within the IDSR system. By assessing the training needs of health workers and stakeholders, capacity-building initiatives can be tailored to address specific areas requiring improvement. Training programs, workshops, and mentoring opportunities can enhance the skills and knowledge of individuals involved in surveillance and response activities, thereby improving the overall effectiveness of the system.

Overall, monitoring and evaluation play a critical role in driving continuous improvement within the IDSR system. By identifying weaknesses, enhancing data quality, strengthening reporting mechanisms, assessing response measures, providing feedback, and supporting evidence-based decision-making, stakeholders can optimize the effectiveness of the system and enhance its ability to detect, respond to, and control infectious diseases effectively.

16.4.2 Measuring progress:

MONITORING AND EVALUATING the implementation of the Integrated Disease Surveillance and Response (IDSR) system is crucial for measuring progress and assessing the extent to which program goals and objectives are being achieved. Here's how monitoring and evaluation contribute to measuring progress within the IDSR system:

16.4.2.1 Goal Tracking:

MONITORING AND EVALUATION provide a framework for tracking progress towards the goals and objectives set for the IDSR system. By establishing clear indicators and targets, stakeholders can systematically measure and assess progress over time. This allows for regular monitoring of key performance areas and enables comparisons against established benchmarks.

16.4.2.2 Outcome Evaluation:

EVALUATION ACTIVITIES within the IDSR system assess the outcomes and impacts of implemented interventions. This includes evaluating the effectiveness of disease surveillance in detecting outbreaks, the efficiency of response measures in controlling disease spread, and the overall impact on public health outcomes.

By measuring these outcomes, stakeholders can gauge the progress made in reducing disease burden and improving public health.

16.4.2.3 Performance Assessment:

MONITORING AND EVALUATION provide a mechanism for assessing the performance of the IDSR system and its various components. This includes evaluating the performance of health workers, laboratories, reporting systems, and response mechanisms. By measuring performance indicators, such as data completeness, timeliness of reporting, and response time, stakeholders can identify areas that require improvement and make necessary adjustments to enhance performance.

16.4.2.4 Identifying Successes and Challenges:

MONITORING AND EVALUATION activities help to identify both successes and challenges within the IDSR system. By examining program outputs and outcomes, stakeholders can identify areas where the system is functioning well and achieving its intended goals. Similarly, challenges and barriers can be identified, allowing for targeted interventions to address those issues and overcome obstacles to progress.

16.4.2.5 Accountability and Transparency:

MONITORING AND EVALUATION contribute to accountability and transparency within the IDSR system. By regularly assessing and reporting on progress, stakeholders can demonstrate their commitment to achieving program goals and be accountable to funders, policymakers, and the public.

Transparency in reporting progress helps to build trust and credibility in the system.

16.4.2.6 Evidence for Decision-Making:

MONITORING AND EVALUATION generate evidence that can inform decision-making processes. By measuring progress, identifying gaps, and assessing program effectiveness, stakeholders can make data-driven decisions to adjust strategies, allocate resources, and prioritize interventions. This evidence-based decision-making enhances the efficiency and effectiveness of the IDSR system.

16.4.2.7 Continuous Improvement:

MONITORING AND EVALUATION activities provide insights for continuous improvement within the IDSR system. By identifying areas of progress and areas requiring attention, stakeholders can refine strategies, strengthen implementation approaches, and adjust targets as needed. This iterative process of improvement ensures that the IDSR system remains responsive and adaptive to evolving public health challenges.

Overall, monitoring and evaluating IDSR implementation play a vital role in measuring progress towards program goals and objectives. By tracking progress, evaluating outcomes, assessing performance, identifying successes and challenges, promoting accountability and transparency, providing evidence for decision-making, and supporting continuous improvement, stakeholders can ensure that the IDSR system remains effective, efficient, and impactful in detecting and responding to infectious diseases.

16.4.3 Accountability and transparency:

MONITORING AND EVALUATION within the Integrated Disease Surveillance and Response (IDSR) system serve as important mechanisms for accountability and transparency. Here's how monitoring and evaluation contribute to accountability and transparency within the IDSR system:

16.4.3.1 Assessing Implementation:

MONITORING AND EVALUATION activities enable stakeholders to assess whether the IDSR program is being implemented as intended. By measuring the adherence to established protocols, guidelines, and standards, stakeholders can determine if the program is being executed correctly. This ensures that the resources allocated to the program are utilized effectively and efficiently.

16.4.3.2 Resource Utilization:

MONITORING AND EVALUATION provide insights into how resources are being utilized within the IDSR system. By assessing the allocation and utilization of financial, human, and material resources, stakeholders can identify any inefficiencies, gaps, or mismanagement. This promotes accountability in resource utilization and helps ensure that resources are used appropriately to support the program's objectives.

16.4.3.3 Performance Evaluation:

MONITORING AND EVALUATION activities assess the performance of various components within the IDSR system, including health workers, laboratories, surveillance systems, and response mechanisms. By evaluating performance indicators such as data quality, timeliness of reporting, and response effectiveness, stakeholders can hold individuals and institutions accountable for their roles and responsibilities within the program.

16.4.3.4 Transparency in Reporting:

MONITORING AND EVALUATION generate data and information that can be shared with relevant stakeholders, including policymakers, funders, and the public. Transparent reporting of monitoring and evaluation findings promotes accountability by providing evidence of program performance and progress. It allows stakeholders to assess the impact of the program, identify areas for improvement, and make informed decisions regarding resource allocation and programmatic adjustments.

16.4.3.5 Stakeholder Engagement:

MONITORING AND EVALUATION involve engaging stakeholders throughout the process, including program implementers, policymakers, communities, and beneficiaries. This participatory approach fosters transparency by involving stakeholders in decision-making, data collection, and evaluation processes. It allows for diverse perspectives to be considered, strengthens accountability to the different stakeholders involved, and builds trust in the program.

16.4.3.6 Learning and Improvement:

MONITORING AND EVALUATION activities provide opportunities for learning and improvement within the IDSR system. By openly discussing evaluation findings and recommendations, stakeholders can collectively identify areas of weakness, address gaps in implementation, and develop strategies for improvement. This promotes transparency in acknowledging challenges and actively working towards resolving them.

16.4.3.7 Adherence to Standards and Guidelines:

MONITORING AND EVALUATION help ensure that the IDSR system adheres to established standards and guidelines. By regularly assessing program performance against these standards, stakeholders can identify deviations or non-compliance, enabling corrective actions to be taken. This accountability to established norms enhances the transparency of the program's operations.

16.4.4 Identifying best practices:

MONITORING AND EVALUATION play a crucial role in identifying best practices and areas for improvement within the Integrated Disease Surveillance and Response (IDSR) system. Here's how monitoring and evaluation contribute to identifying best practices:

16.4.4.1 Comparative Analysis:

MONITORING AND EVALUATION involve collecting and analyzing data from multiple sources and settings. This allows for comparative analysis between different regions, countries, or programmatic approaches. By comparing the performance and outcomes of various interventions and strategies, best practices can be identified and shared.

16.4.4.2 Lessons Learned:

MONITORING AND EVALUATION activities provide opportunities to capture lessons learned from the implementation of the IDSR system. By systematically analyzing successes and failures, stakeholders can identify approaches and interventions that have proven effective in specific contexts. These lessons learned can be shared as best practices, allowing others to benefit from the knowledge and experiences gained.

16.4.4.3 Innovation and Adaptation:

MONITORING AND EVALUATION help in identifying innovative approaches and interventions that have shown promising results. By evaluating new technologies, methodologies, or strategies, stakeholders can identify breakthroughs or adaptations that improve the efficiency and effectiveness of disease surveillance and response. These innovative practices can be shared as best practices to inspire and guide others in their efforts.

16.4.4.4 Collaboration and Networking:

MONITORING AND EVALUATION provide opportunities for collaboration and networking among stakeholders involved in disease surveillance and response. By sharing evaluation findings, experiences, and success stories, stakeholders can learn from each other and identify best practices. This collaborative approach encourages cross-learning and fosters the exchange of ideas, leading to the adoption of successful practices across different countries and regions.

16.4.4.5 Knowledge Exchange:

MONITORING AND EVALUATION contribute to the dissemination of knowledge and information about effective approaches in disease surveillance and response. Evaluation reports, research findings, and case studies highlighting successful interventions can be shared through conferences, workshops, publications, and online platforms. This knowledge exchange facilitates the spread of best practices, enabling countries and regions to learn from each other and improve their own systems.

16.4.4.6 Policy and Programmatic Guidance:

MONITORING AND EVALUATION findings can inform the development of policies, guidelines, and protocols for disease surveillance and response. Successful interventions and best practices identified through evaluation can be integrated into national or regional strategies, providing guidance to health systems and program implementers. This ensures that evidence-based practices are promoted and replicated to enhance the effectiveness of disease surveillance and response efforts.

16.4.4.7 Technical Assistance and Capacity Building:

MONITORING AND EVALUATION activities help identify capacity gaps and areas where technical assistance is needed. By identifying successful practices, stakeholders can develop targeted capacity-building initiatives to support the adoption and implementation of these practices in areas that require improvement. This ensures that countries and regions have the necessary knowledge and skills to implement best practices in disease surveillance and response.

Overall, monitoring and evaluation within the IDSR system contribute to the identification of best practices by enabling comparative analysis, capturing lessons learned, promoting innovation and adaptation, fostering collaboration and networking, facilitating knowledge exchange, informing policy and programmatic guidance, and supporting technical assistance and capacity building. By sharing and implementing these best practices, disease surveillance and response efforts can be strengthened, leading to improved health outcomes and better preparedness for public health emergencies.

16.4.5 Resource allocation:

MONITORING AND EVALUATION play a vital role in informing resource allocation decisions within the Integrated Disease Surveillance and Response (IDSR) system. Here's how monitoring and evaluation contribute to resource allocation:

16.4.5.1 Evidence-Based Decision Making:

MONITORING AND EVALUATION provide evidence on the effectiveness and impact of different interventions, strategies, and activities implemented within the IDSR system. By assessing the outcomes and cost-effectiveness of various approaches, stakeholders can make informed decisions about resource allocation. Evaluation findings help identify interventions that deliver the best results, allowing resources to be directed towards those that have proven to be most effective in terms of disease surveillance, outbreak response, and public health outcomes.

16.4.5.2 Efficiency and Optimization:

MONITORING AND EVALUATION help assess the efficiency and effectiveness of existing resource allocations. By analyzing the utilization and outcomes of allocated resources, stakeholders can identify areas where resources are underutilized, misallocated, or not delivering the expected impact. This information can guide resource reallocation efforts to ensure that resources are optimally used to address priority needs and achieve the desired health outcomes.

16.4.5.3 Prioritization of Interventions:

MONITORING AND EVALUATION provide insights into the relative importance and impact of different interventions within the IDSR system. By assessing the contribution of each intervention to disease surveillance, outbreak detection, and response, stakeholders can prioritize resource allocation based on the interventions that have the greatest potential to reduce morbidity, mortality, and health system burden. This prioritization helps ensure that limited resources are directed towards interventions that have the highest potential for impact.

16.4.5.4 Identification of Funding Gaps:

MONITORING AND EVALUATION activities help identify gaps in funding and resource allocation within the IDSR system. By assessing the resource needs and the actual availability of resources, stakeholders can identify areas where additional funding or resource allocation is required. This information is crucial for advocacy and resource mobilization efforts to secure the necessary funding to support the implementation and strengthening of the IDSR system.

16.4.5.5 Adaptation to Changing Needs:

MONITORING AND EVALUATION provide information on the evolving needs and challenges within the IDSR system. By continuously assessing the performance and outcomes of interventions, stakeholders can identify emerging priorities and allocate resources accordingly. This flexibility in resource allocation allows for the adaptation of the IDSR system to respond effectively to new and emerging diseases, outbreaks, or public health emergencies.

16.4.5.6 Accountability and Transparency:

MONITORING AND EVALUATION contribute to accountability and transparency in resource allocation. By systematically evaluating the use of resources and measuring the outcomes achieved, stakeholders can ensure that resources are allocated efficiently, equitably, and in line with program objectives. This promotes transparency in decision-making processes and enhances public trust in the allocation and utilization of resources.

16.4.5.7 Resource Leveraging:

MONITORING AND EVALUATION findings can be used to leverage additional resources from various sources, including government budgets, development partners, and donor agencies. By demonstrating the effectiveness and impact of interventions, stakeholders can attract additional funding and support for the IDSR system. This allows for the expansion and improvement of disease surveillance and response activities, leading to better health outcomes.

In summary, monitoring and evaluating IDSR implementation is crucial for improving the effectiveness of disease surveillance and response efforts, measuring progress towards program goals, promoting accountability and transparency, identifying best practices, and informing resource allocation decisions.

16.5 Evaluation frameworks for IDSR

THERE ARE DIFFERENT evaluation frameworks that can be used to evaluate the implementation of the Integrated Disease Surveillance and Response (IDSR) system. Some of these frameworks include:

16.5.1 The World Health Organization's (WHO) Framework for Evaluation of Surveillance Systems:

THE WORLD HEALTH ORGANIZATION (WHO) has developed a framework for evaluating surveillance systems, which assesses various attributes of these systems. The framework aims to provide a standardized approach for evaluating the effectiveness of surveillance systems in detecting and responding to disease outbreaks. The attributes considered in the framework are as follows:

16.5.1.1 Simplicity:

SIMPLICITY IS AN IMPORTANT attribute of surveillance systems as it ensures that the system is easily understood and implemented by those involved in reporting and analyzing data. A simple system increases the likelihood of consistent and accurate data collection, which is crucial for effective disease surveillance. Here are some real-world examples that highlight the importance of simplicity in surveillance systems:

1. **Polio Eradication Initiative**: The global effort to eradicate polio relies on a simple surveillance system known as Acute Flaccid Paralysis (AFP) surveillance. AFP is a symptom associated with polio, and the surveillance system focuses on detecting and reporting cases of AFP in children. The simplicity of this system allows for widespread implementation, even in resource-limited settings, enabling early detection and response to polio outbreaks.

2. *Measles Surveillance*: Measles is a highly infectious disease, and timely detection is crucial for effective control and prevention. The surveillance system for measles relies on a simple case definition, which includes fever, rash, and cough. This simplicity allows healthcare providers to easily recognize and report suspected cases, contributing to the early detection and response to measles outbreaks.

3. *Influenza Monitoring*: Influenza surveillance systems are designed to monitor the spread and impact of seasonal flu outbreaks. These systems often employ a simple approach of collecting data on the number of flu cases reported by healthcare facilities. The simplicity of this surveillance system facilitates widespread participation and timely reporting, enabling public health authorities to track the circulation of influenza viruses and guide prevention strategies.

In these examples, the simplicity of the surveillance systems has contributed to their widespread adoption and effectiveness. By focusing on easily recognizable symptoms or outcomes, these systems enable healthcare providers and other stakeholders to participate in data collection and reporting without requiring extensive training or resources. The simplicity of the systems ensures their usability and increases the likelihood of consistent and accurate reporting, leading to timely detection and response to disease outbreaks.

16.5.1.2 Flexibility:

FLEXIBILITY IS A CRUCIAL attribute of surveillance systems as it allows the system to adapt and respond effectively to changes in disease patterns, data sources, and reporting requirements. A flexible system can accommodate emerging diseases, shifting priorities, and evolving surveillance needs. Here are some real-world examples that illustrate the importance of flexibility in surveillance systems:

1. ***COVID-19 Pandemic***: The COVID-19 pandemic highlighted the need for flexible surveillance systems. As the disease rapidly spread across the globe, surveillance systems had to quickly adapt to accommodate the unique characteristics of the virus and the evolving understanding of its transmission. Many countries expanded their surveillance capabilities to include testing, contact tracing, and monitoring of COVID-19 cases. The flexibility of these systems allowed for the rapid implementation of new data sources, such as mobile applications and digital reporting platforms, to capture and analyze real-time information.

2. ***Antimicrobial Resistance (AMR)***: Surveillance systems for AMR require flexibility to monitor the emergence and spread of drug-resistant pathogens. As new resistant

strains emerge and treatment guidelines evolve, surveillance systems must be adaptable to incorporate new laboratory techniques, collect data on resistance patterns, and monitor the effectiveness of antimicrobial stewardship programs. Flexibility enables the integration of diverse data sources, such as laboratory data, clinical records, and antibiotic consumption data, to provide a comprehensive picture of AMR trends.

3. ***Vector-Borne Diseases***: Surveillance systems for vector-borne diseases, such as malaria or dengue fever, require flexibility to respond to changing vector populations, climate patterns, and transmission dynamics. These systems need to adapt data collection strategies, vector control interventions, and case definitions to address the evolving risk factors and emerging hotspots. Flexibility enables the incorporation of new surveillance methods, such as entomological surveillance or geospatial mapping, to improve the understanding of disease transmission and guide targeted interventions.

By being flexible, surveillance systems can effectively respond to emerging diseases, shifting disease patterns, and evolving surveillance needs. They can incorporate new data sources, update reporting requirements, and adopt innovative technologies to enhance data collection, analysis, and dissemination. The ability to adapt quickly to changing circumstances ensures that surveillance systems remain relevant and effective in detecting and responding to public health threats.

16.5.1.3 Data quality:

DATA QUALITY IS A CRITICAL attribute of surveillance systems as it determines the accuracy, completeness, and reliability of the collected data. High data quality ensures that the information used for analysis and decision-making is valid, trustworthy, and representative of the population under surveillance. Here are some real-world examples that highlight the importance of data quality in surveillance systems:

1. *Vaccine Safety Surveillance*: Surveillance systems play a crucial role in monitoring the safety of vaccines. Accurate and reliable data on adverse events following immunization (AEFI) are essential for identifying and responding to potential vaccine-related risks. High data quality in this context means capturing comprehensive information about the timing, severity, and outcomes of AEFI cases. Robust data collection protocols, standardized case definitions, and effective reporting mechanisms contribute to ensuring data accuracy and completeness, which in turn supports evidence-based decision-making regarding vaccine safety.

2. *Notifiable Disease Reporting*: Surveillance systems rely on accurate and timely reporting of notifiable diseases by healthcare providers. Data quality in this context involves the completeness and accuracy of case information, including demographic details, clinical manifestations, and laboratory results. Improving data quality can lead to more accurate disease burden estimates, better understanding of disease trends, and more effective response strategies. For example, the accuracy of surveillance data on sexually transmitted infections

(STIs) is crucial for guiding prevention efforts and monitoring the effectiveness of interventions.

3. ***Global Health Security***: Data quality is a cornerstone of global health security efforts. Surveillance systems that monitor infectious diseases with pandemic potential, such as influenza or coronaviruses, require accurate and reliable data to detect and respond to outbreaks. Ensuring data quality involves validating and verifying data sources, implementing data quality assurance measures, and conducting regular data audits. By maintaining high data quality standards, surveillance systems can facilitate early detection, rapid response, and effective control of public health threats on a global scale.

Efforts to improve data quality in surveillance systems often involve training and capacity-building for data collectors, implementing data validation checks, and promoting data sharing and collaboration among stakeholders. By investing in data quality, surveillance systems can generate robust evidence for public health decision-making, enhance situational awareness, and improve the effectiveness of disease detection, monitoring, and control strategies.

16.5.1.4 Acceptability:

ACCEPTABILITY IS AN important attribute of surveillance systems as it influences the willingness of individuals and organizations to actively participate in the system. When surveillance systems are perceived as valuable, respectful of privacy, and trusted, they are more likely to attract and retain participants. Here are some real-world examples that illustrate the significance of acceptability in surveillance systems:

1. ***Syndromic Surveillance***: Syndromic surveillance systems monitor non-specific health indicators, such as emergency department visits or over-the-counter medication sales, to detect potential outbreaks early. Ensuring the acceptability of these systems involves addressing concerns regarding privacy and data confidentiality. By implementing robust data protection measures, anonymizing data, and clearly communicating the purpose and benefits of syndromic surveillance to healthcare providers and the public, trust in the system can be fostered, encouraging active participation.

2. ***Contact Tracing***: Contact tracing is a crucial surveillance strategy during infectious disease outbreaks, such as the COVID-19 pandemic. To be effective, contact tracing relies on individuals voluntarily providing information about their contacts and movements. Acceptability of contact tracing efforts depends on factors such as clear communication about the purpose and benefits of contact tracing, assurance of data privacy and confidentiality, and the provision of support services to individuals who are identified as contacts. Building trust and addressing concerns can help ensure the willingness of individuals to participate in contact tracing, ultimately enhancing the effectiveness of the surveillance system.

3. ***Behavioral Surveillance***: Surveillance systems that monitor risky behaviors, such as substance abuse or sexual practices, rely on individuals sharing sensitive information. Acceptability plays a vital role in obtaining accurate and reliable data in these contexts. Establishing a safe and confidential environment, maintaining anonymity, and emphasizing the importance of data confidentiality are crucial to encourage individuals to

provide honest and accurate information. This can be achieved through clear communication, informed consent processes, and strict adherence to ethical guidelines.

To enhance the acceptability of surveillance systems, it is important to engage stakeholders, including communities, healthcare providers, and policymakers, in the design and implementation processes. Incorporating feedback, addressing concerns, and highlighting the benefits and public health impact of surveillance efforts can foster trust and increase participation. Additionally, ensuring transparency in data handling and governance, and complying with relevant data protection regulations, can further contribute to the acceptability of surveillance systems among both individuals and organizations.

16.5.1.5 Representativeness:

REPRESENTATIVENESS is a critical attribute in evaluating surveillance systems as it assesses whether the data collected accurately represents the population or region under surveillance. A representative system is essential for understanding the true disease burden, identifying trends, and making informed public health decisions. Here are a few real-world examples that demonstrate the significance of representativeness in surveillance systems:

1. *National Health Surveys*: Many countries conduct national health surveys to gather comprehensive data on various health indicators, including disease prevalence, risk factors, and healthcare utilization. These surveys aim to collect data from a representative sample of the population, ensuring that the findings can be generalized

to the entire country. Through careful sampling techniques, such as random sampling or stratified sampling, these surveys obtain data from diverse demographic groups, geographic regions, and socioeconomic backgrounds. This approach ensures that the collected data accurately reflects the health status and needs of the entire population.

2. ***Sentinel Surveillance Systems***: Sentinel surveillance systems focus on monitoring specific diseases or conditions in selected sentinel sites or sentinel populations. These sites or populations are chosen based on their representativeness of the larger population. For example, sentinel surveillance for influenza may be conducted in selected healthcare facilities or clinics that serve a diverse patient population. By monitoring disease activity in these sentinel sites, public health authorities can make inferences about the disease burden and trends in the broader community.

3. ***Demographic Surveillance Systems***: In some settings, demographic surveillance systems are used to gather longitudinal data on various health outcomes, demographic characteristics, and social determinants of health. These systems typically cover specific geographic areas or populations and collect data through regular household visits or surveys. By collecting data from every individual or household within the surveillance area, demographic surveillance systems strive to achieve a high level of representativeness, enabling accurate assessment of health indicators and trends in the specific population under surveillance.

Ensuring representativeness in surveillance systems requires careful consideration of sampling methods, data collection strategies, and geographic coverage. It is crucial to account for the diversity of the target population in terms of demographics, socioeconomic status, geographic distribution, and other relevant factors. By collecting data from a representative sample or population, surveillance systems can provide valuable insights into the disease burden, identify disparities, and support evidence-based public health interventions.

16.5.1.6 Timeliness:

TIMELINESS IS A CRUCIAL attribute in surveillance systems as it emphasizes the importance of collecting, reporting, and analyzing data in a timely manner. Rapid detection and response to disease outbreaks are vital for effective public health interventions and minimizing the impact of diseases. Here are some real-world examples that highlight the significance of timeliness in surveillance systems:

1. *Notifiable Disease Reporting Systems*: Many countries have established notifiable disease reporting systems, which require healthcare providers and laboratories to report specific diseases or conditions to public health authorities within a specified timeframe. The reporting of notifiable diseases ensures that cases are promptly identified and reported, enabling public health agencies to respond quickly. Timely reporting allows for the implementation of appropriate control measures, such as isolation and quarantine, contact tracing, and targeted public health messaging to prevent further spread of the disease.

2. ***Early Warning Systems***: Timeliness is crucial in early warning systems designed to detect and respond to emerging infectious diseases or public health threats. These systems utilize various data sources, such as syndromic surveillance data, laboratory reports, and social media monitoring, to detect early signs of outbreaks. By analyzing data in near real-time and using advanced algorithms, these systems can identify unusual patterns or spikes in disease activity, triggering timely public health actions. Timely detection enables the deployment of rapid response teams, allocation of resources, and implementation of preventive measures to contain the outbreak.

3. ***Event-based Surveillance***: Event-based surveillance systems monitor media reports, online news, social media platforms, and other sources to identify potential public health events or outbreaks. Timeliness is critical in this type of surveillance as it allows for the early identification of events and facilitates prompt investigation and response. For example, event-based surveillance systems have been used to detect outbreaks of foodborne illnesses, natural disasters, and other public health emergencies. Rapid response based on timely information can help mitigate the impact on public health and facilitate appropriate interventions.

4. ***Real-time Syndromic Surveillance***: Syndromic surveillance involves the monitoring of non-specific health indicators, such as fever or respiratory symptoms, to detect patterns of illness in real-time. Timely collection and analysis of syndromic data allow for the early identification of potential outbreaks or increases in disease activity. This information can be used to guide

public health actions, such as deploying additional healthcare resources, enhancing surveillance in specific areas, or issuing public health advisories.

Timeliness in surveillance systems requires efficient data collection, robust reporting mechanisms, and agile analysis capabilities. Rapid information sharing and collaboration among healthcare providers, laboratories, and public health agencies are essential for timely detection and response to disease outbreaks. By ensuring that data is collected, reported, and analyzed in a timely manner, surveillance systems can facilitate proactive public health interventions, minimize the spread of diseases, and ultimately protect the health and well-being of communities.

16.5.1.7 Stability:

STABILITY IS A CRITICAL attribute in the evaluation of surveillance systems. It refers to the reliability and sustainability of the system over time, ensuring its continuous operation to collect and analyze data consistently. A stable surveillance system offers several advantages for public health authorities and policymakers, as outlined in the real-world examples below:

1. ***Long-term Disease Trend Analysis***: A stable surveillance system allows for the collection of data over extended periods, enabling the analysis of disease trends over time. This longitudinal data is valuable for identifying changes in disease patterns, detecting emerging health threats, and assessing the impact of public health interventions. For example, in the context of infectious diseases, stability in surveillance data can help identify seasonal trends, shifts in pathogen characteristics, or changes in disease

demographics.

2. ***Monitoring Progress of Public Health Initiatives***: Surveillance systems are often employed to monitor the effectiveness of public health initiatives and interventions. Whether it's a vaccination campaign, health promotion efforts, or the implementation of new health policies, stability in data collection ensures that the impact of these measures can be accurately assessed over time. Decision-makers can use this information to fine-tune existing strategies and develop evidence-based policies for the future.

3. ***Early Detection of Reemerging Diseases***: Some diseases may resurface or reemerge after being under control for a period. A stable surveillance system with a long-term focus can help detect the early signs of such diseases, allowing for a rapid response to prevent potential outbreaks. For instance, diseases such as tuberculosis, which can persist in latent form, may reemerge in certain regions. Stable surveillance helps identify such trends and prompts timely interventions.

4. ***Resource Allocation and Planning***: Stable surveillance data provides a foundation for evidence-based resource allocation and public health planning. Governments and health organizations can use this data to identify areas with higher disease burdens and allocate resources accordingly. It also allows them to plan for future healthcare needs, such as ensuring an adequate supply of vaccines and medications based on disease prevalence.

5. **Identification of Risk Factors**: Long-term surveillance data enables the identification of risk factors associated with specific diseases or health conditions. By understanding these risk factors, public health authorities

can implement targeted prevention and control strategies to reduce the burden of the disease. For instance, surveillance data might reveal an increasing trend of diabetes in a particular community, leading to targeted awareness campaigns about healthy lifestyles and regular health check-ups.

6. **Evaluation of Health Policies**: Stable surveillance data plays a crucial role in evaluating the effectiveness of health policies and strategies. Policymakers can assess whether specific interventions have achieved their desired outcomes and adjust their policies accordingly. This process of continuous evaluation and improvement is essential for maintaining an efficient and responsive public health system.

Overall, stability in surveillance systems ensures that data collection is reliable, consistent, and sustainable over time. This attribute enhances the utility of the surveillance system and its ability to support evidence-based decision-making, early detection of health threats, and the implementation of effective public health interventions.

By assessing these attributes, the WHO framework provides a comprehensive evaluation of surveillance systems, enabling policymakers and public health officials to identify strengths, weaknesses, and areas for improvement. This evaluation helps in enhancing the effectiveness and efficiency of disease surveillance and response efforts.

Table 12: The WHO IDSR Evaluation Framework

Component	Description
Simplicity	Simplicity ensures that surveillance systems are easily understood and implemented, leading to consistent and accurate data collection. Examples include the Polio Eradication Initiative, Measles Surveillance, and Influenza Monitoring.
Flexibility	Flexibility allows surveillance systems to adapt to changes in disease patterns, data sources, and reporting requirements. Examples include the COVID-19 Pandemic, Antimicrobial Resistance (AMR) surveillance, and monitoring of vector-borne diseases.
Data Quality	Data quality ensures that collected information is accurate, complete, and reliable. Examples include Vaccine Safety Surveillance, Notifiable Disease Reporting, and global health security efforts.
Acceptability	Acceptability focuses on creating a system that is valued, respectful of privacy, and trusted by participants. Examples include Syndromic Surveillance, Contact Tracing, and Behavioral Surveillance.
Representativeness	Representativeness ensures that surveillance systems collect data that accurately reflects the target population. Examples include National Health Surveys, Sentinel Surveillance Systems, and Demographic Surveillance Systems.
Timeliness	Timeliness emphasizes the importance of collecting, reporting, and analyzing data in a prompt manner. Examples include Notifiable Disease Reporting Systems, Early Warning Systems, Event-based Surveillance, and Real-time Syndromic Surveillance.
Stability	Stability refers to the reliability and sustainability of surveillance systems over time. Examples include Long-term Disease Trend Analysis, Monitoring Progress of Public Health Initiatives, Early Detection of Reemerging Diseases, Resource Allocation and Planning, Identification of Risk Factors, and Evaluation of Health Policies.

The table presents different evaluation frameworks for the Integrated Disease Surveillance and Response (IDSR) system. It includes the attributes assessed in the World Health Organization's framework, along with examples that demonstrate the importance and application of each attribute in real-world surveillance systems.

16.5.2 The Centers for Disease Control and Prevention (CDC) Framework for Program Evaluation:

THE CENTERS FOR DISEASE Control and Prevention (CDC) Framework for Program Evaluation is a comprehensive approach to evaluating public health programs, including the Integrated Disease Surveillance and Response (IDSR) system. The framework consists of six key steps that guide the evaluation process, ensuring a systematic and evidence-based approach. Let's explore each step in more detail:

16.5.2.1 Engaging Stakeholders:

ABSOLUTELY! ENGAGING stakeholders is a fundamental step in the CDC Framework for Program Evaluation. Here's a further expansion on this step:

Engaging stakeholders is essential to ensure that the evaluation process incorporates diverse perspectives and meets the needs of those directly involved or affected by the program. By involving key individuals and organizations, such as program managers, staff members, community representatives, policymakers, and other relevant parties, the evaluation becomes a collaborative effort.

Here are some key aspects of engaging stakeholders in program evaluation:

1. *Identifying Stakeholders*: The first task is to identify the stakeholders who have a vested interest in the program. This includes individuals and organizations that are directly involved in program planning, implementation, or funding, as well as those who are affected by the program's outcomes or have expertise in the program's area. Stakeholders may vary depending on the program's nature, scope, and context.

2. *Involving Stakeholders*: Once stakeholders are identified, it is important to actively involve them in the evaluation process. This can be achieved through regular communication, meetings, workshops, focus groups, or consultations. Involving stakeholders from the beginning helps create a sense of ownership, builds trust, and encourages their active participation in the evaluation activities.

3. *Incorporating Perspectives and Insights*: Engaging

stakeholders ensures that their perspectives, experiences, and insights are taken into account during the evaluation. Stakeholders can provide valuable input on program implementation challenges, contextual factors, potential barriers or facilitators to success, and other relevant considerations. Their involvement helps to broaden the understanding of the program's impact and contributes to a more comprehensive evaluation.

4. ***Collaboration and Co-creation***: The engagement of stakeholders fosters a collaborative approach to evaluation. By involving stakeholders in the design, implementation, and interpretation of the evaluation, their expertise is leveraged, and diverse viewpoints are considered. Collaborative evaluation approaches can include joint planning, shared decision-making, and co-creation of evaluation tools and methods.

5. ***Ensuring Equity and Inclusivity***: Engaging stakeholders also ensures that the evaluation process is equitable and inclusive. It is important to involve individuals and groups representing diverse backgrounds, including those who are historically marginalized or have limited access to decision-making processes. By actively seeking and valuing diverse perspectives, the evaluation becomes more representative and addresses potential biases.

6. ***Building Relationships and Trust***: Effective stakeholder engagement requires building strong relationships and fostering trust. This involves transparent and open communication, active listening, and responsiveness to stakeholder concerns and feedback. Building trust helps create an environment where stakeholders feel comfortable sharing their perspectives, challenges, and suggestions for program improvement.

By engaging stakeholders in program evaluation, the evaluation process becomes more comprehensive, inclusive, and contextually relevant. Stakeholders bring valuable insights, contribute to the interpretation of findings, and help identify actionable recommendations for program improvement. Ultimately, engaging stakeholders increases the likelihood of utilizing evaluation findings and promoting evidence-based decision-making for program enhancement.

16.5.2.2 Describing the Program:

EXACTLY! DESCRIBING the program is a crucial step in the CDC Framework for Program Evaluation. Here's a further expansion on this step:

Describing the program involves providing a clear and detailed overview of the program being evaluated. This step aims to document essential information about the program, including its goals, objectives, activities, target population, and the contextual factors that may influence its implementation and outcomes. By describing the program in depth, evaluators and stakeholders gain a comprehensive understanding of its components and intended impact.

Here are key elements to consider when describing a program for evaluation:

1. ***Program Goals and Objectives***: Start by articulating the program's overarching goals and specific objectives. Program goals reflect the desired long-term outcomes, while objectives outline the measurable targets that the program aims to achieve within a specified timeframe. Clearly stating the goals and objectives provides a

foundation for evaluating the program's effectiveness.

2. ***Program Activities:*** Describe the activities or interventions that the program implements to reach its goals and objectives. These can include specific interventions, services, educational campaigns, policy changes, or community engagement strategies. Detailing the activities helps evaluators understand how the program operates and the strategies employed to bring about the desired outcomes.

3. ***Target Population***: Identify and describe the population or group that the program aims to serve or impact. This includes characteristics such as age, gender, socioeconomic status, geographic location, or specific risk factors. Understanding the target population is crucial for evaluating the program's relevance and effectiveness in addressing their specific needs.

4. ***Program Logic Model or Theory of Change***: A logic model or theory of change illustrates the underlying assumptions and causal pathways through which the program activities lead to the desired outcomes. This graphical representation helps stakeholders visualize the program's theory of how it creates change and provides a framework for evaluation.

5. ***Contextual Factors***: Consider the broader context in which the program operates. This includes factors such as social, economic, cultural, and political influences that may impact the program's implementation and outcomes. Understanding the context helps evaluators identify external factors that may influence program success or challenges.

6. ***Program Implementation***: Describe how the program is implemented, including the roles and responsibilities of

various stakeholders, the resources allocated, and the timeline for implementation. Documenting the implementation process helps evaluators assess whether the program was implemented as intended and identify any implementation challenges or adaptations.

By thoroughly describing the program, evaluators and stakeholders gain a comprehensive understanding of its components, intended outcomes, and the strategies employed. This understanding serves as a foundation for conducting a rigorous evaluation and helps ensure that the evaluation aligns with the program's objectives and context. It also facilitates communication and shared understanding among stakeholders, leading to more meaningful and actionable evaluation findings.

16.5.2.3 Focusing the Evaluation Design:

FOCUSING THE EVALUATION design is a critical step in the CDC Framework for Program Evaluation. Let's delve into it further:

Focusing the evaluation design involves defining the specific evaluation questions and selecting appropriate methods and approaches to answer those questions. This step is crucial as it guides the entire evaluation process and ensures that the evaluation is relevant, meaningful, and aligned with the program's goals and context.

Here are key elements involved in focusing the evaluation design:

1. *Identifying Evaluation Questions*: Evaluation questions are the foundation of the entire evaluation process. They articulate what the evaluation seeks to answer or assess

regarding the program's performance and impact. Evaluation questions may vary depending on the program's goals and stakeholders' information needs. Typical evaluation questions may include:

- *Effectiveness:* To what extent did the program achieve its intended outcomes and objectives?
- *Efficiency*: Were the program's resources utilized effectively in delivering the intended outputs and outcomes?
- *Relevance*: How well does the program address the needs of the target population or community?
- *Sustainability*: What is the likelihood of the program's continued impact and existence after the funding period?

1. **Selecting Evaluation Methods and Approaches**: Once the evaluation questions are defined, appropriate evaluation methods and data collection approaches can be chosen. The choice of methods should align with the evaluation questions and the available resources. Common evaluation methods include:

- **Surveys:** Questionnaires administered to program participants, beneficiaries, or stakeholders to gather quantitative data.
- **Interviews:** Conducting one-on-one or group interviews to gain in-depth insights and perspectives from key informants.
- **Focus Groups:** Group discussions that facilitate a deeper understanding of participants' experiences and perceptions.
- **Observation:** Systematic observation of program activities to assess implementation fidelity or participant

behavior.

- **Document Review:** Analyzing program-related documents, such as reports, records, and data, to extract relevant information.

1. **Data Sources and Data Collection:** Determine the sources of data required to answer the evaluation questions. Data sources can include program records, participant data, existing databases, and external research. Plan how the data will be collected, considering the feasibility, cost, and time constraints.

2. **Sampling Strategy:** If applicable, decide on the sampling strategy for data collection. This involves selecting a representative subset of the target population or program participants for evaluation. The chosen sample should be large enough to provide meaningful insights while being feasible to manage.

3. **Ethical Considerations:** Consider ethical aspects of the evaluation, such as obtaining informed consent from participants, ensuring confidentiality, and protecting vulnerable groups.

4. **Timeline and Resources:** Develop a timeline for the evaluation process and allocate necessary resources, including personnel, budget, and technology.

By focusing the evaluation design, evaluators ensure that the evaluation is purposeful, efficient, and capable of providing relevant and meaningful insights into the program's performance. This step lays the groundwork for data collection and analysis, leading to evidence-based conclusions and actionable recommendations for program improvement and decision making.

16.5.2.4 Gathering Credible Evidence:

IN THIS STEP, DATA is collected to answer the evaluation questions and assess the program's performance. Various data collection methods, both qualitative and quantitative, are employed to gather credible evidence. These may include surveys, interviews, focus groups, document reviews, and data analysis. The data collected should be valid, reliable, and representative of the program's activities and outcomes. Gathering credible evidence provides a solid foundation for drawing conclusions and making informed decisions.

16.5.2.5 Justifying Conclusions:

BASED ON THE EVIDENCE gathered, evaluators analyze the data and draw conclusions about the program's effectiveness, efficiency, and impact. Conclusions are based on the evaluation questions and the evidence collected, and they provide an assessment of the program's achievements and areas for improvement. This step involves critically analyzing the data, considering any limitations or biases, and ensuring the validity and reliability of the conclusions drawn.

16.5.2.6 Ensuring Use and Sharing Lessons Learned:

THE FINAL STEP FOCUSES on ensuring the utilization of evaluation findings and sharing lessons learned. Evaluation results should be communicated effectively to stakeholders, including program managers, policymakers, and the broader public health community. Recommendations for program improvement should be provided based on the evaluation findings. By sharing the lessons learned, stakeholders can incorporate the evaluation results into decision-making processes, program planning, and resource allocation. This step emphasizes the importance of using evaluation findings to enhance program effectiveness and drive continuous improvement.

The CDC Framework for Program Evaluation provides a structured and comprehensive approach to evaluating public health programs. By following these six steps, evaluators can ensure that the evaluation process is rigorous, evidence-based, and aligned with the goals and objectives of the program being evaluated. This framework promotes accountability, transparency, and the utilization of evaluation findings to improve program performance and ultimately contribute to better public health outcomes.

Table 13: The CDC Framework for Program Evaluation:

Step	Description
Engaging Stakeholders	Involving key individuals and organizations in the evaluation process to ensure diverse perspectives, ownership, and collaboration.
Describing the Program	Providing a comprehensive overview of the program, including goals, objectives, activities, target population, and contextual factors.
Focusing the Evaluation	Defining evaluation questions and selecting appropriate methods and approaches to answer them, aligning with program goals and context.
Gathering Credible Evidence	Collecting valid and reliable data through various qualitative and quantitative methods to assess the program's performance and outcomes.
Justifying Conclusions	Analyzing the evidence collected, drawing evidence-based conclusions about the program's effectiveness, efficiency, and impact.
Ensuring Use and Sharing	Communicating evaluation findings effectively, providing recommendations for program improvement, and incorporating lessons learned into decision-making.

The table summarizes the key steps of the CDC Framework for Program Evaluation, a comprehensive approach to evaluating public health programs like IDSR.

16.5.3 The Logical Framework Approach:

THE LOGICAL FRAMEWORK Approach (LFA) is a widely used method in project planning and evaluation, particularly in the field of international development. It provides a systematic and logical framework for designing, implementing, monitoring, and evaluating programs or projects. The LFA consists of several key elements that help structure and guide the planning and evaluation process. Let's further expand on the Logical Framework Approach:

16.5.3.1 Objectives:

IN THE LOGICAL FRAMEWORK Approach (LFA), clearly defining objectives is a fundamental step in program or project planning. Objectives are statements that describe the desired outcomes and impacts that the program aims to achieve. They provide a clear direction and purpose for the project and serve as the foundation for all subsequent planning, implementation, and evaluation activities. Here, we will further expand on the characteristics and categorization of objectives in the LFA:

1. **Clear and specific**: Objectives should be formulated in a clear and specific manner, leaving no room for ambiguity. They should articulate what is intended to be achieved and provide a clear understanding of the desired outcome.
2. **Measurable**: Objectives should be measurable, meaning that their progress and achievement can be quantitatively or qualitatively assessed. This requires the use of indicators and data collection methods to track progress and determine success.
3. **Achievable:** Objectives should be achievable within the given resources, capacity, and timeframe. They should be realistic and consider the limitations and constraints of the project. Setting unattainable objectives can lead to unrealistic expectations and hinder project success.
4. **Relevant**: Objectives should be relevant and aligned with the overall goal of the project. They should address the core issues and needs that the project aims to tackle. Ensuring the relevance of objectives helps maintain

project focus and ensures that resources are allocated effectively.

5. **Time-bound**: Objectives should have a specific time frame or deadline for achievement. This helps create a sense of urgency and provides a clear timeline for planning and implementation. Time-bound objectives enable monitoring and evaluation of progress within defined periods.

In addition to these characteristics, objectives in the LFA are often categorized into different levels to reflect their relationship and contribution to the overall program goals. These levels include:

1. *Immediate objectives*: These are the short-term objectives that are expected to be achieved in the immediate term, often within a few months or a year. They are the initial steps towards reaching the higher-level objectives and contribute directly to the outputs of the program.
2. *Intermediate objectives*: These objectives are typically medium-term goals that are achieved over a longer period, usually spanning several years. Intermediate objectives build upon the immediate objectives and contribute to the attainment of long-term objectives.
3. *Long-term objectives*: These objectives represent the overarching goals of the program or project, reflecting the ultimate desired impacts and outcomes. They are achieved over an extended period, often beyond the project's duration, and embody the desired changes in the target population or sector.

Categorizing objectives into different levels allows for a logical progression and sequencing of activities, ensuring that each level contributes to the higher-level objectives. This hierarchical structure helps maintain focus and track progress throughout the project lifecycle.

By formulating objectives in a clear, specific, measurable, achievable, relevant, and time-bound (SMART) manner, and categorizing them into different levels, the LFA provides a framework for effective project planning and evaluation. This approach enables stakeholders to align their efforts, monitor progress, and measure success in a systematic and structured manner.

Real-world examples of the application of the LFA can be found in various development projects, including health programs, education initiatives, infrastructure projects, and community development efforts. Organizations such as the United Nations Development Programme (UNDP) and the World Bank commonly utilize the LFA as a planning and evaluation tool to enhance project effectiveness and achieve sustainable development outcomes.

16.5.3.2 Outputs:

IN THE LOGICAL FRAMEWORK Approach (LFA), outputs play a crucial role in program planning and evaluation. They represent the specific deliverables or products that a program will produce as a result of its activities. Outputs are directly linked to the immediate objectives and serve as tangible and measurable results of program implementation. Here, we will further expand on the characteristics and significance of outputs in the LFA:

1. **Tangible deliverables**: Outputs are concrete and observable results of program activities. They can include physical products, services, training materials, reports,

infrastructure development, policy changes, or any other measurable outcome that can be directly attributed to program interventions. These deliverables provide evidence of progress and achievement.

2. ***Measurable and observable***: Outputs should be measurable, meaning that their completion and quality can be quantitatively or qualitatively assessed. Measurable outputs allow for objective monitoring and evaluation, enabling stakeholders to track progress, assess performance, and make informed decisions. Observable outputs are easily identifiable and verifiable, providing clear evidence of program implementation.

3. ***Directly linked to objectives***: Outputs are closely connected to the immediate objectives of the program. They represent the intermediate steps necessary to achieve the desired outcomes. By accomplishing the specified outputs, the program moves closer to fulfilling its objectives and ultimately reaching the broader goals.

4. ***Building blocks for outcomes***: Outputs serve as building blocks for achieving program outcomes. When combined, the outputs contribute to the desired changes and impacts in the target population or sector. The successful completion of outputs is essential for the effective implementation of the program and the attainment of higher-level objectives.

5. ***Time-bound***: Similar to objectives, outputs should have a specific timeframe or deadline for completion. Setting clear timelines for output delivery helps ensure accountability and progress monitoring. Time-bound outputs provide a framework for efficient project management and facilitate coordination among stakeholders.

By defining and describing outputs in the LFA, program planners can clearly articulate the tangible results they expect to achieve. This promotes transparency, accountability, and effective communication among stakeholders, as everyone shares a common understanding of what will be produced and how it aligns with program objectives.

Real-world examples of outputs in the LFA can vary depending on the nature of the program. For instance, in a health program, outputs may include the number of health facilities constructed or renovated, the quantity of medical supplies distributed, the percentage increase in healthcare coverage, or the number of trained healthcare workers. In an education program, outputs can be measured by the number of classrooms built, the availability of teaching materials, the percentage improvement in student enrollment rates, or the number of teachers trained.

The LFA helps ensure that programs focus on delivering tangible and measurable outputs that directly contribute to achieving program objectives. By clearly defining and monitoring outputs, stakeholders can assess progress, make informed decisions, and adjust program implementation as necessary to maximize impact.

16.5.3.3 Outcomes:

IN THE CONTEXT OF THE Logical Framework Approach (LFA), outcomes play a critical role in assessing the effectiveness and impact of a program. They represent the observable and measurable changes or benefits that occur as a result of the program's outputs and activities. Here, we will expand on the characteristics and significance of outcomes in the LFA:

1. ***Broader effects and impacts***: Outcomes go beyond the

immediate outputs of a program and focus on the broader effects and impacts on the target population or the environment. They capture the changes in behavior, conditions, or circumstances that result from the program's interventions. Outcomes reflect the ultimate goals and aspirations of the program and demonstrate its ability to bring about meaningful change.

2. *Associated with intermediate and long-term objectives*: Outcomes are closely tied to the intermediate and long-term objectives of the program. They reflect the desired results that are expected to be achieved over a specified period. While outputs represent the tangible products or deliverables, outcomes represent the higher-level changes that are desired in the target population or sector.

3. *Observable and measurable changes*: Outcomes are observable and measurable, meaning they can be quantitatively or qualitatively assessed. They should be specific, measurable, achievable, relevant, and time-bound (SMART) to facilitate monitoring and evaluation. Measurable outcomes allow for the assessment of program impact and enable stakeholders to determine whether the program is achieving its intended goals.

4. *Attribution to program interventions*: Outcomes are directly attributed to the program's activities and interventions. They demonstrate the program's contribution to the observed changes. By establishing a causal link between program interventions and outcomes, stakeholders can determine the program's effectiveness and assess its value in achieving desired results.

5. *Evaluation of program effectiveness*: Outcomes serve as indicators of program effectiveness and impact. By monitoring and evaluating the changes in outcomes,

stakeholders can assess the program's success in achieving its objectives. Evaluation findings provide insights into the program's strengths, weaknesses, and areas for improvement, helping to inform future program planning and decision-making.

Real-world examples of outcomes in the LFA can vary depending on the program's focus. In a poverty alleviation program, outcomes may include a reduction in the poverty rate, an increase in income levels, improved access to basic services, or enhanced economic opportunities for the target population. In an environmental conservation program, outcomes could be measured by the restoration of ecosystems, the reduction of pollution levels, the conservation of biodiversity, or the adoption of sustainable practices.

By clearly defining and monitoring outcomes in the LFA, program stakeholders can assess the broader impact and effectiveness of the program. This allows for evidence-based decision-making, improved accountability, and the identification of best practices for achieving desired changes.

16.5.3.4 Indicators:

INDICATORS ARE SPECIFIC, observable, and measurable criteria that are used to assess progress and achievement of objectives and outcomes. They provide quantitative or qualitative data that help monitor and evaluate the program's performance. Indicators are aligned with each level of objectives and outcomes and serve as the basis for collecting data to track progress and measure success. Indicators should be relevant, reliable, valid, and feasible to measure.

The logical framework is usually presented as a matrix that visually represents the hierarchy of objectives, outputs, outcomes, and indicators. It provides a clear and structured overview of the program's logical framework and allows stakeholders to understand how each component is linked and contributes to the overall program goals.

The use of the Logical Framework Approach helps ensure that programs or projects are well-planned, implemented, monitored, and evaluated. It enables stakeholders to align their efforts, monitor progress, measure results, and make informed decisions for program improvement. The logical framework also facilitates communication and coordination among project stakeholders by providing a common understanding of the program's objectives and expected outcomes.

Real-world examples of the application of the Logical Framework Approach can be found in various development projects, including those related to health, education, infrastructure, and agriculture. International organizations, governments, and non-governmental organizations commonly utilize the LFA as a planning and evaluation tool to enhance program effectiveness and ensure accountability.

In summary, the Logical Framework Approach is a structured and systematic method for project planning and evaluation. By developing a logical framework that outlines objectives, outputs, outcomes, and indicators, stakeholders can effectively plan, monitor, and evaluate programs, leading to improved project design, implementation, and impact assessment.

Table 14: Key elements of the Logical Framework Approach (LFA)

LFA Elements	Description
Objectives	Clearly defined statements describing the desired outcomes and impacts of the program. Objectives are clear, specific, measurable, achievable, relevant, and time-bound (SMART).
Outputs	Tangible deliverables or products that result from program activities. Outputs are measurable and directly linked to the program's objectives. They serve as building blocks for achieving program outcomes.
Outcomes	Observable and measurable changes or benefits that occur as a result of program outputs and activities. Outcomes go beyond the immediate outputs and reflect broader effects and impacts. They are directly attributed to the program's interventions.
Indicators	Specific, observable, and measurable criteria used to assess progress and achievement of objectives and outcomes. Indicators provide quantitative or qualitative data for monitoring and evaluation purposes.

The table summarizes key elements of the Logical Framework Approach (LFA) used in project planning and evaluation. It highlights the importance of clear objectives, tangible outputs, observable outcomes, and relevant indicators in guiding program design, monitoring progress, and assessing impact.

16.5.4 The Results-Based Monitoring and Evaluation Framework:

THE RESULTS-BASED MONITORING and Evaluation (M&E) Framework is a systematic approach to measuring the outcomes and impacts of a program or project. It places a strong emphasis on identifying key performance indicators (KPIs) and tracking progress towards program goals. The framework consists of four stages: planning and design, implementation and data collection, analysis and reporting, and using the results.

16.5.4.1 Planning and Design:

IN THIS STAGE, THE M&E framework is developed during the program planning phase. The objectives and desired outcomes of the program are defined, and specific indicators are identified to measure progress and success. These indicators should be specific, measurable, attainable, relevant, and time-bound (SMART) to ensure they effectively capture the desired results. Additionally, data collection methods and tools are determined, and a monitoring and evaluation plan is established.

16.5.4.2 Implementation and Data Collection:

ONCE THE PROGRAM IS underway, data is collected to measure progress and outcomes. This stage involves implementing the planned activities and interventions, as well as collecting relevant data through various methods such as surveys, interviews, observations, and document reviews. The collected data should align with the identified indicators to provide evidence of program performance.

16.5.4.3 Analysis and Reporting:

IN THIS STAGE, THE collected data is analyzed to assess program performance and determine whether the intended outcomes and impacts are being achieved. The data is evaluated against the predefined indicators, allowing for a comparison between planned targets and actual results. The analysis may involve quantitative data analysis, qualitative data interpretation, and triangulation of different data sources. The findings and conclusions are then compiled into reports or presentations to communicate the results to stakeholders.

16.5.4.4 Using the Results:

THE FINAL STAGE OF the framework focuses on utilizing the evaluation findings to inform decision-making and improve program effectiveness. The results and recommendations generated from the analysis are shared with stakeholders, including program managers, policymakers, and relevant partners. The aim is to facilitate evidence-based decision-making and promote continuous program improvement. The recommendations may lead to program modifications, reallocation of resources, or changes in strategies to better align with the desired outcomes.

Table 15: Results-Based Monitoring and Evaluation Framework:

Stage	Description
Planning and Design	Develop the M&E framework during program planning, define objectives and outcomes, identify specific indicators, and establish data collection methods and a monitoring and evaluation plan.
Implementation and Data Collection	Implement program activities and interventions, collect relevant data through surveys, interviews, observations, and document reviews, ensuring alignment with identified indicators.
Analysis and Reporting	Analyze collected data, evaluate program performance against predefined indicators, compare planned targets with actual results, and compile findings and conclusions into reports for stakeholders.
Using the Results	Utilize evaluation findings to inform decision-making, share results and recommendations with stakeholders, and facilitate evidence-based decision-making, program improvement, and resource allocation.

The table summarizes the four stages of the Results-Based Monitoring and Evaluation Framework. It outlines the key activities involved in each stage, including planning and design, implementation and data collection, analysis and reporting, and using the results to inform decision-making and improve program effectiveness.

By employing the Results-Based M&E Framework, programs and projects can effectively track their progress and assess their impact. This approach provides a structured and systematic method for monitoring and evaluating program performance, ensuring that resources are used efficiently and that program goals are achieved. The framework also promotes accountability and learning, as it enables stakeholders to make data-driven decisions and continuously improve program implementation.

These evaluation frameworks can be adapted to suit the specific context and needs of the IDSR system. They provide a structured approach to evaluating the effectiveness of the system and identifying areas for improvement.

16.6 Case studies of successful monitoring and

evaluation of IDSR in Africa

ONE EXAMPLE OF SUCCESSFUL monitoring and evaluation of IDSR in Africa is the case of Uganda. In Uganda, a comprehensive evaluation of the IDSR system was conducted in 2007. The evaluation used the WHO Framework for Evaluation of Surveillance Systems and assessed the attributes of the IDSR system in terms of simplicity, flexibility, data quality, acceptability, representativeness, timeliness, and stability. The evaluation identified gaps in the system, including inadequate laboratory capacity and poor data management, and made recommendations for improvement.

As a result of the evaluation, the Ugandan government developed a plan to strengthen the IDSR system. The plan included training health workers in disease surveillance and response, establishing a laboratory network for disease diagnosis, and improving data management and reporting.

In Liberia, the IDSR system was also evaluated in 2012 using the WHO Framework for Evaluation of Surveillance Systems. The evaluation identified strengths and weaknesses in the system and made recommendations for improvement. The evaluation found that the system had good timeliness and stability, but had weaknesses in data quality and laboratory capacity.

Following the evaluation, Liberia developed a strategic plan to improve the IDSR system. The plan included strengthening laboratory capacity, improving data management, and enhancing surveillance and response activities.

Overall, these case studies demonstrate the importance of monitoring and evaluating the IDSR system to identify gaps and areas for improvement. The evaluations led to the development of strategic plans for strengthening the system, which ultimately helped to improve disease surveillance and response in Uganda and Liberia.

16.7 Emerging challenges in IDSR implementation in Africa

THERE ARE SEVERAL EMERGING challenges that may affect IDSR implementation in Africa, including:

16.7.1 Weak health systems:

THE PRESENCE OF WEAK health systems in many African countries is a significant challenge when it comes to outbreak response. Here are some real-world examples that highlight the impact of weak health systems on disease surveillance and outbreak response:

1. ***Ebola Outbreak in West Africa (2014-2016):*** The Ebola outbreak that affected Guinea, Liberia, and Sierra Leone in 2014-2016 exposed the weaknesses in the health systems of these countries. The limited resources, infrastructure, and healthcare workforce hindered the ability to detect and respond effectively to the outbreak. Inadequate disease surveillance and weak healthcare systems contributed to the rapid spread of the virus.

2. ***Cholera Outbreaks in Sub-Saharan Africa***: Many countries in sub-Saharan Africa, including Nigeria, Democratic Republic of the Congo, and Zimbabwe, have experienced recurrent cholera outbreaks. Weak health systems, lack of clean water and sanitation infrastructure, and limited access to healthcare services have contributed to the persistence and severity of these outbreaks.

Inadequate surveillance systems and response capacity have made it challenging to control the spread of cholera in affected communities.

3. ***COVID-19 Pandemic***: The COVID-19 pandemic has highlighted the vulnerabilities of weak health systems in Africa. Limited testing capacity, inadequate healthcare infrastructure, and shortages of medical supplies and trained healthcare workers have posed significant challenges in detecting and managing COVID-19 cases. These weaknesses have strained the ability of health systems to respond effectively to the pandemic and mitigate its impact.

Addressing the weaknesses in health systems requires long-term investments in healthcare infrastructure, workforce training, and strengthening surveillance and response capabilities. Building resilient health systems with adequate resources, improved data quality, and enhanced outbreak response capacity is crucial to effectively tackle infectious disease outbreaks in Africa.

16.7.2 Disease outbreaks and epidemics:

THE EMERGENCE AND RE-emergence of infectious diseases in Africa have had a profound impact on the implementation of Integrated Disease Surveillance and Response (IDSR) systems. These outbreaks have strained health systems and diverted resources, impacting the effectiveness of routine surveillance activities. Here are some real-world examples:

1. ***Zika Virus Outbreak (2015-2016):*** The Zika virus outbreak that swept through many countries in Africa, including Cape Verde, demonstrated the challenges faced in implementing IDSR during epidemics. Limited

resources and capacities were diverted to control the outbreak, impacting routine disease surveillance activities.

2. ***COVID-19 Pandemic***: The ongoing COVID-19 pandemic has had a global impact, including in Africa. The rapid spread of the virus has strained health systems, disrupted routine surveillance, and overwhelmed healthcare facilities. The focus on COVID-19 response has diverted resources and attention from other diseases, potentially affecting the timeliness and accuracy of surveillance data.

These examples underscore the challenges faced by health systems in Africa when outbreaks and epidemics occur. Adequate preparedness, including strong surveillance systems, sufficient resources, and effective coordination, is essential to manage these events and ensure the continuity of routine disease surveillance activities.

16.7.3 Inadequate laboratory capacity:

INADEQUATE LABORATORY capacity poses a significant challenge to disease surveillance and response in many African countries. Limited resources, infrastructure, and trained personnel can hinder the timely and accurate detection of disease outbreaks. Here are some real-world examples:

1. ***Cholera Outbreaks***: Cholera outbreaks are a recurring challenge in Africa, particularly in areas with poor water and sanitation infrastructure. Inadequate laboratory capacity in some regions has led to delays in confirming cholera cases, which can impede the implementation of targeted interventions and the timely response to outbreaks.

2. ***Lassa Fever Outbreaks***: Lassa fever is an acute viral hemorrhagic fever that occurs in West Africa. Inadequate laboratory capacity in some affected countries, such as Nigeria and Sierra Leone, has hindered the timely diagnosis and confirmation of Lassa fever cases. This has resulted in delays in implementing appropriate control measures, including contact tracing and isolation of infected individuals.

3. ***Meningitis Outbreaks***: Meningococcal meningitis outbreaks are recurrent in the "meningitis belt" of sub-Saharan Africa. Limited laboratory capacity in some countries within this region has been a challenge in accurately identifying and characterizing the circulating meningococcal strains. This can impact the selection of appropriate vaccines and the implementation of targeted vaccination campaigns.

4. ***Yellow Fever Outbreaks***: Yellow fever is a mosquito-borne viral disease endemic in parts of Africa. Inadequate laboratory capacity in some affected countries has resulted in delays in confirming yellow fever cases, which can impact the implementation of vaccination campaigns and other control measures. It can also contribute to the underreporting of cases and the potential for the disease to spread to other regions.

These examples demonstrate how inadequate laboratory capacity can hinder disease surveillance and response efforts, leading to delays in implementing appropriate control measures, underreporting of cases, and potential outbreaks spreading beyond the affected regions. Strengthening laboratory infrastructure, training laboratory personnel, and improving access to diagnostic tools are crucial for enhancing disease surveillance and response capabilities in Africa.

16.7.4 Poor data quality:

POOR DATA QUALITY IS a significant challenge that hampers the effectiveness of Integrated Disease Surveillance and Response (IDSR) systems in Africa. Incomplete or inaccurate reporting of disease cases can result in delays in detecting and responding to outbreaks. Several factors contribute to poor data quality in disease surveillance:

1. *Underreporting:* Health facilities and personnel may not consistently report all cases of diseases to the surveillance system. This can occur due to various reasons, such as lack of awareness about reporting requirements, inadequate training, or competing priorities in resource-constrained settings.

2. *Inadequate Data Collection and Recording*: Incomplete or inconsistent data collection practices can lead to gaps and inaccuracies in the reported information. This includes missing or incomplete patient demographic details, clinical symptoms, or laboratory results, which are crucial for accurate disease monitoring and response.

3. *Limited Diagnostic Capacity*: In some regions, access to diagnostic tools and laboratory services is limited. This can result in a reliance on clinical diagnoses or presumptive reporting, which may not provide precise and specific information about the disease burden.

4. *Data Entry Errors*: Manual data entry processes are prone to human errors, such as typos, transcription mistakes, or misinterpretation of handwritten records. These errors can introduce inaccuracies into the

surveillance data and compromise the reliability of the system.

Addressing poor data quality requires concerted efforts to strengthen the data collection and reporting processes within the IDSR system. This includes:

1. ***Training healthcare workers***: Providing regular training sessions to healthcare workers on the importance of accurate data reporting, case definitions, and proper data collection techniques.

2. ***Improving data collection tools***: Developing standardized reporting forms and digital data collection tools that prompt for complete and accurate information, reducing the chances of missing or erroneous data.

3. ***Implementing quality assurance measures***: Regular data quality assessments, validation checks, and feedback mechanisms can help identify and correct errors in the surveillance data.

4. ***Enhancing laboratory capacity***: Strengthening laboratory systems to ensure timely and accurate diagnosis, which contributes to more reliable disease reporting and surveillance.

By addressing these challenges and implementing strategies to improve data quality, the IDSR system can become more robust and effective in detecting and responding to disease outbreaks in Africa.

16.7.5 Limited community engagement:

LIMITED COMMUNITY ENGAGEMENT poses a significant challenge to the effectiveness of Integrated Disease Surveillance and Response (IDSR) systems in Africa. Inadequate involvement of communities in disease surveillance and response activities can have several implications for the IDSR system:

1. ***Poor Reporting:*** Without active community participation, there may be underreporting or delayed reporting of disease cases. Community members may not be aware of the importance of reporting diseases or may hesitate to report due to fear, stigma, or mistrust.

2. ***Delayed Detection***: Early detection of disease outbreaks relies on timely reporting of suspected cases. When communities are not actively engaged, there may be delays in recognizing and reporting unusual symptoms or patterns of diseases, which can hinder the rapid response and containment of outbreaks.

3. ***Limited Trust in the Health System***: Effective community engagement builds trust and confidence in the health system. When communities are not involved or feel excluded from disease surveillance and response efforts, they may develop skepticism or distrust towards public health authorities, leading to reluctance in seeking healthcare services or cooperating with response measures.

4. ***Missed Opportunities for Prevention and Control***: Community engagement is crucial for implementing preventive measures such as health education, vaccination campaigns, and vector control activities. Without community participation, these interventions may not reach the target population effectively, resulting in missed opportunities to prevent and control the spread of diseases.

To address limited community engagement in IDSR, it is important to:

1. ***Foster Trust and Communication***: Establish open and transparent communication channels between health authorities and communities. This includes active dialogue, community meetings, and the involvement of community leaders and influencers in disseminating information.

2. ***Promote Health Education and Awareness***: Conduct targeted health education campaigns to raise awareness about the importance of disease reporting, prevention measures, and the role of communities in disease surveillance and response.

3. ***Involve Community Health Workers***: Empower and train community health workers to act as intermediaries between the health system and communities. They can facilitate reporting, provide health education, and address community concerns.

4. ***Participatory Surveillance***: Implement participatory approaches where community members actively participate in disease surveillance activities, such as self-reporting of symptoms, monitoring of disease trends, and reporting of potential outbreaks.

5. ***Tailor Interventions to Cultural Context***: Recognize and respect cultural practices, beliefs, and social norms when designing and implementing community engagement strategies. This ensures that interventions are culturally appropriate and acceptable to the community.

By actively involving communities in disease surveillance and response efforts, the IDSR system can benefit from increased reporting, timely detection of outbreaks, and improved trust and cooperation between communities and the health system.

16.7.6 Climate change and environmental factors:

CLIMATE CHANGE AND environmental factors play a crucial role in the emergence and transmission of infectious diseases, and they can also significantly impact the implementation of Integrated Disease Surveillance and Response (IDSR) systems. Here are some ways in which climate change and environmental factors influence both infectious diseases and IDSR:

1. ***Changes in Vector Distribution***: Climate change can alter the distribution and abundance of disease-carrying vectors like mosquitoes and ticks. As temperatures rise and rainfall patterns change, these vectors may expand their geographical range, bringing diseases like malaria, dengue fever, and Lyme disease to new areas. The shifting distribution of vectors challenges traditional surveillance systems that may not be equipped to detect diseases in regions previously unaffected.

2. ***Seasonal Outbreaks***: Climate variability affects the seasonal patterns of some infectious diseases. For instance, waterborne diseases like cholera may experience increased outbreaks during periods of heavy rainfall and flooding. IDSR systems need to be adaptable to these changing disease patterns to detect and respond to outbreaks effectively.

3. ***Impacts on Water and Foodborne Diseases***: Changes in climate can affect water availability and quality, leading to the contamination of water sources and an increased risk of waterborne diseases such as diarrhea. Additionally, extreme weather events can damage crops and disrupt

food supply chains, increasing the risk of foodborne illnesses. These health threats require vigilant surveillance to prevent and control outbreaks.

4. ***Displacement and Migration***: Climate change-induced environmental disasters, such as hurricanes and droughts, can displace populations, leading to overcrowding and inadequate sanitation in temporary settlements. This scenario creates favorable conditions for infectious diseases to spread rapidly. Migrant populations can also introduce new diseases to regions with susceptible populations.

5. ***Impact on Healthcare Infrastructure***: Climate change can strain healthcare infrastructure and resources. Extreme weather events may damage healthcare facilities, leading to reduced capacity for disease surveillance and response activities. Furthermore, the increased burden of climate-related illnesses can divert resources away from routine disease surveillance efforts.

6. ***Zoonotic Diseases***: Environmental changes can influence the distribution and behavior of animal reservoirs of diseases. This, in turn, impacts the spillover of zoonotic diseases from animals to humans. Diseases like Ebola and COVID-19 have zoonotic origins, and their emergence requires surveillance systems that can detect unusual disease patterns in both human and animal populations.

To effectively address the challenges posed by climate change and environmental factors on IDSR, health authorities need to consider climate resilience in their surveillance strategies. This may involve enhancing early warning systems for climate-related disease outbreaks, integrating environmental data into disease surveillance systems, and strengthening the capacity of healthcare systems to respond to climate-related health emergencies.

Addressing these emerging challenges will require increased investment in health systems, including laboratory capacity, data quality, community engagement, and surveillance and response activities. It will also require a coordinated and integrated approach to disease surveillance and response across all sectors involved in public health, including animal health and the environment.

Table 16: Emerging Challenges in IDSR Implementation in Africa

Challenge	Examples
Weak health systems	- Ebola Outbreak in West Africa (2014-2016)
	- Cholera Outbreaks in Sub-Saharan Africa
	- COVID-19 Pandemic
Disease outbreaks and epidemics	- Zika Virus Outbreak (2015-2016)
	- COVID-19 Pandemic
Inadequate laboratory capacity	- Cholera Outbreaks
	- Lassa Fever Outbreaks
	- Meningitis Outbreaks
	- Yellow Fever Outbreaks
Poor data quality	- Underreporting
	- Inadequate Data Collection and Recording
	- Limited Diagnostic Capacity
	- Data Entry Errors
Limited community engagement	- Poor Reporting
	- Delayed Detection
	- Limited Trust in the Health System
	- Missed Opportunities for Prevention and Control
Climate change and environmental factors	- Changes in Vector Distribution
	- Seasonal Outbreaks
	- Impacts on Water and Foodborne Diseases
	- Displacement and Migration
	- Impact on Healthcare Infrastructure
	- Zoonotic Diseases

This table summarizes the emerging challenges in implementing the Integrated Disease Surveillance and Response (IDSR) system in Africa. The challenges are categorized into six main categories: weak health systems, disease outbreaks and epidemics, inadequate laboratory capacity, poor data quality, limited community engagement, and climate change and environmental factors.

Addressing these challenges requires investments in healthcare infrastructure, laboratory capacity, data quality improvement, community engagement, and climate resilience in disease surveillance strategies. It also calls for a coordinated and integrated approach across sectors involved in public health.

16.8 Opportunities for improvement

DESPITE THE CHALLENGES facing IDSR implementation in Africa, there are several opportunities for improvement, including:

16.8.1 Strengthening health systems:

INVESTING IN HEALTH systems is critical to improving IDSR implementation. This includes increasing funding for public health, improving health infrastructure, and increasing the number and training of health workers.

16.8.2 Enhancing laboratory capacity:

IMPROVING LABORATORY capacity is essential to timely and accurate disease diagnosis and confirmation. This can be achieved through investment in laboratory infrastructure, training of laboratory personnel, and improving the availability of laboratory supplies and reagents.

16.8.3 Increasing community engagement:

ENGAGING COMMUNITIES in disease surveillance and response can improve the effectiveness of the IDSR system. This can be achieved through community education and mobilization, involving community leaders and volunteers in surveillance and response activities, and strengthening community health worker programs.

16.8.4 Leveraging technology:

TECHNOLOGY CAN BE USED to improve the efficiency and effectiveness of IDSR implementation. This includes the use of mobile phone reporting systems, electronic disease surveillance systems, and geographic information systems (GIS) for disease mapping.

16.8.5 Strengthening surveillance and response networks:

BUILDING STRONG SURVEILLANCE and response networks across all sectors involved in public health, including animal health and the environment, can improve the coordination and integration of disease surveillance and response activities.

16.8.6 Increasing research and innovation:

INVESTING IN RESEARCH and innovation can lead to the development of new tools and strategies for disease surveillance and response. This includes the development of new diagnostic tests, vaccines, and drugs, as well as the use of big data analytics and artificial intelligence for disease surveillance and response.

By addressing these opportunities for improvement, countries in Africa can improve their capacity to implement IDSR and effectively prevent, detect, and respond to disease outbreaks.

16.9 Recommendations for the future of IDSR in Africa

BASED ON THE CURRENT state of IDSR implementation in Africa and the opportunities for improvement, the following recommendations can be made for the future of IDSR:

1. **Increase political commitment**: There is a need for strong political commitment and leadership at all levels to ensure the sustained implementation of IDSR. This includes increasing funding for public health, strengthening health systems, and prioritizing disease surveillance and response activities.
2. **Strengthen surveillance and response networks**: Building strong networks across all sectors involved in public health, including animal health and the environment, can improve the coordination and integration of disease surveillance and response activities.
3. **Improve laboratory capacity**: Improving laboratory capacity is critical to timely and accurate disease diagnosis and confirmation. This can be achieved through investment in laboratory infrastructure, training of laboratory personnel, and improving the availability of laboratory supplies and reagents.
4. **Increase community engagement**: Engaging communities in disease surveillance and response can improve the effectiveness of the IDSR system. This can be achieved through community education and mobilization, involving community leaders and volunteers in surveillance and response activities, and strengthening community health worker programs.
5. **Leverage technology**: Technology can be used to improve the efficiency and effectiveness of IDSR implementation. This includes the use of mobile phone reporting systems, electronic disease surveillance systems, and GIS for disease mapping.
6. **Strengthen human resource capacity**: Human resource capacity building is essential to ensure that there are enough trained personnel to carry out IDSR activities at

all levels of the health system. This includes training of health workers in disease surveillance and response, as well as in laboratory and data management.

7. **Increase research and innovation**: Investing in research and innovation can lead to the development of new tools and strategies for disease surveillance and response. This includes the development of new diagnostic tests, vaccines, and drugs, as well as the use of big data analytics and artificial intelligence for disease surveillance and response.

By implementing these recommendations, countries in Africa can improve their capacity to implement IDSR and effectively prevent, detect, and respond to disease outbreaks, ultimately improving public health and saving lives.

16.10 Exercises

1. What is the purpose of monitoring and evaluating the IDSR system? A. To identify gaps and areas for improvement B. To increase the workload of health workers C. To reduce the number of diseases under surveillance D. To decrease the number of laboratory tests performed

Solution: A. Monitoring and evaluating the IDSR system helps to identify gaps and areas for improvement, which can lead to the development of strategic plans for strengthening the system.

1. What evaluation framework is commonly used to assess the attributes of the IDSR system? A. The WHO Framework for Evaluation of Surveillance Systems B. The

Framework for Integrated Disease Surveillance and Response C. The Framework for Capacity Building in Public Health D. The Framework for Monitoring and Evaluation in Health

Solution: A. The WHO Framework for Evaluation of Surveillance Systems is commonly used to assess the attributes of the IDSR system.

1. Which country conducted a comprehensive evaluation of the IDSR system in 2007? A. Liberia B. Uganda C. Kenya D. Nigeria

Solution: B. Uganda conducted a comprehensive evaluation of the IDSR system in 2007.

1. What were the main gaps identified in the Ugandan IDSR system during the 2007 evaluation? A. Inadequate laboratory capacity and poor data management B. Lack of training for health workers and poor communication C. Inadequate funding and poor leadership D. Lack of community involvement and poor surveillance activities

Solution: A. The 2007 evaluation of the Ugandan IDSR system identified inadequate laboratory capacity and poor data management as main gaps in the system.

1. What was the main recommendation for improving the IDSR system in Liberia following the 2012 evaluation? A. Strengthen laboratory capacity B. Increase the number of health workers C. Expand the list of diseases under surveillance D. Improve community involvement in disease surveillance

Solution: A. The main recommendation for improving the IDSR system in Liberia following the 2012 evaluation was to strengthen laboratory capacity.

1. Multiple-choice questions

Why is Integrated Disease Surveillance and Response (IDSR) important in Africa? A. To help prevent and control infectious diseases B. To improve maternal and child health outcomes C. To monitor the burden of non-communicable diseases D. To enhance the capacity of healthcare systems to respond to emergencies

Solution: The correct answer is A, as IDSR is crucial in preventing and controlling infectious diseases, which are a major public health concern in Africa. While improving maternal and child health outcomes, monitoring non-communicable diseases, and enhancing healthcare system capacity are also important, they are not the primary focus of IDSR.

16.11 Call to action for continued improvement and implementation of IDSR in Africa.

AS THE BOOK ON INTEGRATED Disease Surveillance and Response (IDSR) in Africa highlights, the implementation of IDSR is critical to prevent and control disease outbreaks on the continent. While significant progress has been made in many countries, there are still challenges that need to be addressed to ensure the effective implementation of IDSR across the continent. Therefore, it is important for stakeholders at all levels to take action to continue to improve and strengthen IDSR implementation in Africa.

This call to action could include:

1. **Government commitment**: Governments across Africa should continue to demonstrate political will and allocate sufficient resources to support the implementation of IDSR. This includes prioritizing disease surveillance and response in national health policies and budgets.

2. **Capacity building and training**: To ensure the effective implementation of IDSR, there is a need for ongoing capacity building and training for health workers at all levels. This should include training on disease surveillance, laboratory diagnosis, outbreak response, data management, and communication.

3. **Collaboration and coordination**: Collaboration and coordination between different stakeholders, including governments, international organizations, non-governmental organizations, and the private sector, is critical to strengthen the implementation of IDSR. This includes working together to develop and implement effective disease surveillance and response strategies, sharing data and information, and coordinating outbreak response efforts.

4. **Improved laboratory services**: The quality and availability of laboratory services in Africa need to be improved to support disease diagnosis and response. This includes improving laboratory infrastructure, equipment, and staffing, and expanding laboratory networks to ensure access to diagnostic services across the continent.

5. **Continuous monitoring and evaluation**: Continuous monitoring and evaluation of IDSR implementation is

essential to identify areas for improvement and track progress over time. This includes monitoring disease trends, evaluating the effectiveness of outbreak response efforts, and assessing the quality of data collected through the IDSR system.

By taking action to address these challenges and implement these recommendations, stakeholders across Africa can work together to ensure the effective implementation of IDSR and prevent and control disease outbreaks on the continent.

Appendices

Appendix A: List of diseases of public health importance in Africa:

1. Malaria
2. HIV/AIDS
3. Tuberculosis
4. Cholera
5. Measles
6. Lassa fever
7. Yellow fever
8. Ebola virus disease
9. Rift Valley fever
10. Poliomyelitis
11. Onchocerciasis (river blindness)
12. Schistosomiasis
13. Sleeping sickness (African trypanosomiasis)
14. Guinea worm disease
15. Trachoma
16. Chikungunya fever
17. Dengue fever
18. Leishmaniasis
19. Meningococcal meningitis
20. Typhoid fever

It is worth noting that this list is not exhaustive and may vary depending on the region or country within Africa.

Appendix B: Sample data collection and reporting forms

THE FORMS USED MAY vary by country, but some common examples include:

- **Weekly IDSR reporting form**: This is used to report on a weekly basis the occurrence of diseases and conditions that are under surveillance. The form includes information on the number of cases, deaths, and the geographic distribution of the disease.
- **Outbreak investigation form**: This is used when an outbreak is suspected or confirmed. It includes information on the date of onset, the symptoms of the disease, the number of cases, the location of the outbreak, and the results of laboratory tests.
- **Laboratory request form**: This is used to request laboratory testing for suspected cases of disease. The form includes information on the patient, the suspected disease, and the type of testing required.
- **Surveillance evaluation form**: This is used to evaluate the effectiveness of the surveillance system. The form includes information on the surveillance objectives, the methods used, and the results of the evaluation.

These forms are used to collect and report data in a standardized and systematic manner, which allows for timely identification and response to disease outbreaks.

Appendix C: List of national and international organizations involved in IDSR implementation in Africa

HERE ARE SOME EXAMPLES of national and international organizations involved in IDSR implementation in Africa:

- World Health Organization (WHO)
- Centers for Disease Control and Prevention (CDC)
- Africa CDC
- Ministries of Health in various African countries
- International Health Regulations (IHR) National Focal Points
- United States Agency for International Development (USAID)
- United Nations International Children's Emergency Fund (UNICEF)
- Médecins Sans Frontières (MSF)
- The Global Fund
- The World Bank.

Appendix D: Training and capacity building resources

HERE ARE SOME EXAMPLES of training and capacity building resources for IDSR implementation in Africa:

- WHO Integrated Disease Surveillance and Response (IDSR) e-learning course
- CDC Training and Resources for Surveillance and Epidemiology
- Africa CDC Online Training Platform
- Global Health eLearning Center's course on Integrated Disease Surveillance and Response (IDSR)
- USAID ASSIST Project's resources on strengthening disease surveillance and response
- UNICEF's Capacity Building for Improved Service Delivery (CBISD) programme
- The Global Health Security Agenda (GHSA) Training and Learning Centre
- Field Epidemiology Training Programmes (FETP) offered by various African countries and international partners.

Appendix E: List of reference laboratories for disease diagnosis and confirmation

HERE ARE SOME EXAMPLES of reference laboratories for disease diagnosis and confirmation in Africa:

- National Institute for Communicable Diseases (NICD) - South Africa
- African Centre of Excellence for Genomics of Infectious Diseases (ACEGID) - Nigeria
- Kenya Medical Research Institute (KEMRI) - Kenya
- Institut Pasteur de Dakar - Senegal
- National Public Health Laboratory (NPHL) - Ethiopia
- National Institute of Biomedical Research (INRB) - Democratic Republic of the Congo
- Central Public Health Laboratory (CPHL) - Tanzania
- National Institute of Virology (NIV) - South Africa
- Armauer Hansen Research Institute (AHRI) - Ethiopia
- Medical Research Council Unit The Gambia at London School of Hygiene & Tropical Medicine - The Gambia

Note: This is not an exhaustive list, and there may be other reference laboratories in Africa.

Appendix F: Sample outbreak response plans and guidelines

HERE IS AN EXAMPLE of a sample outbreak response plan and guidelines:

Introduction

The purpose of this document is to provide guidance on how to respond to outbreaks of infectious diseases. It outlines the roles and responsibilities of key stakeholders, the steps to be taken in an outbreak response, and the key factors to be considered when implementing a response plan.

Definitions Outbreak:

The occurrence of cases of a particular disease in a population greater than expected. Case: A person who has signs and symptoms of a disease. Confirmed case: A person who has tested positive for the disease. Suspected case: A person who has signs and symptoms of the disease, but has not yet been confirmed. Contact: A person who has been in close proximity to a confirmed or suspected case.

Roles and Responsibilities

National Health Authorities:

- Designate a national focal point for outbreak response.
- Establish mechanisms for coordination and communication with other stakeholders.
- Conduct surveillance to detect outbreaks and monitor the situation.
- Provide guidance and technical support to sub-national health authorities.

- Mobilize resources to support outbreak response activities.

Sub-National Health Authorities:

- Conduct surveillance to detect outbreaks and monitor the situation.
- Report outbreaks to the national health authorities.
- Initiate outbreak response activities in coordination with the national health authorities.
- Provide guidance and technical support to health facilities and other stakeholders in their jurisdiction.

Health Facilities:

- Report suspected and confirmed cases to the sub-national health authorities.
- Implement infection prevention and control measures to prevent the spread of the disease.
- Collect and submit specimens for laboratory confirmation.

Laboratories:

- Conduct laboratory testing to confirm suspected cases.
- Share laboratory results with health authorities.
- Implement biosafety measures to protect laboratory staff.

Other Stakeholders:

- Provide support as needed to health authorities and health facilities.
- Disseminate accurate information to the public.

Steps in an Outbreak Response

Step 1: Detection and Confirmation

- Health facilities and surveillance systems should be vigilant for signs of outbreaks.
- Suspected cases should be tested and confirmed cases should be reported to health authorities.

Step 2: Investigation

- Health authorities should investigate the outbreak to determine the extent of the problem and the source of the infection.
- Contact tracing should be conducted to identify additional cases.

Step 3: Control Measures

- Appropriate control measures should be implemented to prevent the spread of the disease.
- Health facilities should implement infection prevention and control measures.
- Suspected and confirmed cases should be isolated and treated appropriately.
- Contacts should be identified and monitored for signs of infection.

Step 4: Communication

- Accurate and timely information should be disseminated to the public, healthcare workers, and other stakeholders.
- Communication should be clear and concise, and should address concerns and questions from the public.

Step 5: Monitoring and Evaluation

- The outbreak response should be monitored to assess its effectiveness.
- The response plan should be evaluated after the outbreak has been controlled to identify areas for improvement.

Conclusion Outbreaks of infectious diseases can have serious public health consequences. A rapid and effective response is critical to preventing the spread of disease and minimizing the impact on the population. This document provides guidance on the key steps in an outbreak response and the roles and responsibilities of key stakeholders.

Monitoring and evaluation tools and checklists

Here are some examples of monitoring and evaluation tools and checklists that can be used in IDSR implementation in Africa:

- **IDSR Evaluation Tool**: This tool can be used to evaluate the performance of the IDSR system at the district and national levels. It covers key areas such as surveillance, laboratory services, outbreak response, and communication.
- **IDSR Performance Monitoring Checklist**: This checklist can be used by district or national level staff to monitor the performance of the IDSR system on a regular basis. It covers indicators such as timeliness and completeness of reporting, disease case detection rates, and laboratory confirmation rates.
- **IDSR Capacity Building Assessment Tool**: This tool can be used to assess the capacity of IDSR staff at the district and national levels. It covers areas such as

knowledge, skills, and attitudes related to disease surveillance, laboratory services, and outbreak response.

- **IDSR Data Quality Assessment Tool**: This tool can be used to assess the quality of data collected and reported through the IDSR system. It covers areas such as completeness, accuracy, and timeliness of reporting.
- **IDSR Communication and Feedback Assessment Tool**: This tool can be used to assess the effectiveness of communication and feedback mechanisms within the IDSR system. It covers areas such as communication between levels of the health system, feedback to reporting sites, and use of data for decision-making.

These tools and checklists can be customized and adapted to the specific context and needs of each country or district implementing the IDSR system.

Appendix G: List of key stakeholders in IDSR implementation in Africa and their roles

KEY STAKEHOLDERS IN IDSR implementation in Africa and their roles may include:

- National Ministries of Health: responsible for coordinating the implementation of IDSR at the country level, including providing leadership and oversight, setting policies and guidelines, and allocating resources.
- District Health Teams: responsible for the implementation of IDSR at the local level, including data collection, analysis, and reporting, and outbreak response.
- World Health Organization (WHO): provides technical support to countries for IDSR implementation, including developing and disseminating guidelines and training materials, conducting assessments and evaluations, and facilitating communication and coordination among stakeholders.
- Africa Centres for Disease Control and Prevention (Africa CDC): supports countries in developing and implementing IDSR, including providing technical assistance, conducting training and capacity building activities, and coordinating regional and cross-border surveillance and response.
- National Public Health Institutes (NPHIs): responsible for conducting surveillance, laboratory testing, and outbreak response, and for providing technical support to districts and other health facilities.
- Non-governmental organizations (NGOs): support IDSR implementation by providing technical assistance, training, and funding for surveillance and response

activities.

- Development partners: provide financial and technical support for IDSR implementation, including funding for equipment, training, and infrastructure development.
- Community members: play an important role in IDSR by reporting suspected cases of disease, participating in community-based surveillance activities, and supporting outbreak response efforts.

Overall, the key stakeholders in IDSR implementation in Africa work together to strengthen disease surveillance and response systems, detect and respond to outbreaks quickly, and ultimately improve public health outcomes in the region.

Appendix H: Glossary of all key terms and acronyms used in IDSR.

HERE IS A SAMPLE GLOSSARY of key terms and acronyms used in IDSR:

Active case finding: A strategy that involves actively searching for individuals with a particular disease, usually through community-based surveys or screenings.

Acute flaccid paralysis (AFP): A clinical syndrome characterized by sudden onset of weakness or paralysis in one or more limbs.

Adverse event following immunization (AEFI): Any untoward medical occurrence that follows immunization, which may or may not be related to the vaccine.

Aggregated data: Data that has been summarized or grouped together, typically at a higher level than individual cases.

Alert threshold: The level at which a surveillance system is designed to trigger an alarm or alert for a particular disease or event.

Bed net: A mosquito netting used to protect against malaria and other vector-borne diseases.

Biosafety: The principles and practices that ensure the safe handling, storage, and disposal of biological materials to prevent accidental exposure or release into the environment.

Biosafety level: A numerical rating that indicates the level of containment required for working with particular types of biological agents, based on their potential risk to human health and the environment.

Burden of disease: The overall impact of a particular disease on a population, including its morbidity, mortality, and social and economic consequences.

Case definition: A set of criteria used to determine whether an individual is considered to have a particular disease or condition.

Case investigation: The process of identifying and interviewing individuals with a particular disease or condition to determine the source of infection, potential contacts, and other relevant information.

Case management: The medical and supportive care provided to individuals with a particular disease or condition.

Case notification: The process of reporting a confirmed or suspected case of a particular disease to the appropriate authorities.

Case reporting: The collection and transmission of data on confirmed or suspected cases of a particular disease from health facilities to public health authorities.

Contact tracing: The process of identifying and monitoring individuals who have been in close contact with a confirmed case of a particular disease to prevent further transmission.

Cross-border collaboration: Cooperation between neighboring countries to address common health issues, such as disease outbreaks, that cross national borders.

Data analysis: The process of transforming raw data into meaningful information that can be used for decision-making.

Data quality: The accuracy, completeness, and timeliness of data.

Disease outbreak: The occurrence of cases of a particular disease in excess of what is normally expected within a given population or geographical area.

District health team: A multidisciplinary team responsible for the planning, implementation, and monitoring of health activities at the district level.

Early warning system: A system designed to detect and alert public health authorities to potential disease outbreaks or other public health emergencies.

Epidemic: An increase in the number of cases of a particular disease in a particular population or geographical area, usually above what is normally expected.

Epidemiology: The study of the distribution and determinants of health and disease in populations.

Essential medicines: Medicines that are considered necessary and cost-effective for meeting the priority health needs of a population.

Focal person: An individual designated to oversee a specific area or activity within a public health program, such as disease surveillance or laboratory services.

Field epidemiology: The application of epidemiological methods to investigate and control outbreaks of disease in the field.

Formative research: Research conducted to inform the development or implementation of public health programs or interventions.

Health information system: A system designed to collect, process, analyze, and disseminate information related to health and healthcare.

Health promotion: The process of enabling individuals and communities to increase control over and improve their health.

Health facility: A place where health services are provided, including hospitals, clinics, health posts, and dispensaries.

Health information system (HIS): A system that collects, analyzes, and uses health-related data and information.

IDSR: Integrated Disease Surveillance and Response.

Incidence: The number of new cases of a disease occurring within a specific population over a defined period of time.

Indicator: A variable or measure that is used to assess or describe a particular aspect of a health system, disease, or population.

Infectious disease: A disease caused by a microorganism, such as a bacterium, virus, parasite, or fungus, that can be transmitted from one person to another.

Integrated surveillance system: A system that combines data from different sources to provide a comprehensive picture of a disease or health event.

Laboratory: A facility where diagnostic tests are conducted on samples of bodily fluids, tissues, or other substances to identify the presence or absence of a disease or condition.

Morbidity: The occurrence of illness or disease within a population.

Mortality: The occurrence of death within a population.

Outbreak: The occurrence of cases of a disease in excess of what is normally expected within a specific geographic area and time period.

Passive surveillance: A system in which health workers report cases of disease to health authorities when they occur.

Population: A group of individuals living in a defined geographic area.

Prevalence: The proportion of individuals in a population who have a specific disease or condition at a specific point in time.

Real-time surveillance: A system that provides data and information on a disease or health event as it occurs.

Reporting: The process of notifying health authorities of the occurrence of a disease or health event.

Sentinel surveillance: A system in which a representative sample of health facilities or population groups report data on a disease or health event.

Surveillance: The ongoing systematic collection, analysis, interpretation, and dissemination of data on a disease or health event.

Threshold: The level of incidence or prevalence that triggers a response to a disease or health event.

Underreporting: The failure to report cases of a disease or health event to health authorities.

Vector: An organism, such as a mosquito or tick, that can transmit a disease from one host to another.

WHO: World Health Organization.

Bibliography

ACT-ACCELERATOR. (2021). Access to COVID-19 Tools Accelerator. Retrieved from https://www.who.int/initiatives/act-accelerator

Adam DC, et al. (2020). Clustering and superspreading potential of SARS-CoV-2 infections in Hong Kong. Nature Medicine, 26(11), 1714-1719.

Adams, L. V., Perin, D. M., Prado, M. R., de Queiroz, T. L., & Ribeiro, G. S. (2018). Community engagement and Zika virus control in Brazil: Lessons learned and the way forward. Tropical Medicine and International Health, 23(12), 1314-1320. doi: 10.1111/tmi.13159

Adekolu-John, E. O., et al. (2015). Schistosoma haematobium infection in schoolchildren in Abeokuta, Nigeria: Urine microscopy and serologic test comparison. Asian Pacific Journal of Tropical Biomedicine, 5(7), 584-589. doi:10.1016/j.apjtb.2015.03.012

Africa Centres for Disease Control and Prevention (Africa CDC). (n.d.). About Africa CDC. Retrieved from https://africacdc.org/about-us/

African Field Epidemiology Network. (n.d.). About AFENET. Retrieved from https://www.afenet.net/index.php/en/about-afenet

African Society for Laboratory Medicine. (n.d.). About ASLM. Retrieved from https://www.aslm.org/about/

African Union. (n.d.). Africa CDC COVID-19 Response Fund. Retrieved from https://africacdc.org/donate/

Aguemon, B., Taha, M. K., & Mueller, J. E. (2017). Laboratory diagnosis of meningococcal meningitis. The Lancet Infectious Diseases, 17(10), e368-e377. doi: 10.1016/S1473-3099(17)30319-1

Akpede, G. O., Asogun, D., Okogbenin, S. A., Akpede, N., Agbonlahor, D., & Okokhere, P. (2018). Lassa fever: Epidemiology, clinical features, diagnosis, management, and prevention. Infectious Disease Reports, 10(2), 24-28. doi: 10.4081/idr.2018.7581

Allegranzi B, et al. (2011). The First Global Patient Safety Challenge "Clean Care is Safer Care": From launch to current progress and achievements. Journal of Hospital Infection, 79(3), 1-6.

Altizer, S., Ostfeld, R. S., Johnson, P. T., Kutz, S., & Harvell, C. D. (2013). Climate change and infectious diseases: from evidence to a predictive framework. Science, 341(6145), 514-519.

Andersen, K. G., Rambaut, A., Lipkin, W. I., Holmes, E. C., & Garry, R. F. (2020). The proximal origin of SARS-CoV-2. Nature Medicine, 26(4), 450-452.

Anderson, R. M., & May, R. M. (1991). Infectious diseases of humans: dynamics and control. Oxford University Press.

Anderson, R. M., May, R. M. (1992). Infectious Diseases of Humans: Dynamics and Control. Oxford University Press.

Andrews JR, et al. (2014). Transmission dynamics of tuberculosis in Tijuana, Mexico: Modeling community-based interventions to reduce transmission. Journal of Infectious Diseases, 210(4), 504-514.

Aral SO, et al. (2012). Sexual mixing patterns in the spread of HIV/AIDS: A review. Sexually Transmitted Infections, 88(Suppl 2), i82-i87.

Bawo, L., Faye, O., & Ndiaye, M. (2016). Enhancing surveillance and response to emerging zoonotic diseases in East Africa through digital surveillance. BMC Veterinary Research, 12(1), 13.

Bergman, A. (2020). Jacinda Ardern's leadership style: Empathy, reassurance and straight talk. The Guardian. Retrieved from https://www.theguardian.com/world/2020/dec/13/jacinda-arderns-leadership-style-empathy-reassurance-and-straight-talk

Biswas, A., & Rahman, A. (2020). Climate Change and Food Security: Implications for Sustainable Agriculture. Journal of Agricultural Extension and Rural Development, 12(1), 1-10.

Black, R., Adger, W. N., Arnell, N. W., et al. (2011). The effect of climate change on migration and displacement. Global Environmental Change, 21(Supplement 1), S3-S11.

Butler, C. D., & Friel, S. (2006). Food, water, and population health: security and scarcity. The Lancet, 365(9458), 540-541.

Bwire, G., Ali, M., Sack, D. A., & Mogasale, V. (2017). Challenges and opportunities for cholera control in sub-Saharan Africa: the case of Uganda. Journal of Infectious Diseases, 216(Supplement_1), S27-S32. doi: 10.1093/infdis/jiw617

Cairncross, S., & Feachem, R. (1993). Environmental Health Engineering in the Tropics: An Introductory Text (2nd ed.). Wiley.

Campbell-Lendrum, D., Manga, L., Bagayoko, M., Sommerfeld, J., & Menne, B. (2015). Climate change and vector-borne diseases: what are the implications for public health research and policy?. Philosophical Transactions of the Royal Society B: Biological Sciences, 370(1665), 20130552.

Centers for Disease Control and Prevention (CDC). (2019). Parasites - Toxoplasmosis. Retrieved from https://www.cdc.gov/parasites/toxoplasmosis/index.html

Centers for Disease Control and Prevention (CDC). (2020). Human Papillomavirus (HPV). Retrieved from https://www.cdc.gov/std/hpv/

Centers for Disease Control and Prevention (CDC). (2020). Parasites - Lice. Retrieved from https://www.cdc.gov/parasites/lice/index.html

Centers for Disease Control and Prevention (CDC). (2021). Genital Herpes. Retrieved from https://www.cdc.gov/std/herpes/

Centers for Disease Control and Prevention (CDC). (2021). Gonorrhea. Retrieved from https://www.cdc.gov/std/gonorrhea/

Centers for Disease Control and Prevention (CDC). (2021). Handwashing: Clean Hands Save Lives. Retrieved from https://www.cdc.gov/handwashing/index.html

Centers for Disease Control and Prevention (CDC). (2021). HIV Testing. Retrieved from https://www.cdc.gov/hiv/testing/index.html

Centers for Disease Control and Prevention (CDC). (2021). HIV/AIDS. Retrieved from https://www.cdc.gov/hiv/basics/whatishiv.html

Centers for Disease Control and Prevention (CDC). (2021). Isolation and Quarantine. Retrieved from https://www.cdc.gov/quarantine/index.html

Centers for Disease Control and Prevention (CDC). (2021). Lyme Disease. Retrieved from https://www.cdc.gov/lyme/index.html

Centers for Disease Control and Prevention (CDC). (2021). Sexually Transmitted Diseases (STDs) - Testing. Retrieved from https://www.cdc.gov/std/testing/default.htm

Centers for Disease Control and Prevention (CDC). (2021). Tuberculosis (TB) Testing. Retrieved from https://www.cdc.gov/tb/topic/testing/default.htm

Centers for Disease Control and Prevention (CDC). (2021). West Nile Virus. Retrieved from https://www.cdc.gov/westnile/index.html

Centers for Disease Control and Prevention (CDC). (2021). Zika Virus. Retrieved from https://www.cdc.gov/zika/index.html

Centers for Disease Control and Prevention (CDC). Fungal Diseases. Retrieved from https://www.cdc.gov/fungal/index.html

Centers for Disease Control and Prevention (CDC). Group A Streptococcal (GAS) Disease. Retrieved from https://www.cdc.gov/groupastrep/diseases-public/index.html

Centers for Disease Control and Prevention (CDC). Infectious Diseases. Retrieved from https://www.cdc.gov/ncezid/index.html

Centers for Disease Control and Prevention (CDC). Infectious Disease Laboratory Testing. Retrieved from https://www.cdc.gov/csels/dls/locs/2020/laboratory-testing-infectious-diseases.html

Centers for Disease Control and Prevention (CDC). Influenza (Flu). Retrieved from https://www.cdc.gov/flu/index.htm

Centers for Disease Control and Prevention (CDC). Principles of Epidemiology in Public Health Practice. Retrieved from https://www.cdc.gov/csels/dsepd/ss1978/index.html

Centers for Disease Control and Prevention. (2019). Pandemic Influenza Storybook: International Responses to the H1N1 Influenza 2009. Retrieved from https://www.cdc.gov/flu/pandemic-resources/pdf/2009-storybook-web-508.pdf

Centers for Disease Control and Prevention. (2021). Antiviral agents for the treatment and chemoprophylaxis of influenza: Recommendations of the Advisory Committee on Immunization Practices (ACIP). MMWR Recommendations and Reports, 70(1), 1-28.

Centers for Disease Control and Prevention. (2021). Interim Public Health Recommendations for Fully Vaccinated People. Retrieved from https://www.cdc.gov/coronavirus/2019-ncov/vaccines/fully-vaccinated-guidance.html

Centers for Disease Control and Prevention. (2021). National Notifiable Diseases Surveillance System (NNDSS). Retrieved from https://www.cdc.gov/nndss/index.html

Centers for Disease Control and Prevention. (2021). People who need extra precautions. Retrieved from https://www.cdc.gov/coronavirus/2019-ncov/need-extra-precautions/index.html

Cetron, M., Hamer, D. H., & Perl, T. M. (2003). The "Hong Kong" flu: The global response to the pandemic of 1968-1969. Clinical Infectious Diseases, 37(6), 829-837.

Chen, S., Tevi-Benissan, C., Wong, G., Leung, A., & Fairley, C. K. (2018). Yellow fever vaccine: Why do we need it? Journal of Travel Medicine, 25(suppl_1), S20-S26. doi: 10.1093/jtm/tay044

Confalonieri, U., Menne, B., Akhtar, R., Ebi, K. L., Hauengue, M., Kovats, R. S., & Revich, B. (2007). Human health. Climate Change 2007: Impacts, Adaptation, and Vulnerability. Contribution of Working Group II to the Fourth Assessment Report of the Intergovernmental Panel on Climate Change.

Corbett EL, et al. (2003). The impact of HIV infection on TB transmission in high HIV prevalence settings: A systematic review. Journal of Infectious Diseases, 188(7), 1151-1157.

Curtis V, Cairncross S. (2003). Effect of washing hands with soap on diarrhoea risk in the community: A systematic review. The Lancet Infectious Diseases, 3(5), 275-281.

Denecke, K., & Velasco, E. (2015). Monitoring online media reports for early detection of unknown infectious diseases: Proposal for a digital early warning system. Journal of Medical Internet Research, 17(12), e215.

Department of Health. (2013). National Action Plan to Prevent and Control Healthcare Associated Infections in Ireland. Retrieved from https://assets.gov.ie/22136/6d3eb02d736f4b2ea3be38307a40b5c4.pdf

Dhillon, R. S., Kelly, J. D., Schwartz, R., & Nshom, E. (2017). Ebola epidemic in Liberia: Courage, quick response, and resilience of the society. Surgery, 161(6), 1574-1580. doi: 10.1016/j.surg.2016.12.026

Drummond, M. F., Sculpher, M. J., Claxton, K., Stoddart, G. L., & Torrance, G. W. (2015). Methods for the Economic Evaluation of Health Care Programmes. Oxford University Press.

Dzinamarira, T., Dzobo, M., & Chitungo, I. (2020). COVID-19: A perspective on Africa's capacity and response. Journal of Medical Virology, 92(11), 2465-2472. doi: 10.1002/jmv.25904

East African Integrated Disease Surveillance Network. (n.d.). About EAIDSNet. Retrieved from https://eac.int/health/index.php?option=com_content&view=article&id=192&Itemid=539

Ebi, K. L., & Nealon, J. (2016). Dengue in a changing climate. Environmental Research, 151, 115-123.

European Centre for Disease Prevention and Control (ECDC). (n.d.). Coordination mechanisms. Retrieved from https://www.ecdc.europa.eu/en/about-us/who-we-cooperate/coordination-mechanisms

European Centre for Disease Prevention and Control (ECDC). (n.d.). About us. Retrieved from https://www.ecdc.europa.eu/en/about-us

European Centre for Disease Prevention and Control (ECDC). (n.d.). Mission and vision. Retrieved from https://www.ecdc.europa.eu/en/about-us/who-we-are/mission-vision

European Centre for Disease Prevention and Control. (2021). About ECDC. Retrieved from https://www.ecdc.europa.eu/en/about-us

European Centre for Disease Prevention and Control. (2021). European Surveillance System (TESSy). Retrieved from

https://www.ecdc.europa.eu/en/about-us/what-we-do/
surveillance-and-disease-data/european-surveillance-system-tessey

European Centre for Disease Prevention and Control. (2021).
European Influenza Surveillance Network (EISN). Retrieved from
https://www.ecdc.europa.eu/en/seasonal-influenza/surveillance-
and-disease-data/european-influenza-surveillance-network-eisn

European Centre for Disease Prevention and Control. (2021).
European Antimicrobial Resistance Surveillance Network
(EARS-Net). Retrieved from https://www.ecdc.europa.eu/en/
about-us/what-we-do/surveillance-and-disease-data/european-
antimicrobial-resistance-surveillance

European Commission. The Logical Framework Approach.
Retrieved from https://ec.europa.eu/europeaid/sites/devco/files/
methodological_guide_-_logical_framework_en.pdf

European Commission. The Logical Framework Approach.
Retrieved from https://ec.europa.eu/europeaid/sites/devco/files/
methodological_guide_-_logical_framework_en

European Commission. The Logical Framework Approach.
Retrieved from https://ec.europa.eu/europeaid/sites/devco/files/
methodological_guide_-_logical_framework_en

FAO/OIE/WHO. (2019). Contributing to One World, One
Health: A Strategic Framework for Reducing Risks of Infectious
Diseases at the Animal-Human-Ecosystems Interface. Retrieved
from http://www.fao.org/3/i1323e/i1323e00.pdf

FAO/OIE/WHO. (2019). Contributing to One World, One
Health: A Strategic Framework for Reducing Risks of Infectious
Diseases at the Animal-Human-Ecosystems Interface. Retrieved
from http://www.fao.org/3/i1323e/i1323e00.pdf

Federal Ministry of Health Nigeria. (2017). Nigeria National Action Plan for Health Security (NAPHS) 2018-2022. Retrieved from https://extranet.who.int/sph/docs/file/3287

Fichet-Calvet, E., & Rogers, D. J. (2009). Risk maps of Lassa fever in West Africa. PLoS Neglected Tropical Diseases, 3(3), e388. doi: 10.1371/journal.pntd.0000388

Fitzpatrick, G. (2015). The West Africa Ebola outbreak: What lessons were learned? The Lancet Infectious Diseases, 15(3), 252-253.

Fitzpatrick, G. (2015). The West Africa Ebola outbreak: What lessons were learned? The Lancet Infectious Diseases, 15(3), 252-253.

Fleming-Dutra, K. E., Hersh, A. L., Shapiro, D. J., et al. (2016). Prevalence of Inappropriate Antibiotic Prescriptions Among US Ambulatory Care Visits, 2010-2011. JAMA, 315(17), 1864-1873.

Fleming-Dutra, K. E., Hersh, A. L., Shapiro, D. J., et al. (2016). Prevalence of Inappropriate Antibiotic Prescriptions Among US Ambulatory Care Visits, 2010-2011. JAMA, 315(17), 1864-1873.

Ford, J. D., Berrang-Ford, L., & Paterson, J. (2011). A systematic review of observed climate change adaptation in developed nations: Adaptation to climate change in developed nations. Climatic Change, 106(2), 327-336.

Ford, J. D., Berrang-Ford, L., & Paterson, J. (2011). A systematic review of observed climate change adaptation in developed nations: Adaptation to climate change in developed nations. Climatic Change, 106(2), 327-336.

Freifeld, C. C., Chunara, R., Mekaru, S. R., Chan, E. H., Kass-Hout, T., Ayala Iacucci, A., Brownstein, J. S. (2010). Participatory epidemiology: use of mobile phones for community-based health reporting. PLoS Medicine, 7(12), e1000376. doi: 10.1371/journal.pmed.1000376

Freimuth, V. S., Musa, D., & Hilyard, K. (2009). Strategies for Effective Communication during Public Health Emergencies: Lessons Learned from Controversies in Public Health Crises. Journal of Health Communication, 14(5), 415-431. doi: 10.1080/10810730903032947

Friedman, E. A., Gostin, L. O., Buse, K., & Sridhar, D. (2018). Ebola in the Democratic Republic of the Congo: time to sound a global alert? The Lancet, 392(10149), 449-451. doi: 10.1016/S0140-6736(18)31374-3

Garelli, F. M., Espinosa, M. O., Weinberg, D., Coto, H. D., & Gaspe, M. S. (2009). Usefulness of generalized additive models for predicting complex biological processes: The case of Aedes aegypti (Diptera: Culicidae) pupal development. Environmental Entomology, 38(3), 458–466. doi: 10.1603/022.038.0303

GPHIN. (n.d.). Global Public Health Intelligence Network. World Health Organization. Retrieved from https://www.who.int/csr/alertresponse/gphin/en/

Grace, D., Mutua, F., Ochungo, P., Kruska, R. L., Jones, K., Brierley, L., ... & Ogutu, F. (2012). Mapping of poverty and likely zoonoses hotspots. Zoonoses Project 4. Report to the UK Department for International Development. Nairobi, Kenya: ILRI.

Gulland, A. (2014). Ebola outbreak is a "public health emergency of international concern," WHO warns. BMJ, 349, g5089.

Gyawali, N., & Bradbury, R. S. (2019). Strengthening health systems for global health security: insights from a systematic review. BMJ Global Health, 4(4), e001637.

Hales, S., de Wet, N., Maindonald, J., Woodward, A. (2002). Potential effect of population and climate changes on global distribution of dengue fever: an empirical model. The Lancet, 360(9336), 830-834.

Hassell, J. M., Begon, M., Ward, M. J., & Fèvre, E. M. (2017). Urbanization and disease emergence: dynamics at the wildlife–livestock–human interface. Trends in ecology & evolution, 32(1), 55-67.

Hastings, R., Kidd, M., & Cai, M. (2019). Surveillance Outbreak Response Management and Analysis System (SORMAS): A new way of detecting and responding to public health threats in Nigeria. Public Health Action, 9(Suppl 1), S18-S21.

Health Protection Surveillance Centre. (2021). Infectious Disease Surveillance Reports. Retrieved from https://www.hpsc.ie/a-z/respiratory/coronavirus/novelcoronavirus/surveillance/infectiousdiseasesurveillance/

Hethcote, H. W. (2000). The mathematics of infectious diseases. SIAM Review, 42(4), 599-653.

Higgins, J. P., Thomas, J., Chandler, J., Cumpston, M., Li, T., Page, M. J., & Welch, V. A. (Eds.). (2019). Cochrane Handbook for Systematic Reviews of Interventions. John Wiley & Sons.

International Organization for Migration. (2017). Migration, Environment and Climate Change: Evidence for Policy. IOM.

International Society for Infectious Diseases. (2021). ProMED-mail. Retrieved from https://www.promedmail.org/

Jefferson T, et al. (2008). Physical interventions to interrupt or reduce the spread of respiratory viruses. Cochrane Database of Systematic Reviews, 2, CD006207.

Joint United Nations Programme on HIV/AIDS (UNAIDS). (2020). Country Fact Sheets 2020. Retrieved from https://www.unaids.org/en/resources/fact-sheet

Keeling, M. J., & Rohani, P. (2008). Modeling infectious diseases in humans and animals. Princeton University Press.

Keusch, G. T., Pappaioanou, M., Gonzalez, M. C., & Scott, K. A. (2010). Global health through global disease surveillance and response: the GHS Initiative. In Global health in times of violence (pp. 73-98). Springer, Boston, MA.

Khan, K., Arino, J., Hu, W., Raposo, P., Sears, J., Calderon, F., ... & Gardam, M. (2009). Spread of a novel influenza A (H1N1) virus via global airline transportation. New England Journal of Medicine, 361(2), 212-214.

Khan, K., McNabb, S. J. N., Memish, Z. A., Eckhardt, R., Hu, W., Kossowsky, D., & Sears, J. (2012). Infectious Disease Surveillance and Modelling Across Geographic Frontiers and Scientific Specialties. The Lancet Infectious Diseases, 12(3), 222-230. doi: 10.1016/S1473-3099(11)70252-6

Köck R, Becker K, Cookson B, et al. Methicillin-resistant Staphylococcus aureus (MRSA): burden of disease and control challenges in Europe. Euro Surveill. 2010;15(41):19688.

Kolbe, A. R., Hutson, R. A., Shannon, H., Trzcinski, E., Miles, B., Levitz, N., ... & James, L. (2010). Mortality, crime and access to basic needs before and after the Haiti earthquake: a random survey of Port-au-Prince households. Medicine, Conflict and Survival, 26(4), 281-297.

Koonin, L. M., Beauvais, D. R., Shimabukuro, T., & Wortley, P. M. (2011). The 2009 H1N1 pandemic response: a case study of local public health agency coordination with the health care delivery system in New York City. Journal of Public Health Management and Practice, 17(2), 161-169. doi: 10.1097/PHH.0b013e3181e9a112

Kraemer, M. U., & Reiner Jr, R. C. (2019). Vector-borne diseases and climate change: a European perspective. FEMS microbiology letters, 366(10), fnz057.

Kruk, M. E., Myers, M., Varpilah, S. T., Dahn, B. T., & Raviglione, M. (2015). What is a resilient health system? Lessons from Ebola. The Lancet, 385(9980), 1910-1912. doi: 10.1016/S0140-6736(15)60755-3

Kucharski AJ, et al. (2020). Early dynamics of transmission and control of COVID-19: A mathematical modelling study. The Lancet Infectious Diseases, 20(5), 553-558.

Kucharski, A. J., Edmunds, W. J., & Piot, P. (2015). Containing Ebola virus infection in West Africa. PLoS Biology, 13(1), e1002057. doi: 10.1371/journal.pbio.1002057

Le Masson, V., & Schwarz, A. M. (2018). Climate change, migration and health in the Sahel. Global Health Action, 11(sup3), 1546694.

Lederberg, J., Shope, R. E., & Oaks, S. C. (Eds.). (2008). Emerging infections: microbial threats to health in the United States. National Academies Press.

Lessler J, et al. (2016). Measuring the impact of Ebola control measures in Sierra Leone. PNAS, 113(48), 13936-13941.

Lipp, E. K., Huq, A., & Colwell, R. R. (2008). Effects of global climate on infectious disease: the cholera model. Clinical Microbiology Reviews, 15(4), 757-770.

Luby SP, et al. (2004). Effects of handwashing on child health: A randomised controlled trial. The Lancet, 364(9451), 1896-1901.

Luquero, F. J., Grout, L., Ciglenecki, I., Sakoba, K., Traore, B., Heile, M., ... & Page, A. (2014). Use of Vibrio cholerae vaccine in an outbreak in Guinea. New England Journal of Medicine, 370(22), 2111-2120. doi: 10.1056/NEJMoa1312680

Machalaba, C. C., Salerno, R. H., Barton Behravesh, C., et al. (2017). Health and climate change: policy responses to protect public health. Environmental Health Perspectives, 125(8), 085001.

Madoff, L. C., & Woodall, J. P. (2005). The internet and the global monitoring of emerging diseases: Lessons from the first 10 years of ProMED-mail. Archives of Medical Research, 36(6), 724-730.

Mateus, A. L. P., Otete, H. E., Beck, C. R., Dolan, G. P., Nguyen-Van-Tam, J. S., & Effectiveness of Travel Restrictions in the Rapid Containment of Human Influenza: A Systematic Review. Bulletin of the World Health Organization, 92(12), 868-880. doi: 10.2471/BLT.13.124800

Mawudeku, A. (2007). GPHIN. In N. G. Dedrick (Ed.), Disease surveillance: A public health informatics approach (pp. 245-259). John Wiley & Sons.

Mazigo, H. D., et al. (2018). Prevalence of schistosomiasis in Tanzania: A systematic review and meta-analysis. PLOS Neglected Tropical Diseases, 12(8), e0006902. doi:10.1371/journal.pntd.0006902

McEwen, S. A., & Collignon, P. J. (2018). Antimicrobial resistance: a One Health perspective. Microbiology spectrum, 6(2), ARBA-0009-2017.

McMichael, A. J., Woodruff, R. E., Hales, S. (2006). Climate change and human health: present and future risks. The Lancet, 367(9513), 859-869

McMichael, C., Barnett, J., & McMichael, A. J. (2012). An ill wind? Climate change, migration, and health. Environmental Health Perspectives, 120(5), 646-654.

Ministry of Health - Ghana. (2017). National Action Plan for Health Security (NAPHS) Ghana. Retrieved from http://moh.gov.gh/wp-content/uploads/2019/01/NAPHS-Ghana.pdf

Ministry of Health - Liberia. (2017). National Action Plan for Health Security (NAPHS) Liberia. Retrieved from https://www.who.int/ihr/publications/Liberia_NAPHS.pdf

Monath, T. P. (2008). Yellow fever: An update. The Lancet Infectious Diseases, 8(11), 691-702. doi: 10.1016/S1473-3099(08)70288-

Morse, S. S. (1995). Factors in the Emergence of Infectious Diseases. Emerging Infectious Diseases, 1(1), 7-15.

Morse, S. S., Mazet, J. A., Woolhouse, M., Parrish, C. R., Carroll, D., Karesh, W. B., ... & Daszak, P. (2012). Prediction and prevention of the next pandemic zoonosis. The Lancet, 380(9857), 1956-1965.

Mossong J, et al. (2008). Social contacts and mixing patterns relevant to the spread of infectious diseases. PLoS Med, 5(3), e74.

Mueller, J. E., Borrow, R., Gessner, B. D., & von Gottberg, A. (2004). Laboratory confirmation of meningococcal disease in Africa: Surveillance matters. PLoS Medicine, 1(1), e6. doi: 10.1371/journal.pmed.0010006

Myers, S. S., Gaffikin, L., Golden, C. D., Ostfeld, R. S., Redford, K. H., Ricketts, T. H., ... & Osofsky, S. A. (2013). Human health impacts of ecosystem alteration. Proceedings of the National Academy of Sciences, 110(47), 18753-18760.

National Health Service. (2020). Exercise Cygnus report published. Retrieved from https://www.england.nhs.uk/2020/10/exercise-cygnus-report-published/ U.S. Department of Health and Human Services. (2020). Strategic National Stockpile. Retrieved from https://www.phe.gov/about/sns/Pages/default.aspx World Health Organization. (2016). Lessons learned from the 2014-2016 Ebola outbreak in Guinea, Liberia, and Sierra Leone. Retrieved from https://www.who.int/csr/disease/ebola/lessons-learned/en/ World Health Organization. (2021). Global Influenza Programme. Retrieved from https://www.who.int/teams/global-influenza-programme

National Institute for Communicable Diseases. (2015). Integrated Disease Surveillance and Response: Implementation Manual.

Retrieved from https://www.nicd.ac.za/wp-content/uploads/2019/03/IDSR-Manual-2015_FINAL.pdf

National Institute for Public Health and the Environment (RIVM). (n.d.). Surveillance. Retrieved from https://www.rivm.nl/en/surveillance

National Institute for Public Health and the Environment (RIVM). (n.d.). Research and Development. Retrieved from https://www.rivm.nl/en/research-and-development

National Institute for Public Health and the Environment (RIVM). (n.d.). Advice and Guidelines. Retrieved from https://www.rivm.nl/en/advice-and-guid

Ngbede, E. O., Raji, M. A., & Ameh, J. A. (2018). Detection of antibiotic residues in poultry products in Jos, Nigeria. Veterinary World, 11(2), 161-166.

Nigeria Centre for Disease Control. (2018). Nigeria National Action Plan for Health Security 2018-2022. Retrieved from https://ncdc.gov.ng/themes/common/docs/protocols/56_1526420139.pdf

Ostfeld, R. S., & Brunner, J. L. (2015). Climate change and Ixodes tick-borne diseases of humans. Philosophical Transactions of the Royal Society B: Biological Sciences, 370(1665), 20140051.

Otte Im Kampe, E., Lehfeld, A.-S., Buda, S., Buchholz, U., Haas, W., & Wichmann, O. (2020). Estimating the effects of non-pharmaceutical interventions on the spread of COVID-19 using statistical modelling. Bundesgesundheitsblatt, Gesundheitsforschung, Gesundheitsschutz, 63(6), 688-694.

Overseas Development Institute (ODI). The Logical Framework Approach (LFA): A Summary of Key Concepts and Steps. Retrieved from https://www.odi.org/sites/default/files/resource-documents/odi_10172.pdf

Pawlotsky, J. M. (2014). Treatment of chronic hepatitis C: Current and future. Current Topics in Microbiology and Immunology, 369, 321-342.

Petersen, E., Wilson, M. E., Touch, S., McCloskey, B., Mwaba, P., Bates, M., & Dar, O. (2016). Rapid spread of Zika virus in the Americas: Implications for public health preparedness for mass gatherings at the 2016 Brazil Olympic Games. International Journal of Infectious Diseases, 44, 11-15. doi: 10.1016/j.ijid.2016.02.001

Pittet D, et al. (2000). Effectiveness of a hospital-wide programme to improve compliance with hand hygiene. The Lancet, 356(9238), 1307-1312.

Polgreen, P. M., Chen, Y., Pennock, D. M., Nelson, F. D., & Weinstein, R. A. (2008). Using internet searches for influenza surveillance. Clinical Infectious Diseases, 47(11), 1443-1448.

ProMED-mail. (n.d.). About ProMED-mail. Retrieved from https://www.promedmail.org/aboutus/

ProMED-mail. (n.d.). ProMED mail: The Program for Monitoring Emerging Diseases. International Society for Infectious Diseases. Retrieved from https://promedmail.org/

Public Health Agency of Canada. (2015). Global Public Health Intelligence Network. Retrieved from https://www.canada.ca/en/public-health/services/reports-publications/canadian-pandemic-influenza-preparedness-planning-guidance/appendix-b.html

Public Health Agency of Canada. (2020). Global Public Health Intelligence Network (GPHIN). Retrieved from https://www.canada.ca/en/public-health/services/reports-publications/canada-communicable-disease-report-ccdr/monthly-issue/2020-46/global-public-health-intelligence-network.html

Reference: World Health Organization. (2020). Global Tuberculosis Report 2020. Retrieved from https://www.who.int/teams/global-tuberculosis-programme/tb-reports/global-tuberculosis-report-2020

Robert Koch Institute. (2021). About Us. Retrieved from https://www.rki.de/EN/Content/Institute/Institute_node.html

Robert Koch Institute. (2021). Infectious Disease Epidemiology - Epidemiological Bulletins. Retrieved from https://www.rki.de/EN/Content/Institute/Institute_node.html

Robert Koch Institute. (2021). Infectious Disease Epidemiology - Guideline. Retrieved from https://www.rki.de/EN/Content/Institute/Institute_node.html

Robert Koch Institute. (2021). National Reference Centre for Influenza. Retrieved from https://www.rki.de/EN/Content/Institute/Institute_node.html

Robine, J. M., Cheung, S. L. K., Le Roy, S., et al. (2008). Death toll exceeded 70,000 in Europe during the summer of 2003. Comptes Rendus Biologies, 331(2), 171-178.

Shively, M., Stoddard, G. J., Scott, R. D., & Holmes, H. K. (2017). Role of antiviral use during the 2009-2010 influenza outbreak in preventing influenza-like illness after influenza vaccination. Infection Control & Hospital Epidemiology, 38(3), 302-309.

Shrivastava, S. R., Shrivastava, P. S., & Ramasamy, J. (2013). Strengthening Integrated Disease Surveillance and Response in the African Region. Annals of African Medicine, 12(4), 225-226. doi: 10.4103/1596-3519.122708

Shumba, C., Mazambani, D., Mawere, K., & Shoko, E. (2020). The COVID-19 pandemic and challenges for Africa: An evidence-based review. Pan African Medical Journal, 37(Supplement 1), 1. doi: 10.11604/pamj.supp.2020.37.1.24503

Sridhar, D., Majumder, M. S., Liu, Y., & Roser, M. (2021). Learning from the past: Did experiences with previous outbreaks help mitigate the impact of COVID-19? PLOS ONE, 16(1), e0245675.

Tarnagda, Z., et al. (2019). Prevalence and risk factors of schistosomiasis among school-aged children in Burkina Faso, West Africa. Parasites & Vectors, 12(1), 19. doi:10.1186/s13071-018-3256-0

Tuite, A. R., Ng, V., Rees, E., Fisman, D., & Ontario COVID-19 Modelling Collaborative. (2020). Estimation of COVID-19 outbreak size in relation to epidemic interventions in Ontario, Canada. Canadian Medical Association Journal, 192(20), E497-E504.

U.S. Department of State. (2020). Global Health Security Agenda (GHSA). Retrieved from https://www.state.gov/global-health/global-health-security-agenda/

UNAIDS. (2021). Global AIDS Update 2021. Retrieved from https://www.unaids.org/sites/default/files/media_asset/2021-global-aids-update_en.pdf

United Nations Development Programme (UNDP). The Logical Framework Approach (LFA) Handbook for Objectives-oriented Planning. Retrieved from https://www.undp.org/publications/logical-framework-approach-lfa-handbook-objectives-oriented-planning

Ventola, C. L. (2015). The antibiotic resistance crisis: Part 1: Causes and threats. Pharmacy and Therapeutics, 40(4), 277-283.

Verity, R., Okell, L. C., Dorigatti, I., Winskill, P., Whittaker, C., Imai, N., ... Ferguson, N. M. (2020). Estimates of the severity of coronavirus disease 2019: A model-based analysis. The Lancet Infectious Diseases, 20(6), 669-677.

Weaver, S. C., Charlier, C., Vasilakis, N., & Lecuit, M. (2018). Zika, chikungunya, and other emerging vector-borne viral diseases. Annual review of medicine, 69, 395-408.

WHO Regional Office for Africa. (2014). Early warning, alert, and response system (EWARS) in the African Region: A framework for implementation. World Health Organization Regional Office for Africa.

Woolhouse, M. E., & Gowtage-Sequeria, S. (2005). Host range and emerging and reemerging pathogens. Emerging infectious diseases, 11(12), 1842-1847.

World Bank. (2020). Liberia: Health Systems Strengthening for Resilience Project. Retrieved from https://projects.worldbank.org/en/projects-operations/project-detail/P167111 World Health Organization. (2021a). Polio Eradication Initiative. Retrieved from https://www.who.int/teams/polio-eradication World Health Organization. (2021b). Integrated Disease Surveillance and Response (IDSR). Retrieved from https://www.afro.who.int/health-topics/integrated-disease-surveillance-and-response

World Bank. (2021). Pandemic Emergency Financing Facility. Retrieved from https://www.worldbank.org/en/topic/pandemics/brief/p

World Health Organization (WHO) - Chikungunya: https://www.who.int/news-room/fact-sheets/detail/chikungunya

World Health Organization (WHO) - Dengue and Severe Dengue: https://www.who.int/news-room/fact-sheets/detail/dengue-and-severe-dengue

World Health Organization (WHO) - Malaria: https://www.who.int/news-room/fact-sheets/detail/malaria

World Health Organization (WHO) - Yellow fever: https://www.who.int/news-room/fact-sheets/detail/yellow-fever

World Health Organization (WHO) - Zika virus: https://www.who.int/news-room/fact-sheets/detail/zika-virus

World Health Organization (WHO). (2016). Ebola situation report - 30 March 2016. Retrieved from https://www.who.int/csr/disease/ebola/situation-reports/archive/en/

World Health Organization (WHO). (2016). Sri Lanka certified malaria-free by WHO. Retrieved from https://www.who.int/news/item/05-09-2016-sri-lanka-certified-malaria-free-by-who

World Health Organization (WHO). (2020). Advice on the use of masks in the context of COVID-19: Interim guidance, 5 June 2020. Retrieved from https://www.who.int/publications/i/item/advice-on-the-use-of-masks-in-the-community-during-home-care-

and-in-healthcare-settings-in-the-context-of-the-novel-
coronavirus-(2019-ncov)-outbreak

World Health Organization (WHO). (2020). COVID-19 strategic preparedness and response plan: Operational planning guidelines to support country preparedness and response. Retrieved from https://www.who.int/publications-detail-redirect/WHO-2019-nCoV-Strategic_Preparedness_and_Response_Plan-2020.4

World Health Organization (WHO). (2020). COVID-19: A public health emergency of international concern. Retrieved from https://www.who.int/docs/default-source/coronaviruse/transcripts/who-audio-emergencies-coronavirus-press-conference-full-23jul2020.pdf

World Health Organization (WHO). (2021). MERS-CoV global summary and assessment of risk. Retrieved from https://www.who.int/publications/i/item/mers-cov-global-summary-and-assessment-of-risk

World Health Organization (WHO). (2020). Dengue and Severe Dengue. Retrieved from https://www.who.int/news-room/fact-sheets/detail/dengue-and-severe-dengue

World Health Organization (WHO). (2020). Report of the WHO-China Joint Mission on Coronavirus Disease 2019 (COVID-19). Retrieved from https://www.who.int/docs/default-source/coronaviruse/who-china-joint-mission-on-covid-19-final-report.pdf

World Health Organization (WHO). (2021). Coronavirus disease (COVID-19) testing. Retrieved from https://www.who.int/news-room/feature-stories/detail/coronavirus-disease-(covid-19)-testing

World Health Organization (WHO). (2021). Global Health Observatory (GHO) data: HIV/AIDS. Retrieved from https://www.who.int/data/gho/data/themes/hiv-aids

World Health Organization (WHO). (2021). Global Outbreak Alert and Response Network (GOARN). Retrieved from https://www.who.int/initiatives/global-outbreak-alert-and-response-network

World Health Organization (WHO). (2021). Hepatitis B. Retrieved from https://www.who.int/news-room/fact-sheets/detail/hepatitis-b

World Health Organization (WHO). (2021). Malaria. Retrieved from https://www.who.int/health-topics/malaria

World Health Organization (WHO). (2021). Quarantine and isolation. Retrieved from https://www.who.int/health-topics/quarantine#tab=tab_1[1]

World Health Organization (WHO). (2021). Schistosomiasis. Retrieved from https://www.who.int/health-topics/schistosomiasis

World Health Organization (WHO). (2021). Soil-transmitted helminth infections. Retrieved from https://www.who.int/news-room/fact-sheets/detail/soil-transmitted-helminth-infections

World Health Organization (WHO). (2021). Syphilis. Retrieved from https://www.who.int/health-topics/syphilis

World Health Organization (WHO). (2021). WHO guidelines on ethical issues in public health surveillance. Retrieved from

---

1. https://www.who.int/health-topics/

quarantine#tab_43ec3e5dee6e706af7766fffea512721_tab_1

https://www.who.int/publications/i/item/who-guidelines-on-ethical-issues-in-public-health-surveillance

World Health Organization (WHO). Cholera. Retrieved from https://www.who.int/health-topics/cholera#tab=tab_1[2]

World Health Organization (WHO). Communicable Disease Surveillance and Response Systems. Retrieved from https://www.who.int/csr/resources/publications/surveillance/ CSR_ISR_2000_1/en/

World Health Organization (WHO). Communicable Diseases. Retrieved from https://www.who.int/topics/infectious_diseases/ en/

World Health Organization (WHO). Ebola virus disease. Retrieved from https://www.who.int/health-topics/ ebola#tab=tab_1[3]

World Health Organization (WHO). Evaluation in Public Health: Interventions and Best Practices. Retrieved from https://www.who.int/healthinfo/topics/evaluation/en/

World Health Organization (WHO). Fungal diseases. Retrieved from https://www.who.int/news-room/fact-sheets/detail/ fungal-diseases

World Health Organization (WHO). HIV/AIDS. Retrieved from https://www.who.int/health-topics/hiv-aids#tab=tab_1[4]

---

2. https://www.who.int/health-topics/

   cholera#tab_43ec3e5dee6e706af7766fffea512721_tab_1

3. https://www.who.int/health-topics/

   ebola#tab_43ec3e5dee6e706af7766fffea512721_tab_1

4. https://www.who.int/health-topics/

   hiv-aids#tab_43ec3e5dee6e706af7766fffea512721_tab_1

World Health Organization (WHO). Introduction to Epidemiology. Retrieved from https://www.who.int/publications/i/item/introduction-to-epidemiology

World Health Organization (WHO). Laboratory testing for infectious diseases. Retrieved from https://www.who.int/infection-prevention/publications/laboratory-testing/en/

World Health Organization (WHO). Tuberculosis. Retrieved from https://www.who.int/health-topics/tuberculosis#tab=tab_1[5]

World Health Organization Regional Office for Africa. (2013). Technical Guidelines for Integrated Disease Surveillance and Response in the African Region. Retrieved from https://www.afro.who.int/sites/default/files/2017-06/b2315.pdf

World Health Organization Regional Office for Africa. (2015). Good practices in health sector response to HIV/AIDS, Tuberculosis and Malaria in Uganda. Retrieved from https://www.afro.who.int/sites/default/files/2017-06/Good%20Practices%20in%20Health%20Sector%20Response%20to%20H

World Health Organization Regional Office for Africa. (2017). Integrated Disease Surveillance and Response: Strategy and Plan of Action 2016-2020. Retrieved from https://apps.who.int/iris/bitstream/handle/10665/258680/9789290233847-eng.pdf

World Health Organization Regional Office for Africa. (2018). Integrated Disease Surveillance and Response (IDSR) in the African Region: A Decade of Progress 2001-2010. Retrieved from https://www.afro.who.int/publications/integrated-disease-

---

5. https://www.who.int/health-topics/
   tuberculosis#tab_43ec3e5dee6e706af7766fffea512721_tab_1

surveillance-and-response-idsr-african-region-decade-progress-2001

World Health Organization. (2014). Quantitative risk assessment of the effects of climate change on selected causes of death, 2030s and 2050s. WHO.

World Health Organization. (2015). Antimicrobial resistance: Global report on surveillance. Geneva: World Health Organization.

World Health Organization. (2015). Climate change and health: Fact sheet. Retrieved from https://www.who.int/news-room/fact-sheets/detail/climate-change-and-health

World Health Organization. (2015). Outbreaks and emergencies: Ebola outbreak 2014-2016. Retrieved from https://www.who.int/csr/disease/ebola/en/

World Health Organization. (2015). Outbreaks and emergencies: Ebola outbreak 2014-2016. Retrieved from https://www.who.int/csr/disease/ebola/en/

World Health Organization. (2016). Ebola outbreak 2014-2016. Retrieved from https://www.who.int/emergencies/ebola/en/

World Health Organization. (2016). Learning from the Ebola response in Liberia. Retrieved from https://apps.who.int/iris/bitstream/handle/10665/204134/9789241510054_eng.pdf

World Health Organization. (2016). Learning from the Ebola response in Liberia. Retrieved from https://apps.who.int/iris/bitstream/handle/10665/204134/9789241510054_eng.pdf

World Health Organization. (2016). The Global Public Health Intelligence Network (GPHIN). Retrieved from https://www.who.int/activities/tracking-disease-outbreaks-global-public-health-intelligence-network

World Health Organization. (2016). WHO Response to the Ebola Outbreak in West Africa: Lessons Learned for Public Health Emergency Preparedness. Retrieved from https://apps.who.int/iris/bitstream/handle/10665/251781/WHO-WHE-IHM-GAR-16.1-eng.pdf

World Health Organization. (2017). Integrated Disease Surveillance and Response: A Regional Strategy for Communicable Diseases 2016–2020. Retrieved from https://apps.who.int/iris/bitstream/handle/10665/258681/B4681.pdf

World Health Organization. (2017). Laboratory Quality Management System: Handbook. Retrieved from https://www.who.int/ihr/publications/lqms_2017/en/

World Health Organization. (2018). Climate change and health. Retrieved from https://www.who.int/news-room/fact-sheets/detail/climate-change-and-health

World Health Organization. (2018). Competency Framework for Health Workers' Education and Training on Antimicrobial Resistance. Retrieved from https://apps.who.int/iris/bitstream/handle/10665/272135/9789241514663-eng.pdf

World Health Organization. (2018). Emergency Response Framework. Retrieved from https://www.who.int/ihr/publications/WHO_HSE_GCR_2018_2/en/

World Health Organization. (2018). Financing Preparedness: Essential Interventions for a Harmonized Approach. Retrieved from https://apps.who.int/iris/bitstream/handle/10665/326344/9789241516162-eng.pdf

World Health Organization. (2018). International Health Regulations (2005). Retrieved from https://www.who.int/health-topics/international-health-regulations#tab=tab_1[6]

World Health Organization. (2018). Strengthening Health Systems for Emergency Preparedness: Tool for Assessing Health System Capacity. Retrieved from https://apps.who.int/iris/bitstream/handle/10665/259847/9789241513505-eng.pdf

World Health Organization. (2019). Cholera. Retrieved from https://www.afro.who.int/health-topics/cholera

World Health Organization. (2019). Consolidated guidelines on the use of antiretroviral drugs for treating and preventing HIV infection. Geneva: World Health Organization.

World Health Organization. (2019). Consolidated guidelines on tuberculosis: Module 4: Treatment - Drug-resistant tuberculosis treatment. Geneva: World Health Organization.

World Health Organization. (2019). Disease surveillance for public health: Surveillance systems. Retrieved from https://www.who.int/immunization/monitoring_surveillance/burden/vpd/surveillance_type/passive/disease_surveillance_type_intro/en/

World Health Organization. (2019). Everybody's business: strengthening health systems to improve health outcomes: WHO's framework for action. Retrieved from https://www.who.int/healthsystems/strategy/everybodys_business.pdf

---

6. https://www.who.int/health-topics/international-health-regulations#tab_43ec3e5dee6e706af7766fffea512721_tab_1

World Health Organization. (2019). Global health security. Retrieved from https://www.who.int/health-topics/global-health-security#tab=tab_1[7]

World Health Organization. (2019). Guidelines for the prevention, care and treatment of persons with chronic hepatitis B infection. Geneva: World Health Organization.

World Health Organization. (2019). World malaria report 2019. Retrieved from https://www.who.int/publications/i/item/world-malaria-report-2019

World Health Organization. (2019). Zoonoses: Diseases that spread from animals to humans. Retrieved from https://www.who.int/news-room/fact-sheets/detail/zoonoses

World Health Organization. (2020). Antimicrobial Resistance. Retrieved from https://www.who.int/news-room/fact-sheets/detail/antimicrobial-resistance-(amr)

World Health Organization. (2020). Coronavirus disease (COVID-19) outbreak. Retrieved from https://www.who.int/emergencies/diseases/novel-coronavirus-2019

World Health Organization. (2020). COVID-19 Strategic Preparedness and Response Plan. Retrieved from https://www.who.int/publications/m/item/covid-19-strategic-preparedness and response plan

World Health Organization. (2020). COVID-19: Resources, tools, and publications. Retrieved from https://www.who.int/emergencies/diseases/novel-coronavirus-2019/resources publications

---

7. https://www.who.int/health topics/

global-health-security#tab_43ec3e5dee6e706af7766fffea512721_tab_1

World Health Organization. (2020). Early warning, alert, and response system for major public health events. Retrieved from https://www.who.int/health-topics/early-warning-alert-and-response-system-for-major-public-health-events

World Health Organization. Global tuberculosis report 2020. Geneva: World Health Organization; 2020.

Yang Y, et al. (2009). The transmissibility and control of pandemic influenza A (H1N1) virus. Science, 326(5953), 729-733.

Zinsstag, J., Schelling, E., Waltner-Toews, D., Whittaker, M., & Tanner, M. (2015). One Health: The Theory and Practice of Integrated Health Approaches. CABI.

Don't miss out!

Visit the website below and you can sign up to receive emails whenever Mogana S. Flomo, Jr. publishes a new book. There's no charge and no obligation.

https://books2read.com/r/B-A-JCHY-TIJVC

BOOKS 2 READ

Connecting independent readers to independent writers.

About the Author

Dr. Mogana S. Flomo, Jr. is a versatile and accomplished individual, known for his extensive experience in education and diverse roles. He founded the Center for Environmental and Public Health Research (CEPRES) Inc. and CEPRES International University in Liberia, boasting over 26 years as an educator in subjects like Chemistry, Mathematics, and Physics. Beyond academia, Dr. Flomo is a politician, farmer, environmentalist, and public health professional. His leadership includes serving as the Minister of Agriculture in Liberia and establishing the Liberia Commodities and Smallholder Farmers Empowerment Enterprise (LICSFEE), significantly impacting food security. In addition to his wide-ranging contributions, Dr. Flomo is also an accomplished author of several books.

Dr. Flomo is deeply committed to youth-focused initiatives, collaborating with local and international organizations and universities. He has an impressive skill set, including proficiency in statistics and music software, as well as expertise in setting up and managing distance education platforms. His unwavering passion lies in enhancing Liberia's food security and educational system, and he has played vital roles as both Board Chairman and member in numerous organizations and government agencies.